THE STORY OF
MEDICINE IN AMERICA

BY THE SAME AUTHORS

The Medical Garden
Women in White

The Story of

Medicine

in America

GEOFFREY MARKS

AND

WILLIAM K. BEATTY

Illustrated with photographs

CHARLES SCRIBNER'S SONS · New York

FOR GINNY

*who has helped with ideas, inspiration,
and common sense*

CONTENTS

PREFACE   *xi*

Part I.   *Medical Practices and Practitioners from*
           Colonial Times to the Early Republic

           1. The Virginia Colony   *3*
           2. The New England Colonies   *15*
           3. Indigenous Remedies and Practices   *29*
           4. Cotton Mather, Medical Polemicist   *40*
           5. Hospitals: Care of the Sick Poor and
              the Mentally Ill   *55*

Part II.   *The Development of Medical Education*

           6. Dissection and Anatomy   *73*
           7. The Early Medical Schools   *98*
           8. Medicine and War   *114*

Part III. *Progress in the Nineteenth Century*

           9. Medicine beyond the Alleghenies   *141*
          10. The Phenomenon of Specialization   *159*
          11. The Sectarians   *181*
          12. Reforms in Medical Practice and Education   *194*

CONTENTS

Part IV. *The Problems of Public Health*

    13. The Smallpox Epidemics   *213*

    14. The Scourge of Yellow Fever   *234*

    15. The Battle against Widespread Diseases   *246*

    16. Toward a Public Health Service   *262*

Part V. *Advances on Several Fronts*

    17. Research on a Sound Foundation   *273*

    18. The Fight against Polio   *284*

    19. Investigation of the Brain   *292*

Part VI. *Into the Modern Age*

    20. In Defiance of Obsolescence   *309*

    21. Aerospace Medicine   *332*

    22. Nuclear Medicine   *342*

    23. The Future of Medical Practice   *349*

    REFERENCE NOTES   *365*

    SELECTED BIBLIOGRAPHY   *388*

    ILLUSTRATION CREDITS   *402*

    INDEX   *404*

ILLUSTRATIONS

	PAGE
Thomas Thacher	25
Cotton Mather	41
Thomas Bond	60
Samuel Bard	67
Thomas Cadwalader	76
John Morgan	100
John Warren	108
Joseph Warren	118
William Shippen, Jr.	122
James Thacher	128
James Tilton	133
John Jones	136
Daniel Drake	149
William Beaumont	154
James Marion Sims	162
William S. Halsted	173
S. Weir Mitchell	176
Samuel Thomson	183
Andrew Taylor Still	189

ILLUSTRATIONS

Abraham Flexner   *203*

Mathew Carey   *237*

Walter Reed   *242*

Stephen Smith   *266*

Charles A. Hufnagel   *329*

FOLLOWING PAGE *138*

The tobacco plant, used in medical treatment

Apothecary's indenture

Admission card, Pennsylvania Hospital

The Pennsylvania Hospital

Statue of Benjamin Rush

Bill for chains, Pennsylvania Hospital

Jefferson Medical College

The Indian Doctor's Dispensatory, title page

Manuscript home remedy book, title page

"Thomson's patent"

First public demonstration of surgical anesthesia

Ephraim McDowell, commemorative mdeal

Massachusetts General Hospital

Daniel Hale Williams

Harvey Cushing and Walter Dandy

William H. Welch and colleagues

The Mayos

PREFACE

⎯⎯⎯⎯⎯⎯⎯⎯⎯⎯⎯⎯⎯⎯⎯⎯⎯

The story of medicine in America in terms of space, time, and people is a vast one. America, after all, in the broadest geographic sense of the word, covers North, Central, and South America as well as the adjacent islands. In terms of time and people the story begins thousands of years before Columbus and embraces a variety of native peoples, succeeded by Spanish, Portuguese, Dutch, and many other colonists. The full story would be unmanageable within the covers of a book of this size.

For this reason we have limited the story to the area now encompassed by the United States, the time to the three and a half centuries since 1600, and the peoples to the original British colonists and those that followed them. *The Story of Medicine in America* illustrates within this framework the medical problems of a new and growing country and the ways in which these problems have been met and, for the most part, overcome by developments in medical practice, education, and research—developments that have often had profound effects throughout the medical world.

THE STORY OF
MEDICINE IN AMERICA

Part I

MEDICAL PRACTICES AND
PRACTITIONERS FROM
COLONIAL TIMES
TO THE EARLY REPUBLIC

$\{(1)\}$

The Virginia Colony

The first permanent English settlement in North America was established in what would be Jamestown, Virginia, in May 1607. The undertaking was sponsored by the London Company, a private enterprise set up to develop new opportunities for the overseas trade that was essential to England's prosperity.

The colonization of Virginia was a carefully planned venture. The professions, crafts, and trades dominant in the mother country were reflected in the skills of those the Company sent out—except for medicine.

Medical practice in England at the beginning of the seventeenth century was divided among the members of three guilds—the physicians, the surgeons, and the apothecaries.

The physicians, who usually possessed a university degree, were the elite. They preferred studying, teaching, and debating the various theories of disease to dealing directly with the sick. Addressed as "doctor," they limited such practice as they might engage in to treating the upper classes.[1]

Next in line, but socially quite inferior to the physicians, were the surgeons, divided sometimes into the Surgeons of the Long Robe and the more humble barber-surgeons. Few surgeons held university degrees. They were trained through apprenticeships and hospital instruction. They were addressed as "mister," a practice that has been continued to this day (now as a mark of distinction) by English surgeons. The designation surgeon (originally "chirurgeon") came from the Greek *cheir,* meaning "hand," and *ergon,* "work." Barber surgeons used their razors to open veins and let out blood, as well as for trimming beards.

Apothecaries were tradesmen and, until 1617, shared a guild with the grocers. As tradesmen, they were permitted to charge only for merchandise—the drugs they prescribed, concocted, and sold. In reality, they were the general practitioners of medicine for the masses, learning their skills through apprenticeships and sometimes in hospital wards.

Two other groups offered medical services to the public. The midwives, who were often ignorant, superstitious, but well-meaning women, held almost exclusive sway over childbirth. The ever-present quacks, who imitated the regular practitioners, were unscrupulous predators.

The London planners seemingly anticipated wounds and injuries but no sickness, for there was no physician accompanying the first Virginia settlers. A gentleman-surgeon, Thomas Wotton, served as physician to the fleet of three little ships. Listed as a surgeon on the ship's roster among the indentured servants was Will Willkinson, but nothing more is known about him. Among his fellow passengers was "Thos. Cowper the Barber." At that time there was little distinction between surgery and barbering, and the fact that the term "barber-surgeon" did not appear in the ship's records, nor did it appear subsequently in the records of Virginia, would indicate that from the beginning these were separate professions in the colony.[2]

On the voyage out shipboard deaths from improper diet, disease, and epidemics were frequent. On landing, despite instructions from the Company to avoid low, moist places, a fortified trading post was established on marshy lowlands, where disease flourished. It is hard to comprehend why Wotton did not effectively oppose this unhealthy site. In any event, the marshland was not the sole cause of ill health—the unfavorable climate, the hostile Indians, and near starvation took their toll.

There was trouble with the Indians from the start. Early in the summer of 1607 Captain John Smith, the military adventurer without whose various skills the colony would have failed, wrote: "Smith newly recovered, Martin and Ratcliffe was by his care preserved and relieved, and the most of the soldiers recovered, with the skillful diligence of Mr. Thomas Wotton, our Chirurgeon generall." [3]

The annals of the period record disputes between Wotton and colonial authorities over money with which to obtain drugs and necessities and the surgeon's preference for living aboard ship away from the Indian tomahawks and arrows that made Jamestown life hazardous. Nothing further is known of his activities.

During the first summer more than half the settlers—60 out of 105—died. Help for those remaining came around New Year's Day, 1608. A supply ship brought over a hundred new settlers, including a few women, and medical reinforcements—Walter Russell, the first physician (as distinct from surgeon), Post Ginnat, a surgeon, and two apothecaries, Thomas Field and John Harford.

Over the next few years the London Company continued to send out settlers and supplies. The ships, boarded in the epidemic centers of England, were overcrowded, dogs and other domestic animals sharing with humans the scant space left by the cargo; sanitation was primitive; provisions, particularly citrus fruits needed to prevent scurvy, were inadequate; and it took the sailing vessels two to three months to cross the Atlantic. It is not altogether surprising that on one voyage thirty-two persons from two ships were thrown overboard, and another vessel lost 130 out of 185 passengers.[4] If the ship was routed through the Antilles to allow for "restitution of our sick people into health by the helpes of Fresh ayre, diet, and the baths," [5] passengers and sailors were exposed to tropical diseases, which they carried with them to the Virginia colony.

Those who arrived in the "sickly season"—June, July, and August—were also vulnerable to the "seasoning" or "summer sickness." It was therefore considered best to arrive in the fall or winter so as to become "hardened" before the next year's "sickly season." The "seasoning" was attributed to a variety of causes—undernourishment and disease on the trip, poor food, and not least the hot sun of the Virginia summer to which the immigrants were unaccustomed.[6]

Famine was more than a direct cause of death. It invited the attack, in epidemic proportions, of food-deficiency diseases. Beriberi seems to have been common among the Indians. Early settlers were warned to avoid localities in which the natives showed large bellies and strange swellings, often characteristic of beriberi.[7] Eggs, vegetables, fruit, and vitamin B could prevent beriberi. The first three the colonists did not have. Indeed, their sustenance per man per day was half a pint of wheat and half a pint of barley boiled in water in a common pot. What little vitamin B there might have been was boiled out.

Scurvy, a disease characterized by mental apathy, lassitude, and painful joints, attacked the immigrants during their long voyage to America (as it had been attacking mariners from earliest times) and persisted on their arrival.

Medical care was at best minimal, when there was any. No account of Walter Russell's services to the colony at large has survived, but it is known that he accompanied Captain John Smith on a trip of exploration into Chesapeake Bay in June 1608. In fact some islands from which a supply of fresh water was obtained were named Russell's Isles. During the expedition Russell rendered valuable professional service to Captain Smith. Russell's account of the incident (written with an Amos Todkill) must be considered the first case report by an American physician:

> But it chanced, the Captaine taking a fish from his sword (not knowing her condition), being much of the fashion of a Thornebacke with a longer taile whereon is a most poysoned sting 2 or 3 inches long, which shee strooke an inch and halfe into the wrist of his arme; the which in 4 houres, had so extremely swolne his hand, arme, shoulder, and part of his body, as we all with much sorrow concluded his funerall, & prepared his grave in an Ile hard by (as himselfe appointed) which then wee called Stingeray Ile, after the name of the fish. Yet by the helpe of a precious oile, Doctour Russel applyed, ere night his tormenting paine was so wel asswaged that he eate the fish in his supper; which gave no

less joy and content to us, then ease to himselfe. Having neither Surgeon nor surgerie but that preventative oile we presently set saile for James Towne.[8]

Stingray Point at the mouth of the Rappahannock River still appears on maps of Virginia.

Nothing is known of the activities of the surgeon Ginnat or of the apothecaries Field and Harford.

Later in 1608 Anthony Bagnall, a surgeon, appeared. The only record of him is in a report by Captain Smith that Bagnall went along on a second expedition up the bay. In an encounter with Indians, Smith wrote, "none were hurt only Anthony Bagnall was shot in his Hat and another in his sleeve." In the course of the expedition they came across an Indian almost dead from a shot in the knee. Bagnall "so dressed this Salvage [sic] that within an hour he looked somewhat chearfully and did eate and speake." [9]

Evidently none of these doctors remained long in the colony. When Smith suffered a gunpowder burn in 1609 he had to go to England for treatment "because there was neither chirurgeon or chirurgerye in the fort." [10]

Conditions were so bad by then that the undertaking would have failed but for the timely arrival of Lord De La Warr in June 1610, with supplies and more settlers. Lord De La Warr had been sent out by the now reorganized Company to rule the colony and put it on a solid footing, for it was nothing more than a poor trading post—and the Indians had little to trade except corn.

It is likely that Lawrence Bohun (d. 1621), "doctor in phisick," arrived in the company of Lord De La Warr. On July 7 his lordship wrote to London of "Mr. Dr. Boone [Bohun] whose care and industrie for the preservation of our men's lives (assaulted with strange fluxes and agues), we have just cause to commend unto your noble favours." [11]

Faced by widespread sickness and exhausted medicine chests, Bohun investigated the medical potentials of native plants. He experimented with sassafras and other vegetation that grew abundantly in the Jamestown area. He also tried the gums of local trees and found that the clear gum of the white poplar resembled turpentine. He claimed that, made into a balsam, it would heal any fresh wound. A medicine derived from a tree resembling the myrtle proved a specific for dysentery, and Bohun used it to combat an epidemic of diarrhea. He had great faith in what he named *Terra Alba Virginensis,* a white clay to which he attributed poison-expelling properties. He used it to fight serious fevers.

In March 1611 Lord De La Warr, suffering from scurvy, had Bohun accompany him on a trip to the West Indies in search of a cure. It is unlikely that his lordship again set foot on Virginia soil. He was succeeded by Sir Thomas Dale, who maintained strict military discipline and ruled with an iron hand. The colony still led a precarious existence—no profitable product for export had been developed; the settlers had no stake in the country, and English liberty had not been extended to them.

Under these conditions it is understandable why so few men with medical degrees settled in the colony. They "were gentry" and "upper classes in general did not emigrate." Then, too, there were "no opportunities worthy of their prestige." [12]

Following the appointment of Sir George Yeardley, first as acting governor in 1616 and then as governor in 1619, prospects brightened. He was ordered by the Company to abolish arbitrary rule, introduce English common law, encourage private property (no individual had been allowed to own land heretofore), and summon a representative assembly. The economic problems were being solved by the cultivation and export of tobacco.

During these years Dr. Bohun must have been back in Virginia, at least from time to time. At the beginning of 1620 he and a John Swifte were given the right to transport three hundred persons to Virginia, and later that year he was appointed physician-general to the colony with a grant of five hundred acres of land. In 1621 Bohun and his company, sailing in the West Indies, were attacked by two Spanish ships-of-war. The English ship escaped, but a random shot mortally wounded Bohun.

On July 16, 1621, the Company decided:

> For so much as the physicians place to the Company was now become void by reason of the untimely death of Dr. Bohune . . . [on] 19th of March last; Doctor Gulstone did now take occasion to recommend unto the Company for the said place one Mr. Pottes, a Master of Arts and as he affirmed well practised in Chirurgerie and Phisique, and expert allso in distilling of waters and that he had many other ingenious devices so as he supposed his service would be of great use unto the Colony of Virginia.[13]

A month later the Company wrote Governor Yeardley that "Dr. John Potts [had been sent] for the phisition's place with two chirurgions and a chest of Physicke and Chirurgery." [14]

John Pott (d. c. 1642), a man with business acumen and

a bent for politics, was very ready to settle in Virginia. He was frequently the center of controversy. He quickly gained a seat on the council of the colony, only to lose it when word reached England that he had been the ringleader in poisoning Indians with whom the colonists had concluded a treaty.

In 1625 a Mrs. Blany (or Blainie) brought suit against Dr. Pott, charging that she had miscarried because he had refused her a piece of hog's flesh that she had requested of him. The case was dismissed by the court because "it no way appereth, and it is barbarows to Imagine, that he had any conceipt that she had A longing to it." [15] A year later he was again in court, fighting with the secretary of the colony over some cows that, he claimed, went with his post of physician-general. Again he won, and at about the same time his council seat was restored to him.

In 1629 he became temporary governor, serving until the arrival of Sir John Harvey in March 1630. During his short tenure, important regulations for the defense of the colony were adopted and the export trade was expanded, with no less than twenty-three ships visiting Virginia waters in 1629.

Harvey, taking an immediate dislike to Pott, had him arrested for, allegedly, pardoning a willful murderer, killing other people's hogs, and placing his mark on other people's cattle. A jury handpicked by Harvey found him guilty on all counts, and his estates were ordered confiscated. Appeal to the king, with Harvey quite inconsistently supporting clemency on the grounds that Pott was the only physician in the colony capable of treating epidemic diseases, produced a pardon, and Pott returned to the active practice of medicine.

In 1634–35 he headed a movement to get Harvey removed from office in redress of grievances. The governor had

Pott arrested and placed in irons, but public feeling ran so high that Harvey was deposed and sent home to England. Dr. Pott sailed on the same ship to present the colony's side of the case. He remained in England until 1639, when he had the satisfaction of seeing Harvey replaced by Sir Francis Wyatt.

The little evidence that survives suggests that Pott was a good physician. Records of the council and general court contain a number of orders that he be paid for services rendered, and even Harvey paid tribute to his skill in treating epidemic diseases.

Nothing is known of the two surgeons who accompanied Pott to Virginia, beyond the fact that the name of one of them was Cloybourne. However, Pott trained and left behind him a remarkable apprentice in Richard Townshend (c. 1606–1650).

Townshend was fifteen when he became apprenticed to Pott to learn the art of an apothecary. Six years later he sued Pott, alleging that the physician was neglectful in his teaching. The court

> hereuppon ordered yt Mr. Doctor Pott doe henceforth from time to time endeavor to teach & instruct the said Richard Townshend in ye art of an Apothecary by all convenient wayes & means he can or may, that soe hee may prove at ye end of his service a sufficient Apothecarye, wch if ye said Mr. Doctor Pott shall neglect or refuse, the Court hath ordered yt he shall pay the said Richard Townshend for his servive fro ye daye of ye date hereof unto the end and expiration thereof.[16]

However neglectful the master, Townshend learned more than medicine from Dr. Pott. The latter appears to have been well versed in Latin, Greek, and Hebrew, and study under him for six years could not fail to produce an individual better educated than his fellows, many of whom could neither read nor write. The pupil followed the master into politics. By 1628 he was a member of the House of Burgesses; in 1633 he was a justice for York County, and thirteen years later became presiding justice; in the interim he served as a member of the council.

There are records of a few other early doctors. Robert Pawlett functioned as a preacher, physician, and surgeon from 1619 until his death around 1623. Captain John Smith mentioned a Captain William Norton who was killed in the Indian massacre of 1622 and was "a valiant, industrious Gentleman, adorned with many good qualities besides Physicke and Chirurgery, which for the public good he freely imparted to all gratis, but most bountifully to the poore." [17]

William Rowsley, a surgeon, arrived in the colony in 1623 but, along with his wife and servants, died shortly thereafter.

A tombstone found near the site of an Indian village on Potomac Creek is the only surviving evidence that Edmond Hiller (1542–1618) practiced "Physick and Chirurgery" there.

In 1623 William Green, a ship's surgeon, remained ashore for seventeen months, and another, Henry Hitch, practiced for about five months. A Samuel Mole practiced surgery from 1620 to 1623. Edward Gibson, seemingly a physician, cured a number of persons at a settlement at Falling Creek not long before the Indian massacre of 1622, which took 347 victims through the colony.

The charter of the London Company was annulled in

1624, and Virginia became a royal colony. In the following years there were probably no physicians or surgeons comparable in training and education to men like Russell, Bohun, Pott, and Pawlett, who had been sent out by the Company.[18] Medical men were mostly home-grown, self-educated, or products of local apprenticeship.

An apprentice was an indentured servant, a young man who served as house- and stable-boy and at the same time learned from his master how to bleed and cup, to prepare drugs and apply them. These were the basic elements of medicine in that day. Many apprentices became successful physicians.

Sometimes ship's surgeons, having served their apprenticeships or obtained some hospital experience in England, simply established themselves in practice. They also took on apprentices. In this way a body of indigenous doctors began to emerge.

Prior to 1700 there were only three or four physicians with medical degrees in Virginia. Physicians and surgeons practiced side by side—the only difference between them was the extent of education, with no specialties to confuse the public. When women began to number among the immigrants, some served as midwives, nurses, and doctresses. There were no obstetricians.[19]

At the time of the Revolution there were probably four hundred physicians with medical degrees throughout the colonies, while the number of physicians was over thirty-five hundred.[20]

{(2)}

The New England
Colonies

The small band of Puritan Separatist families who disembarked at Plymouth in December 1620 were bound together by their determination to practice their religion freely. They were not chosen for specific qualifications, as the early immigrants to Virginia had been.

The Pilgrim Fathers, led by William Brewster, intended to set up a trading post near the mouth of the Hudson, a region granted in 1606 to a Northern Virginia Company, similar to the London Company that had started Jamestown. The crossing was rough and navigation difficult, and they landed on Cape Cod. This area seemed inhospitable, and after investigation they decided to settle at Plymouth, so named by Captain John Smith, who in 1614 had been employed by the Northern Virginia Company to chart the coast.

Since this area was not in Virginia, the leaders drew up their own plan of government, known as the Mayflower Compact. When in a few years the North Virginia Company was reorganized as the Council of New England and granted this region, the Plymouth Colony was able to obtain a patent.

Other Puritan groups were also granted patents. In 1628, under John Endecott, a group settled at Salem. Their organization was taken over by other Puritans who gained control and formed the "Governor and Company of the Massachusetts Bay in New England." By 1650 there were five Puritan colonies under royal charter.

In 1684 Charles II revoked the charter of the Massachusetts Bay Company and with Maine and New Hampshire, two proprietary colonies, formed the Dominion of New England. In 1686 James II added Plymouth Colony, which had until then been a corporate colony ruled by freemen.

The *Mayflower* carried a ship's surgeon, Giles Heale. He had served as an apprentice in the Guild of Barber Surgeons and had received his right to practice in 1619. But he remained in the area only about six months—until the ship sailed.

In any event, Deacon Samuel Fuller (1580-1633) was the physician of record among the passengers. He was followed into medicine by other members of the cloth.

The clergyman-physician, whether trained in medicine or not, largely limited himself to what could be described as the public-health aspects of medicine. He circulated medical information, generally by printing pamphlets. He dealt with such deficiency diseases as scurvy. He established quarantines during epidemics of contagious diseases. Into "internal medicine" he ventured little, believing that man had an appointed time to live on earth and that any attempt to upset the timetable was sacrilegious.

DEACON-DOCTOR FULLER

Samuel Fuller, then, was the earliest practitioner of medicine in New England. He was born in Norfolk County, England, and completed his theological studies at the Dutch University of Leyden, also the great medical center of the day. It seems probable that Fuller acquired some medical knowledge as a sideline. His third wife, Bridget Lee, whom he met and married in Leyden, was a capable and respected midwife.

In Leyden, Fuller became a close friend of William Bradford, a Puritan Separatist, who persuaded him to join the *Mayflower* expedition.

On arrival, Fuller became a deacon of the church at Plymouth. He found that the local Indians had been almost wiped out by a disease that turned their skins yellow. This may have been bubonic plague.[1] Whatever it was, it does not seem to have been responsible for the death rate of around 50 per cent in the winter of 1620-21. This was generally attributed to scurvy and other diseases brought on by the long voyage in totally inadequate accommodations. No detailed account of Fuller's ministrations to the sick of Plymouth has survived, but it is clear that he served the colonists during the epidemics of typhus and smallpox in 1621.

In 1628 Endecott asked Fuller to come to Salem, where the recently arrived colonists were dying from scurvy and lack of proper food and shelter. The following year, Fuller was again in Salem, dealing with an outbreak of sickness. One of these visits was extended to Charlestown, an unfortunately situated settlement, from where he wrote back to Plymouth: "Many are sick, and many are dead, the Lord in mercy look down on them . . . I here but lose time and long to be home." [2]

Deacon Fuller exhibited more than medical skill in Salem. His skill in matters spiritual closed a rift developing between the two Puritan leaders, Endecott of Salem and Bradford, who had become the second governor of Plymouth Colony in 1621.

On June 28, 1630, Fuller reported by letter to Governor Bradford: "I have been to Matapan [Dorchester], and let some twenty of those people blood." [3]

Plymouth, Salem, Charlestown—for almost a decade Deacon Fuller appears to have been the only physician practicing in the region. He was even in Wessagusset (Weymouth), "although the settlers at that place had behaved in a most unneighborly manner towards those at Plymouth." [4]

His professional services were not restricted to his fellow colonists. When the English dispatched a punitive expedition against Indian chief Corbitant (allegedly to avenge the death of an interpreter named Tisquantum) and returned with two wounded Indians, Fuller took care of their injuries.

In 1828 James Thacher, a physician and medical historian, wrote:

> In his medical character, and for his christian virtues and unfeigned piety, Dr. Fuller was held in the highest estimation, and was resorted to as a father and wise counsellor during the perils of his day. He was finally one of several heads of families who died of a fever which pre-

vailed in Plymouth in the summer of 1633, and was most deeply lamented by all the colonists.[5]

INDIAN NEIGHBORS

Kindness to the Indians did not go unrewarded. When Massasoit, friendly chief of the Wampanoag Indians, was gravely ill and was expected to die, the Plymouth colonists decided to observe Indian custom and send representatives to express sympathy. Edward Winslow (1595-1655), John Hamden, and an Indian named Hobbamock were selected.

Winslow obtained Massasoit's permission to dose him. He gave him "a confection of many comfortable conserves, etc., on the point of my knife . . . which I could scarcely get through his teeth. When it was dissolved in his mouth, he swallowed the juice of it; whereat those that were about him much rejoiced, saying, he had not swallowed any thing in two days before. Then I desired to see his mouth, which was exceedingly furred, and his tongue swelled in such a manner, as it was not possible for him to eat such meat as they had, his passage [esophagus] being stopped up. Then I washed his mouth, and scraped his tongue, and got abundance of corruption out of the same. After which I gave him more of the confection, which he swallowed with more readiness. Then he desiring to drink, I dissolved some of it in water, and gave him thereof. Within half an hour this wrought a great alteration in him, in the eyes of all that beheld him. Presently after his sight began to come to him, which gave him and us good encouragement. In the mean time I inquired how he slept, and when he went to stool. They said he had not slept in two days before and had not had a stool in five." Then Winslow prepared a chicken broth that so greatly strengthened the Indian chief that the next day he asked Winslow to go ". . . amongst those that were sick in the town, requesting me to wash their mouths also, and give to each of them some of the same I gave him, saying they were good folk. This pains I took with willingness."[6]

Massasoit's gratitude for the medical care extended to him was manifested when he subsequently warned Winslow that Indians were planning to massacre the Plymouth settlers.

GILES FIRMIN, JR.

Although, in April 1629, a surgeon, Lambert Wilson, contracted to treat the colonists at Salem and the neighboring Indian tribes for three years and "to educate and to instruct in his art one or more youths," it is unlikely that medical instruction progressed very far, if it was ever begun, because Wilson left the colony about a year after his arrival.[7] Credit for being the first teacher of medicine in New England goes to Giles Firmin, Jr. (1615-1697).

The senior Giles (d. 1634), who had been an apothecary in Sudbury, England, served as a deacon of Boston Church, and at the same time was highly esteemed as a physician. The son, who first came to Massachusetts in 1632, had been educated at Cambridge, a hotbed of Puritanism in England. He studied under Dr. John Clerk (1582-1653) of London, who would be president of the College of Physicians from 1645 to 1649. This tutelage may have occurred around 1634; in *The Real Christian,* published in 1670, Firmin wrote that he was far distant when his father passed away.

While well trained in medicine, Firmin also had a strong bent toward the church. In a pamphlet entitled *A Serious*

Question Stated, he was to write: "Being broken from my study in the prime of my years, from eighteen years of age to twenty-eight, and what time I could get in them years I spent in the study and practise of physic in that wilderness till these times changed, and then I changed my studies to divinity." [8]

Firmin was in Boston in March 1638 and may have practiced there. He is first mentioned in the archives of Ipswich, Massachusetts, on January 4, 1639, when he was granted a hundred acres of land conditional on his remaining in Ipswich for three years. In 1644 he sailed for England, where he spent his remaining years.

A romanticized account of Firmin making rounds accompanied by an apprentice named Luke was penned by Dr. Oliver Wendell Holmes (1809–1894), a prominent physician and writer in his own time.

In the first dwelling they come to, a stout fellow is bellowing with colic.

"He will die, Master, of a surety, methinks," says the timid youth in a whisper.

"Nay, Luke," the Master answers, " 'tis but a dry belly-ache. Didst thou not mark that he stayed his roaring when I did press hard over the lesser bowels? Note that he hath not the pulse of them with fevers, and by what Dorcas telleth me there hath been no long shutting up of the *viœ naturales.* We will steep certain comforting herbs which I will shew thee, and put them in a bag and lay them on his belly. Likewise he shall have my cordial julep with a portion of this confection which we do call *Theriaca Andromachi,* which hath juice of poppy in it, and is a great stayer of anguish. This fellow is at his prayers to-day, but I warrant thee he shall be swearing with the best of them to-morrow."

They jog along the bridle-path on their horses until they come to another lowly dwelling. They sit a while with a delicate looking girl in whom the ingenuous youth naturally takes a special interest. The good physician talks cheerfully with her, asks her a few questions. Then to her mother: "Good-wife, Margaret hath somewhat profited, as she telleth, by the goat's milk she hath taken night and morning. Do thou pluck a maniple—that is an handful—of the plant called Maidenhair, and make a syrup therewith as I have shewed thee. Let her take a cup full of the same, fasting, before she sleepeth, also before she riseth from her bed." And so they leave the house.

"What thinkest thou, Luke, of the maid we have been visiting?"

"She seemeth not much ailing, Master, according to my poor judgment. For she did say she was better. And she had a red cheek and a bright eye, and she spake of being soon able to walk unto the meeting, and did seem greatly hopeful, but spare of flesh, methought, and her voice something hoarse, as of one that hath a defluxion, with some small coughing from a cold, as she did say. Speak I not truly, Master, that she will be well speedily?"

"Yea, Luke, I do think she shall be well, and may-hap speedily. But it is not here with us she shall be well. For that redness of the cheek is but the sign of the fever which, after the Grecians, we do call the hectical; and that shining of the eyes is but a sickly glazing, and they which do every day get better and likewise thinner and weaker shall find that way leadeth to the church-yard gate. This is the malady which the ancients did call *tabes,* or the wasting disease, and some do name the consumption. A disease whereof most that fall ailing do perish. This Margaret is not long for earth—but she knoweth it not, and still hopeth."

"Why, then, Master, didst thou give her of thy medicine, seeing that her ail is unto death?"

"Thou shalt learn, boy, that they which are sick must have somewhat wherewith to busy their thoughts." [9]

On September 24, 1647, the missionary John Eliot (1604–1690), known as the Apostle to the Indians, wrote to Thomas Shepard, a minister at Cambridge:

Our young students in Physick may be trained up better than yet they bee, who have only theoreticall knowledge, and are forced to fall to practise before ever they saw an Anatomy made, or duely trained up in making experiments, for we never had but one Anatomy [skeleton] in the Countrey, which Mr. Giles Firman (now in England) did make and read upon very well, but no more of that now.[10]

HARVARD'S MEDICAL PRESIDENTS

Charles Chauncy (1592–1672), of good English stock, was a student at the Westminster School at the time of Guy Fawkes' attempt to blow up the Parliament building in 1605. Charles almost lost his life in the adventure but lived to obtain several degrees from Cambridge—a B.A. in 1613, an M.A. in 1617, and an S.T.B. in 1624—and to become a fellow of Trinity College. Between 1627, when he left Cambridge to become vicar of Ware, and 1637, when he was forced to emigrate to America, Chauncy's puritanical proclivities kept him in constant trouble with the ecclesiastic authorities, including the Archbishop of Canterbury, William Laud.

After landing at Plymouth in January 1638, he served for three years as assistant to a Mr. Raynor, then moved on to Scituate, where he was pastor of a church for thirteen years. In 1654 he was in Boston, preparing to return to England, when Henry Dunster, first president of Harvard College, was ejected from his post. Chauncy was offered and accepted the position, and held it until his death. He was one of Harvard's early instructors in medicine. He had six sons, all of whom studied medicine; several returned to England to practice.

Leonard Hoar (1629?–1675), who succeeded Chauncy in 1672, had obtained his bachelor's degree from Harvard in 1650 and had gone on to study medicine at Cambridge. Although he introduced technical education by adding a workshop and a chemical laboratory, the "students were too much indulged in their prejudices against him, and he was obliged to resign." [11]

THOMAS THACHER

On January 21, 1678, a broadside entitled *Brief Rule to guide the Common People of New-England How to order themselves and theirs in the Small Pocks, or Measels* appeared. Printed as a poster in double column on one side of a sheet 15½ by 10 inches in size, it was the first medical publication by an author in the colonies. The author was Thomas Thacher (1620–1678), an elderly minister of the Old South (Third) Church.

Thacher was born in England, the son of the Reverend

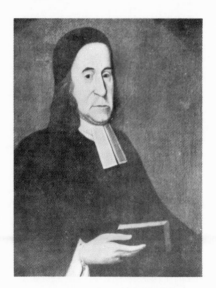

THOMAS THACHER

Peter Thacher, a fellow of Corpus Christi College, Oxford. Young Thomas was destined to go to Oxford or Cambridge, but at the age of fifteen he elected to join his uncle, Anthony Thacher, who was about to sail for New England.

Thomas Thacher's introduction to the New World was marred by disaster. About two months after their arrival, his uncle Anthony, Anthony's cousin Joseph Avery, and their families set sail out of Ipswich for Marblehead, where Avery had agreed to establish a church. Luckily Thomas, who seemingly had had enough of the sea during the two-month voyage from Southampton to Boston, decided to travel overland with a friend. There were twenty-three persons aboard the pinnace when, on August 15, 1645, it was wrecked in a severe storm off the rocky coast of Salem. Only Anthony Thacher and his wife survived.

Thomas had received a sound grammar-school education

in England and he appears to have been a quick and unusual student. "He studied not only what is common for youth to acquire, but also the oriental languages. He afterwards composed a Hebrew lexicon, and . . . he was a scholar in Arabic, the best the country afforded. Dr. Mather tells us that he was a great logician, that he understood mechanics in theory and practice, and he would make all kinds of clock work to admiration." [12]

His religious instruction was at the hands of Charles Chauncy, who may also have provided his medical education; "under the Conduct of that eminent Scholar, [Thacher] became such an one himself." [13]

Thacher was "eminent in two professions. He was pastor of a church, and was ordained at Weymouth, where he practised physic as well as preached, and was an eminent physician in Boston. He was considered as a great divine, and when a third church was founded in the town he was chosen their minister." [14]

He died the same year his broadside appeared, as a result of "visiting a *Sick* Person; after his going out of the Assembly, he got some Harm, which turned into a *Fever,* whereof he did, without any *Hour and Power of Darkness* upon his Holy Mind, expire on *October* 15, 1678." [15]

OTHER PRACTITIONERS

The first strictly medical men to practice in New England were appointed by the London Court of Assistants on March 5, 1628, to serve for a period of three years. Mr. Pratt, a surgeon, practiced in Cambridge until his death in 1645. Of Robert Morly, a barber-surgeon, nothing more is known.

There is no record of William Gager's arrival in Boston,

but it was presumably after Fuller's visit to Charlestown in 1628 or 1629. He died in September 1630 and was described by Governor John Winthrop as "a godly man, skillful chirurgeon, and one of the deacons of the congregation." [16]

A John Wilson is on record as being the first physician in Braintree, practicing there prior to his death in 1627.

John Fisk, a cleric-physician, settled in Salem in 1637.

Another John Wilson (1621–1691), son of the pastor of the first church built in Boston, was graduated from Harvard at its first commencement in 1642 and settled in Medfield as pastor, schoolmaster, and physician. Two of his classmates went on to Europe for their medical education, Samuel Bellingham and Henry Saltonstall.

Henry Greenland (b. 1628) is referred to in a letter to John Winthrop, Jr., first governor of the Connecticut Colony: "Mr. Eliot is under Mr. Greenland's mercuriall administrations, with some encouragement in its operations, yet the issue is all with God." [17]

Matthew Fuller (d. 1678) settled at Plymouth in 1640 and moved on to Barnstable in 1652. In 1673 he was appointed surgeon-general to the provincial forces raised by Plymouth. His estate included a surgeon's chest and drugs valued at sixteen pounds and a library worth ten pounds.

Thomas Starr, who lived at Yarmouth from 1640 to 1670, is referred to many times in the town records as a surgeon. A Comfort Starr (d. 1663) practiced surgery in Newton, Duxbury, and Boston.

∾

This was the picture in Plymouth and the Massachusetts Bay colonies a hundred years before the Declaration of Independence. In the other colonies established along the eastern seaboard the medical development in some colonies followed the New England pattern of clergyman-physician and the haphazard arrival of the medical man, and in others the Virginia planned pattern of physician and surgeon practicing side by side. Either way, medicine was facing and adjusting to the medical needs of the New World.

⸹(3)⸹

Indigenous Remedies
and Practices

Research began as a matter of necessity in the colonies. When medicine chests brought from England were exhausted, enterprising medical men turned to local botanical sources for replacements. Much was learned from Indian practices.

As early as 1610 Lawrence Bohun, as we have seen, was experimenting with native plant remedies. In 1634–35 a Dutch surgeon who had arrived in New Amsterdam in 1630 made a trip into Iroquois country. He noted that "Indian medicine was not all hocus pocus," pointing out that the Iroquois used sulphur to treat many maladies, "but principally for their legs when they were sore from long marching." [1]

A quarter of a century later a visitor from England investigated remedies developed by New England Indians and the practices of the colonists. Between 1684 and 1686 John Clayton, a minister at Jamestown, produced a detailed account of the practices of Virginia Indians.

In 1700 John Lawson, as surveyor-general of North Carolina, traveled through the Carolinas, and nine years later published in London an account of what he had seen.

JOHN JOSSELYN, MEDICAL OBSERVER

John Josselyn (fl. 1675) paid two visits to America and spent considerable time in the Massachusetts settlements. In the chronicle of his visits, first published in 1674, he wrote of the diseases afflicting the Indians:

> The great pox is proper to them, by reason (as some do deem) that they are *Man-eaters*. . . . In *New-England* the *Indians* are afflicted with pestilent Feavers, Plague, Black-pox, Consumption of the Lungs, Falling-sickness, Kings-evil, and a Disease called by the *Spaniard* the Plague in the back, with us *Empyema,* their physicians are the *Powaws* or *Indian* Priests who cure sometimes by charms and medicine, but in a general infection they seldom come amongst them, therefore they use their own remedies, which is sweating, &c. Their manner is when they have plague or small pox amongst them to cover their *Wigwams* with Bark so close that no Air can enter in, lining them (as I said before) within, and making a great fire they remained there in a stewing heat till they are in a top sweat, and then run out into the Sea or River, and presently after they come into their Hutts again they either recover or give up the Ghost.[2]

Josselyn learned from the Indians of a tree growing far inland, big as an oak, that was considered an infallible cure for the falling-sickness. To his lasting regret, he was never able to see a sample or learn whether the bark, the wood, the leaf, or the fruit was used in the cure. The Indians also used white helle-bore as a substitute for opium, which did not grow in America, a habit adopted by the English settlers.

Of the afflictions of the colonists and preferred remedies, he said:

> The Diseases that the *English* are afflicted with, are the same that they have in *England,* with some proper to *New-England,* griping of the belly (accompanied with Feaver and Ague) which turns to the bloudy-flux, a common disease in the Countrey, which together with the small pox hath carried away abundance of their children, for this the common medicines amongst the poorer sort are Pills of Cotton swallowed, or Sugar and Sallet-oyl boiled thick made into Pills, Alloes pulverized and taken in the pap of an Apple. I helped many of them with a sweating medicine only. Also they are troubled with a disease in the mouth or throat which hath proved mortal to some in a very short time, Quinsies, and Imposthumations of the Almonds, with great distempers of cold. Some of our *New-England* writers affirm that the *English* are never or very rarely heard to sneeze or cough, as ordinarily they do in *England,* which is not true. For a cough or stitch upon cold, Wormwood, Sage, Marygolds, and Crabs-claws boiled in posset-drink and drunk off very warm, is a soverign medicine. Pleurisies and Empyemas are frequent there, both cured after one and the same way; but the last is a desperate disease and kills many. For the Pleurisie I have given *Coriander*-seed prepared, *Carduus* seed, and *Harts-horn* pulverized with good suc-

cess, the dose one dram in a cup of wine. The Stone terribly afflicts many, and the Gout, and Sciatica, for which take Onions roasted, peeled and stampt, then boil them with neats-feet oyl and Rhum to a plaister, and apply it to the hip. Head-aches are frequent, Palsies, Dropsies, Worms, Noli-me-tangeres, Cancers, pestilent Feavers. Scurvies, the body corrupted with Sea-diet, Beef and Pork tainted, Butter and Cheese corrupted, fish rotten, a long voyage, coming into the searching sharpness of a purer climate, causes death and sickness amongst them. Men and Women keep their complexions, but lose their Teeth: The Women are pitifully Tooth-shaken; whether through coldness of the climate, or by sweet-meats of which they have store, I am not able to affirm.[3]

Josselyn found in use a plant "called for want of a name *Clownes wound wort,* by the *English,* though it be not the same, that will heal a green [fresh?] wound in 24 hours, if a wise man have the ordering of it." [4]

He had nothing but praise for tobacco:

The vertues of tobacco are these, it helps digestion, the Gout, the Tooth-Ach, prevents infection by scents, it heats the cold, and cools them that sweat, feedeth the hungry, spent spirits restoreth, purgeth the stomach, killeth nits and lice; the juice of the green leaf healeth green wounds, although poysoned; the Syrup for many diseases, the smoak for the Phthisick, cough of the lungs, distillations of Rheume, and all diseases of a cold and moist cause, good for all bodies cold and moist taken upon an emptie stomach, taken upon a full stomach it precipitates digestion, . . . [but] immoderately taken it dryeth the body, enflameth the blood, hurteth the brain, weakens the eyes and sinews.[5]

THE CLAYTON LETTER

Very little is known about the Reverend John Clayton beyond his writings, which include a lengthy letter directed in 1687 to Dr. Nehemiah Grew of the Royal Society, in response to "several Quaerys sent to him by that learned Gentleman." Clayton wrote:

Their *Wiochist,* that is, their Preist [sic] is generally their Physician. And is a person of great honour and esteem among [the Indians], next to the King, or their great War-Captain. . . . Nature is their great Apothecary, each Physician furnishing himself, according to his skill, with Herbs or the leaves, fruit roots or bark of trees. . . .

The means whereby they convey their art to Posterity, I take to be this. They lodge in the Wiochisan houses, i.e. their temples, certain kinds of reliques, such as mens skulls some certain grains or pulse, and several herbs which are dedicated to the Gods. Viz the skulls in memory of their fights and Conquests. The pulse by way of thank-offering for their provisions, and the Herbs upon the same account for some special cure performed thereby. For when any one is cured by any herb he brings part thereof and offers it to his God, whereby the remembrance of this herb and its virtue is not only preserved: But the Preist also becomes best instructed thereby and knowing in the art of Medicine. For otherwise they are mighty reserved of their knowledge even among themselves. Whether the Preist takes certain persons to instruct or teaches only his own Children I know not. Often when they are abroad hunting in the woods, and fall sick, or come by any hurt, they then are forced to make use of any herbs which are nearest at hand, which they are not timorous in venturing upon though they know not the virtue or qualitys thereof. And thus by making many trials and experiments, they find out the virtues of Herbs and by using simple remedys, they certainly know what it is that effects the cure.[6]

The Wiochists employed a sweating process similar to that described by Josselyn, "and they have [herbs in] great plenty and seldom prescribe any thing else." For the most part, their therapy was based on symptoms. "The Indians mind neither the pulse nor Urine only judge by the common most remarkable symptoms, and some pretend to form a judgement from the Countenance." [7]

Clayton credited the Wiochists with "various good wound-herbs." These included *"Indian-weed,"* a member of the genus *Valeriana, white Plantain* (catfoot), and *"Englishmans foot* (or Whiteman's foot)," which, they claimed, was unknown until the English came and only grew where Englishmen had trodden.

The great success they have in curing wounds and sores, I apprehend mostly to proceed from their manner of dressing them: For they first cleanse them by sucking, which though a very nasty, is no doubt the most effecheal and best way imaginable; then they take the *biting Persi-*

cary [probably one of the smartweeds], and chaw it in their mouths, and thence squirt the Juice thereof into the wound, which they will do as if it were out of a Syringe. Then they apply their salve-herbs, either bruised or beaten into a salve with grease, binding it on with bark and silk grass.[8]

While Clayton found no evidence of bloodletting, the Indians clearly believed in purging and induced vomiting. A number of plant-cathartics were used, including *"Poakesroot* [pokesweed] . . . a strong purge, and by most deemed poison" and "wild Ipecac." To produce vomiting they took "the leaves of a certain curious odoriferoys shrub, that grows in the swamps, which I take to be the *lesser sassafras,* they bruise them in water, and then express the juice, which they drink warm."

Native herbs were the mainstay of their *materia medica.* "I have collected about 300 several sorts that were no European plants," he wrote, and then mentioned those "whose virtues I take to be most remarkable."

The morals and social habits of the Indians were also noted by Clayton, and he recounted one of their legends of particular interest:

I have been told that one of their famous Wiochists prophecyed that bearded men (for the American Indians have no beards) should come and take away their Country and that there should none of the original Indians be left, within a certain number of years, I think it was an hundred and fifty. This is very certain that the Indian inhabitants of Virginia are now very inconsiderable as to their number; and seem insensibly to decay though they

35

live under the English protection and have no violence offered them. They are undoubtedly no great breeders.[9]

In the course of his letter Clayton discoursed on the "distempers amongst the English-Natives (for I cannot give so particular an account of the distempers most prominent among the Indians)." These were:

> scorbital-Dropsys, Chachexies [rickets], Lethargys, Seasonings [probably malaria], griping of the guts [intestinal spasms], Sore throats which . . . unless early prevented became a cancerous humour [and] Pains in the Limbs, which I apprehend to have proceeded partly from the same humour floating up and down the body. . . . The oyl of a fish called a Drum [probably the fish now called the sea drum] was found very effecheal to cure these pains. . . . [There are] 3 sorts of oyls in that Country, whose virtues if fully proved might not be found despicable; The oyle of Drums, the oyle of Rattlesnakes, and the oyl of Turkey Bustards [probably the turkey vulture]. The oyl of Sassafras leaves may be deservedly considered too, for they will almost entirely dissolve into an oyle.[10]

JOHN LAWSON, SURVEYOR

Lawson's account of what he found in the Carolinas seems to be overly dramatic, and it is hard to believe in the primitive "medicine" he described.

In the case of a young woman suffering from fits, the medicine man placed her "on her belly and made a small incision with rattlesnake teeth; then laying his mouth to the place he sucked out near a quart of black conglutinated blood and serum."

When a member of Lawson's party became lame in one knee, treatment involved "an instrument something like a comb, which was made of split reed, with fifteen teeth of rattle-snakes, set at much the same distance as in a large horn comb. With these [the operator] scratched the place where the lameness chiefly lay till the blood came, bathing it both before and after incision with warm water spurted out of his mouth; this done, he ran into his plantation and got some sassafras root, which grows there in great plenty, dried it in the embers, scraped off the outward rind, and having beat it between two stones, applied it to the part afflicted, binding it up well. Thus in a day or two the patient became sound."

The treatment performed in this case suggests some medical soundness behind the dramatic façade; less so is the description of methods in vogue among the Indian medicine men:

As soon as the doctor comes into the cabin, the sick person is set on a mat or skin stark naked, except some trifle that covers their nakedness when ripe, otherwise, in very young children there is nothing about them. In this manner the patient lies when the conjurer appears, and the King of that nation comes to attend him with a rattle made of a gourd with peas in it. This the King delivers into the doctor's hand, whilst another brings a bowl of water and sets it down. Then the doctor begins and utters some few words very softly; afterwards he smells of the patient's navel and belly; and sometimes scarifies him a little with a flint, or an instrument made of rattlesnake teeth for this purpose; then he sucks the patient and gets out a mouthful of blood and serum, but serum chiefly, which perhaps may be a better method in many cases than to take away great quantities of blood, as is commonly practised, which he spits in the bowl of water. Then he begins to mutter and talk apace, and at last to cut capers and clap his hands on his breech and sides, till he gets into a sweat, so that a stranger would think that he was running mad, now and then sucking the patient, and so at times keeps sucking till he has got a great quantity of very ill-colored matter out of the belly, arms, breast, forehead, temples, neck and moist parts, still continuing his grimaces and antic postures, which are not to be matched in Bedlam. At last you will see the doctor all over of a dropping sweat, and scarce able to utter one word, having quite spent himself; then he will cease for awhile, and so begin again till he comes in the same pitch of raving and seeming madness as before; all this time the sick body never so much as moves, although doubtless the lancing and sucking must be a great punishment to them, but they certainly are the patientest and most steady people under any burden that I ever saw in my life. At last the conjurer makes an end, and tells the patient's friends whether the patient will live or die.[11]

Lawson did not have much interest in botany, and he provided only scant information about the therapeutic agencies employed. A favorite remedy involved the oil of acorns, "but from what sort of oak I am not certain." Burns were cured "beyond credit," but no mention was made of the medicine used. Pox was cured by "a berry that salivates as mercury does," and they used "decoctions very much," and so on, but he rarely identified Indian plant medicines. He did, however, agree with Josselyn and Clayton about the practice of "sweatings," indicating that "when they are thoroughly heated they leap into the river." [12]

It is a pity that John Lawson did not combine his flair for romantic description with the meticulous observation and devotion to investigatory detail that made John Clayton's account of the medical practice of the Virginia Indians an invaluable document.

❴(4)❵

Cotton Mather, Medical Polemicist

It is hard to reconcile the evaluation of Cotton Mather (1663–1728) as an "intelligent and able [man], but also vain, quarrelsome, excitable, moody, and a fanatical believer in witches," [1] with the description of him as "the first significant figure in American medicine," [2] yet there is justification for both points of view.

There is ample evidence that the young Cotton Mather was a prig. When he entered Harvard at the age of twelve (the youngest student ever to have been admitted there) he already viewed himself "as by birth appointed to carry on [his family's] leadership in the church," [3] and he set about reforming his less pious comrades. While popular with his tutors, he was considerably less acceptable to his classmates. The situation was aggravated when his father, Increase Mather (1639–

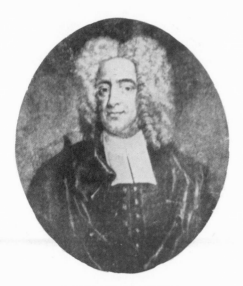

COTTON MATHER

1723), assumed the presidency of Harvard in Cotton's final year.

In 1685 Cotton was ordained at his father's Second Church in Boston, where he served for the rest of his life. The two Mathers came to be regarded by their contemporaries as Puritan saints. This veneration, which continued through several generations, did much to enlarge the retrospective picture of Cotton Mather as a pompous, reactionary theologian, especially when the swing away from the blue laws of Puritan theocracy came.

Cotton's position in regard to witchcraft was to say the least equivocal. The 1692 trials of the Salem witches were ordered by Sir William Phips, who had just been appointed governor of Massachusetts on the nomination of Increase Mather. The son, undoubtedly seeing in this appointment an opportunity for the exercise of political influence, became a staunch supporter of Phips, defending his acts in *Political Fables,* which he circulated in manuscript in 1693, and in his 1697 biography of Phips, *Pietas in Patriam.*

Earlier, Cotton Mather had concluded that "persons molested by the Devil might best be treated by fasting and prayer, and he . . . decided . . . to study cases of diabolical possession in order to combat Satan's wiles. His fervent introspection, coupled with his taste for scientific investigation, led him not only to scrutinize everything which might tend to demonstrate the reality of the world of the spirits but also to exaggerate the importance of his observations." Between 1689 and 1691 he wrote at least three works expressing his views on witchcraft. Just before the Salem trials he warned one of the judges against relying on "spectral evidence" unfavorable to the accused and proposed that whatever punishments might be meted out be less severe than execution. However, presumably out of loyalty to Phips, when executions followed, he failed to protest them.[4]

It is said that Cotton Mather stammered so badly at the time of his graduation from Harvard in 1678 that, believing himself incapable of preaching, he undertook the study of medicine.[5] Undoubtedly his stammering influenced young Mather in the direction of an alternative career, but his interest in medicine predated his Harvard matriculation. In his manuscript autobiography, *Paterna,* he spoke of the "Power of Melancholy," which attacked him between the ages of eleven and fourteen, and "studying Physick at the time, I was unhappily led away with Fancies, that I was myself troubled, with almost every Distemper that I read of, in my Studies; which caused me to use Medicines upon myself, that I might cure my Imaginary maladies." [6]

Mather's education in medicine must have been almost exclusively acquired through book learning. The only basic scientific subject offered at Harvard in the 1670s was physics, and this was at best an introductory course; substantial instruction in the subject was not available until 1687.

The first catalogue of the Harvard College library was not issued until 1723, but many of the medical works listed in it may well have been on hand fifty years earlier. In addition to the works of Galen, these included books by Felix Plater, a sixteenth-century professor of medicine at the University of Basel (Switzerland) and a strong advocate of the study of anatomy through dissection; by Francis de Le Boë (also known as Sylvius), a seventeenth-century professor at the University of Leyden, who established the difference between the organic and inorganic processes in chemistry and who introduced ward instruction in medical education; by William Harvey, who worked out the manner in which blood circulates; by Nicholas Culpeper, the famous herbalist who translated the *Pharmacopoeia Londinensis* into English in 1649 and whose *English Physician* was printed in the colonies in 1708; by Thomas Willis, an unusually successful London practitioner, who was the leading English exponent of chemistry in medicine, a careful clinical observer, and the author of several works including the *Pharmaceutice rationalis* (1674), a valuable summary of the medical writings of his day.

Beyond the Harvard library, Cotton had access to his father's collection of books, which included medical and scientific works, and to other collections, such as that of President Leonard Hoar of Harvard.

In modern times it has become customary to discount book learning, but in the seventeenth century most universities had little else to offer, so much so that at ancient institutions

43

like Oxford and Cambridge students down to the present century were said to "read" their subject of choice. Thus, unless Cotton Mather had followed William Harvey to the University of Padua in Italy or attended another rare school of medicine that offered some practical instruction, he would have gained no more from the typical European and British schools than from his self-teaching, except for an M.D. degree that was no guarantee of empirical knowledge or manual dexterity.

In February 1686 Cotton noted in his diary that he had given up all thought of becoming a physician, but he was to return time and time again to his medical interests, integrating them into his spiritual beliefs.

There is no concrete evidence that Mather ever practiced medicine in the full sense of the word. This may have been because there were enough physicians in Boston at the beginning of the eighteenth century, and Mather seems to have held the true professional in high regard. In his *Essays to do Good* (*Bonifacius*), which appeared in 1710, he urged urban clergy to unite their counsels with physicians on medical problems. Nevertheless, he was firm in his belief that clergymen-physicians should serve their flock medically as well as physically when regular physicians were not available. In issuing a series of medical pamphlets, starting with one on measles published anonymously in 1713, he made it clear that these were only intended to serve "the Poor, and such as may want [i.e., lack] the help of Able Physicians." [7]

In 1711 Mather decided to train his daughter Katy in "Knowledge of Physic, and the Preparation, and the Dispensation of noble Medicines." [8] Free dispensaries did not generally appear in the New World until later in the eighteenth century. In training Katy, Mather almost certainly had in mind the need for dispensing medicines to the poor. While Mather may have refrained from the public practice of medicine, he seemingly did not hesitate to prescribe for his family and friends. In 1713 he recommended that his seventy-four-year-old father take frequent doses of *Sal Volatile* and continue to do so as long as he might live. Nor did he hesitate to make recommendations to physicians. In 1718 he proposed that doctors treating "distracted persons" employ baths, a type of therapy that is still used in some cases of mental illness.

In the seventeenth century serious attempts were made to throw off the superstitions inherited from the Middle Ages and put medicine on a scientific basis. The extent to which these new ideas penetrated the colonies in America is questionable. No local school taught medicine, there were no general hospitals, and there was no scientific society (other than the short-lived Philosophical Society founded in Boston in 1683, which may or may not have discussed medical matters). There was little locally produced medical literature to encourage an interchange of knowledge, techniques, and ideas.

Cotton Mather, however, read European medical literature throughout his life and wrote as prolifically as he read and preached. So great were his output on scientific subjects and his growing scientific reputation—not to mention a voluminous if somewhat one-sided correspondence with Richard Waller, one of the secretaries of the Royal Society of London—that in 1713 he was elected to that body.

The *Angel of Bethesda,* Mather's only full-scale medical work, was written toward the end of his life—between 1720 and 1724. As a physician of the body as well as of the soul, at least in theory, he saw little reason to differentiate between his vocations. His religious teachings made full use of medical metaphor; his medical thinking embraced religious concepts. Christ was the great and glorious physician; *The Great Physician, Inviting Them that are Sensible to their Internal Maladies To Repair Unto Him for His Heavenly Remedies* was published in Boston in 1700. Disease came into the world through original sin seeded in man by Adam. The sinner suffers from "the Palsey of an unsteady Mind . . . the Feavour of Unchastity . . . the Cancer of Envy . . . the Tympany of Pride." His audience was "a Congregation of Sick Souls: Where am I preaching, Sirs, but in an Hospital?" [9]

Because of their sin, sinners could become more than metaphorically diseased. Since such illness must be relieved by prayers for divine intercession and forgiveness, who could better guide the sufferer than his pastor?

This soul medicine was in a sense a forerunner of Christian Science and of psychosomatic medicine as it is known today. It is just possible that the ministrations of the clergy were as effective as the bleedings, the sweatings, and other procedures that were the stock-in-trade of the typical medical practitioner. Though the bedside manner of the clergy was undoubtedly impressive, emphasis on inborn depravity as a cause of disease may have inspired patients with fear rather than hope.

Mather's *Magnalia Christi Americana: or the Ecclesiastical History of New England from its First Planting* (1702) has been described as "a more considerable literary achievement than any previously produced in Massachusetts." [10] In this work Mather frequently included details of illnesses, particularly of the final illness, of those about him. Some of his descriptions are picturesque.

Nathaniel Rogers survived youthful attacks of *Flatus Hypocondria* (whatever that may be) and a subsequent spitting of blood, which led him to believe he was at death's door, only to succumb to a "flood of rheum, occasioned partly by his disuse of tobacco." [11]

Brother Nathaniel Mather's weak constitution allowed ill humors to collect where "the *os ileon* and the *os sacrum* join," at the base of the spine, and form a tumor. When an operation failed to disperse the "putrid juices," the patient developed a fever and died.[12]

A fascinating example of early brain surgery involved Abigail Eliot, who had lost part of her brain in an accident. What remained swelled in synchrony with the tides. After a silver plate had been inserted in her head, Abigail resumed her normal way of life. It is somewhat hard to credit Mather's account of Sarah Wilkinson, who, after her death of a dropsy, was found to have lived for years with, essentially, no internal organs.[13]

In 1712, ten years after the *Magnalia*, Mather completed his *Biblia Americana*, which was never published.

Between 1713 and 1725 he directed about one hundred communications to the Royal Society. Medicine and related subjects were well represented. There were comments on the medical properties of native plants and animals. He mentioned a valuable drug derived from the gall of rattlesnakes that produced sweating and was used to reduce fevers and alleviate the difficulties of childbirth. There was an antidote for snakebite. And while Mather regarded the native Indians as children of the devil rather than noble red men, he was satisfied that God had devised remedies appropriate to each part of the world and that the original Americans had resided in theirs long enough to uncover His local blessings.

His medical letters drew heavily on Indian medical lore. There was the plant fagina, which was believed to have some of the properties of the Peruvian plant coca, but of which Mather was frank to admit: "All that I yet know from my experience of my own, is that it is a tea, it has a mighty invigorating and exhilirating vertue. It refreshes the spirits with an uncommon Brightnesse, . . . It prevents and removes Lassitude when great Fatigues are to be encountered." [14] There were partridgeberry with which to cure dropsy, throat-weed to relieve a sore throat, bleeding root, which could cure jaundice in six days, and cranesbill (geranium), which, brewed into a tea, was a specific for syphilis.

The letters show a lessening dependence on divine intervention as the basis for remarkable cures. In the *Magnalia,* Mather's answer to the question of what wounds may be considered mortal was, ". . . such as he shall in his holy providence actually make so." [15] Facing the same question in writing to the Royal Society, he found the problem "almost impossible to be decided." [16]

In *The Christian Philosopher,* published in London in 1720, Mather brought together his accumulated scientific knowledge. While less attention was given to medicine than to the natural sciences, there was some discussion of the skeleton, the muscles, the nerves, the sense organs, and the teeth—in short, the chief features of anatomy and physiology. The book clearly revealed how Mather's preoccupation with medicine and other sciences had influenced his seemingly unshakable Puritan religious views and beliefs. He no longer regarded nature as a manifestation of God's dread power; nature, in its wondrous beauty, was the symbol of God's goodness and mercy.

His writing on medical subjects had also been considerable but largely scattered through pamphlets and unpublished letters to members of the Royal Society. As he approached his sixtieth year he felt it was time to bring these together. An announcement of the forthcoming work was made by "Your Servants, the BookSellers," but the book was not published. In the "Proposals for printing a BOOK entituled:—THE ANGEL OF BETHESDA," they described the work as "An Essay upon the Common Maladies of Mankind: offering, first, The Sentiments of Piety, whereto the Invalids are to be awakened in and from their bodily Maladies. And then, a rich Collection of plain but potent and approv'd Remedies for the Maladies." [17]

The Angel of Bethesda had been the title of one of Mather's pamphlets. He had also applied the phrase to John Winthrop, Jr., who was famous throughout New England for his medical knowledge and skill: "Wherever he came, still the diseased flocked about him, as if the Healing Angel of Bethesia [sic] had appeared in the place." [18]

In his last major work Mather again presents sickness as divine punishment for original sin. Sin, he says, brings on "a Sickness in the Spirit [which] will naturally cause a Sickness in the Body." Sin begins in the mind, causing a sickness of the spirit, which in turn takes the form of physical illness. Cure is dependent on the activity of "The Breath of Life" but most "certainly, the Physician that can find out Remedies (particularly in the Mineral or Vegetable Kingdome) that shall have a more immediate Efficacy to brighten, and strengthen, and comfort . . . will be the most successful Physician in the World. Especially, if he can irradiate the Spirit in the Stomach, he will do wonderfully. The things also, which fortify the Blood, and restore a volatil Ferment, in the vapid and languid Blood, will do wonders for us. It is impossible to kill a Man, . . . till the Circulation of his Blood be ruined." [19]

Mather next turns to mental factors in bodily health. "A

cheerful Heart does Good like a Medicine, but a broken Spirit dries the Bones," he says, and goes on to quote Giorgio Baglivi (1669–1707), the outstanding Roman clinician: " 'That a great part of our Diseases, either do rise from, or are fed by a Weight of Cares, lying on the Minds of Men. Diseases that seem incureable, are easily cured by agreeable Conversation. . . .' " Therefore, says Mather, "Lett the Physician with all possible Ingenuity of Conversation, find out, what Matter of Anxiety there may be upon the Mind of the Patient; what there is that has made his Life uneasy to him. Having discovered the Burden, lett him use all the Ways he can devise, to take it off. Offer him such Thoughts of the Righteous, and the Ways to a Composure with religious Principles. Give him a Prospect, if you can, of sound Deliverance from his Distresses, or some Abatement of them. Raise in him as bright Thoughts as may be; and scatter the Clouds, remove the Loads, which his Mind is perplexed withal; especially, by representing and magnifying the Mercy of God in Christ unto him." [20]

Of particular significance is Chapter VII, *"Conjecturalies, or, some Touches upon, A New Theory of many Diseases."* Mather starts from a conclusion that a distempered stomach is the origin of all diseases, and then asks how such distempering of the stomach comes about.

Mather was well acquainted with and relied on the works of such men as the English physician Benjamin Marten (fl. 1720); the Jesuit priest Athanasius Kircher (1602–1680), one of the earliest of the microscopists; the pathologist August Hauptman (1607–1674); the Dutch lexicologist Stephen Blancard, or Blankaart (1650–1702); and the Dutch merchant with a hobby of grinding lenses and constructing microscopes, Anton van Leeuwenhoek (1632–1723). Among Mather's conclusions were:

> Every Part of Matter is peopled. Every green Leaf swarms with Inhabitants. The Surfaces of Animals are covered with other Animals. Yea, the most solid Bodies, even Marble itself, have innumerable Cells, which are Crouded with imperceptible Inmates. As there are infinite Numbers of these, which the Microscopes bring to our View, so there may be inconceivable Myriads yett smaller than these, which no Glasses have yett reach'd unto. The Animals that are much more than thousands of times less than the finest Grain of Sand, have their Motions; and so, their Muscles, their Tendons, their Fibres, their Blood, and the Eggs wherein their Propogation is carried on. The Eggs of these Insects (and why not the living Insects too!) may insinuate themselves by the Air, and with our Aliments, yea, thro' the Pores of our Skin; and soon gett into the Juices of our Bodies. They may be convey'd into our Fluids, with the Nourishment which we received, even before we were born; and may ly dormant until the Vessels are grown more capable of bringing them into their Figure and Vigour for Operations. Thus may Diseases be convey'd from the Parents unto their Children, before they are born into the World. . . .

> As for the Distempers in humane Bodies, Kircher and Hauptman assert, the Malignant Fevers never proceed from any other Cause than little Animals. Blancard affirms, that the Microscope discovers the Blood in Fevers to be full of Animals. . . .[21]

He goes on to illustrate how the migration of what would later be called bacteria explains epidemic diseases in man. He quotes from Dr. Marten to the effect that "great Quantities of these Animals . . . may . . . find a Nest" in our blood or vessels and reproduce themselves there, but if our bodily functions are normal, the animals may be cast out as fast as they are bred there.[22]

Although there was considerable European acceptance of the germ theory in the seventeenth and eighteenth centuries, there was little knowledge of it in the colonial medical fraternity. This makes it more amazing that an American clergyman who had started out so closely wedded to the concept of soul medicine should so wholeheartedly have endorsed the theory. Unfortunately, because *The Angel* did not achieve publication until 1973, Mather exerted little influence on eighteenth-century American physicians.

While much of what Cotton Mather wrote was based on reading rather than practical experience, he was not hesitant in criticism. Chapter XL, "A Pause made upon, The Uncertainties of PHYSICIANS," begins:

> When we are upon a Consumption it may be a proper Time and Place as any to make a Remark upon, The Uncertainties of Physicians, on whose Advice the Patients depend so much for their Lives, and Comfort of them. Their Uncertainties appear notoriously and sufficiently in their Contradictions to one another: which indeed are very conspicuous in this Distemper . . . but also to be found in all Diseases. . . . A famous Physician, who shall be nameless, died of a Disease, which at that very Time, he had a Book in the Press, to teach the Cure of.

We will single out, the Consumption, for our Experiment; because it is one of those Maladies . . . upon which more has been written than upon many others. And here we will not concern ourselves with the Differences among the Physicians, about the Cause of this Distemper; (whereupon, who can read the Collection made by [Johann] Dolaeus [(1651–1707)], and not cry out, The Diviners are mad!) but only see, how they differ about the Cure of it. . . .[23]

Mather is driven to a desperate, if not untypical, conclusion:

The Result of this Discourse is, to take off our Dependence on Arm of Flesh, and show what Cause we have to depend on the glorious God alone, for the Cure of our Diseases. What should be the Motto on the Curtains of every sick Bed, but this: *My Help cometh from the Lord who made Heaven and Earth!*

All this, without the least Intention to depreciate the skilful and faithful Physician.

The Words in the thirty eighth Chapter of Ecclesiasticus, deserve as good a Reception with us, as the most oraculous that ever fell from the Pen of Hippocrates.

Honour a Physician with the Honour due him, for the Uses you may have of him. Inasmuch as the Lord hath created him; for of the Most High cometh Healing; and the Skill of the Physician shall lift up his Head.

Give Place to the Physician for the Lord hath created him; lett him not go from thee for thou hast Need of him. There is a Time when in their Hands there is good Success.[24]

Had Cotton Mather done no more than theorize, as he largely did in *The Angel* and his other works, he might have become the forgotten man of medicine. Fortunately there was one area in which his theories were put to practical use so successfully that he may justly be regarded as the first significant figure in American medicine. That area was inoculation.

❧(5)❧

Hospitals: Care of the Sick Poor and the Mentally Ill

Until the nineteenth century hospitals were for the poor, the homeless, the stranger, and the mentally ill—not for private patients. It is generally thought that the Pennsylvania Hospital, chartered in 1751, was the first in the American colonies, with the New York Hospital, twenty years later, the second. Actually the first American hospital was built in 1612 at Henricopolis, Virginia, fifty miles upriver from Jamestown.

This hospital boasted eighty beds, with "keepers"—probably male nurses—on hand to take care of the patients and speed their recovery. Since nothing more is on record about this hospital, it may be assumed that it was burned to the ground in the 1622 Indian massacre.

From 1620 until its regime ended in 1624, the London Company provided "guest houses" with accommodations for sick men as well as strangers. For fifty years thereafter, patients were "hospitalized" in the homes of physicians and the houses of Virginians who, while not doctors, had acquired some reputation for nursing and found the care of the sick profitable.

In December 1658 Jacob Hendricksen Varrevanger, a New Amsterdam surgeon, became concerned about the lack of proper medical care for ailing soldiers and other employees of the Dutch West India Company; under prevailing practices, they suffered much "through cold, inconveniences, and the untidiness of the people who have taken the poor fellows into their houses where bad smells and filth counteract all health producing medicaments." Varrevanger petitioned the Provincial Council, and as an outcome the first hospital on Manhattan Island was established. The Old Hospital, as it came to be known, was opened prior to July 1660, with Hilletze Wilbruch, the wife of Condil Tubias Wilbruch, serving as matron at an annual salary of one hundred florins. In 1680 the Old Hospital was rated unserviceable and pulled down by order of Governor Andros. People were thereafter attended in their homes by doctors provided by the municipality.

There is no further mention of a hospital in New York until 1736, when a Workhouse and House of Correction was erected where New York's City Hall now stands. The designation of this poorhouse as a hospital was based on a directive "that the Upper Room at the West End of the said House be suitable furnished for an infirmary and for no other use whatsoever." It did not have a regular medical attendant prior to the Revolution, and probably its chief claim to remembrance is the fact that out of its one room evolved New York's Bellevue Hospital.[1]

Whether the pesthouses or quarantine stations set up in the seaports in the eighteenth century should be rated as hospitals—they were sometimes known as isolation hospitals—is questionable. Their purpose, after all, was to protect the well, with care of the sick a secondary consideration.

On May 15, 1717, the selectmen of Boston authorized the acquisition of not more than an acre of land on Dere Island for the erection of a pesthouse. Charleston, South Carolina, had a pesthouse on Sullivan's Island prior to 1752, when a hurricane carried the shelter several miles up the Cooper River, drowning nine people. On February 3, 1743, Fisher's Island became the site of the Philadelphia pesthouse. Fifteen years later Bedloe's Island, on which the Statue of Liberty would be erected in the 1880s, was purchased for the construction of a pesthouse. There was also a pesthouse in Salem, Massachusetts.

In 1734, the vestry of St. Philip's Parish in Charleston obtained permission from the governor to raise money to build a "good, substantial, and convenient Hospital, workhouse and House of Correction." (The construction of adjacent buildings to house patients, paupers, and prisoners was then a common if undesirable practice.) The hospital seems to have been opened in 1738 (fourteen years before the Pennsylvania Hospital) and to have continued in operation at least until 1789, when care of the poor passed from religious hands and hospital entries in the account book of St. Philip's vestry ceased.[2]

The Philadelphia Hospital has also challenged the Pennsylvania Hospital's claim to first place. In 1742, "ten years before the founding of the Pennsylvania Hospital," the Philadelphia Hospital "was dispensing its blessings in a varied routine of beneficial operations, giving employment and support to the poor; a hospital for the sick, an asylum for the insane, the idiotic, and the orphan. It was dispensing its acts of mercy . . .

57

more than twenty years before a school of medicine was founded in Philadelphia. . . ." [3]

Whatever the claims and counterclaims, it is clear that the Pennsylvania Hospital was not the first hospital established in the American colonies. It is, however, "generally recognized as the oldest [surviving] institution for the care of the sick in the United States." [4]

THE PENNSYLVANIA HOSPITAL

A contemporary account of the conception of the Pennsylvania Hospital and the first few years of existence had as its author Benjamin Franklin. In 1754 he wrote:

About the end of the year 1750, some persons, who had frequent opportunities of observing the distress of such distempered poor as from time to time come to Philadelphia, for the advice and assistance of the physicians and surgeons of that city; how difficult it was for them to procure suitable lodgings, and other conveniences proper to their respective cases, and how expensive the providing good and careful nurses, and other attendants, for want whereof, many must suffer greatly, and some probably perish, that might otherwise have been restored to health and comfort, and become useful to themselves, their families, and the publick, for many years after; and considering moreover, that even the poor inhabitants of this city, though they had homes, yet were therein but badly accommodated in sickness, and could not be so well and so easily taken care of in their separate habitations, as they might be in one convenient house, under one inspection, and in the hands of skilful practitioners; and several of the inhabitants of the province, who unhappily became disordered in their senses, wandered about, to the terror of their neighbours, there being no place (except the house of correction) in which they might be confined, and subjected to proper management for their recovery, and that house was by no means fitted for such purposes; did charitably consult together, and confer with their friends and acquaintances, on the best means of relieving the distressed, under those circumstances; and an Infirmary, or Hospital, in the manner of several lately established in Great Britain, being proposed, was so generally approved, that there was reason to expect a considerable subscription from the inhabitants of this city, towards the support of such a Hospital; but the expense of erecting a building sufficiently large and commodious for the purpose, it was thought would be too heavy, unless the subscription could be made general through the province and some assistance could be obtained from the assembly. . . .[5]

The prime movers in the project were Dr. Thomas Bond (1712–1784) and Benjamin Franklin, neither of whom was native to Pennsylvania. Franklin had moved from Boston to Philadelphia early in life and was a keen organizer of the philanthropic, cultural, and scientific activities of his adopted city. By 1750, as editor and publisher of a local newspaper, he was regarded as its most distinguished and influential citizen.

Bond, born in Calvert County, Maryland, studied under Dr. Alexander Hamilton at Annapolis. Then, since there were no domestic schools, or hospitals in which to serve an internship, he studied in England, Scotland, and France at medical schools that were affiliated with hospitals. In these Bond

59

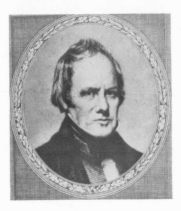

THOMAS BOND

learned the value of institutional care of the sick. Back in this country, and in practice in Philadelphia, he recognized the need for a local hospital and tried to interest his friends and acquaintances. He made little progress in securing the necessary money until he turned to Benjamin Franklin.

Franklin wrote in his autobiography:

> In 1751, Dr. Thomas Bond, a particular friend of mine, conceived the idea of establishing a hospital in Philadelphia, (a very beneficial design, which has been ascribed to me, but was originally and truly his) for the reception and cure of poor sick persons, whether inhabitants of the province or strangers. He was zealous and active in endeavoring to procure subscriptions for it; but the proposal being a novelty in America, and at first not well understood, he met with little success.
>
> At length he came to me with the compliment, that he found there was no such thing as carrying a public-spirited project through without my being concerned in it.

"For," he said, "I am often asked by those to whom I propose subscribing 'Have you consulted Franklin on this business? And what does he think of it?' And when I tell them I have not, (supposing it to be rather out of your line) they do not subscribe, but say they will consider it." I inquired into the nature and probable utility of the scheme, and receiving a very satisfactory explanation, I not only subscribed to it myself, but engaged heartily in the design of procuring subscriptions from others. Previously, however, to the solicitation, I endeavored to prepare the minds of the people by writing on the subject in the newspapers, which was my usual custom in such cases, but which he had omitted.

The subscriptions afterwards were more free and generous; but beginning to flag, I saw they would be insufficient without some assistance from the Assembly, and, therefore, proposed to petition for it; which was done. . . .[6]

When the bill was before the Assembly, passage was in question because some members were afraid "that the expense of paying physicians and surgeons, would eat up the whole of any fund that could be reasonably expected to be raised; but three of the profession, viz. doctors Lloyd Zachary, Thomas Bond, and Phineas Bond, generously offered to attend the Hospital gratis for three years, . . . the bill on the seventh of the same month passed the house." [7] On May 11, 1751, "An ACT to encourage the establishing of an Hospital for the Relief of the Sick Poor of this province, and for the Reception and Cure of Lunaticks" was approved by the governor.[8]

Before the hospital opened the doors of its temporary quarters in February 1752, the services of other well-known physicians were secured. "Rules to be observed in the choice of Physicians and Surgeons" were already established.

The ninth rule read: "No person shall be received hereafter as a candidate to be employed in the said Hospital, as a physician or surgeon, until he be a member of this corporation, and of the age of twenty seven years, hath served a regular apprenticeship in this city or suburbs, hath studied physick and surgery seven years or more, and hath undergone an examination of six of the practitioners of the Hospital, in the presence of the managers, and is approved by them: And with respect to strangers, they shall have resided three years or more in this city, and shall be examined and approved of in the manner, and under the restrictions aforesaid." [9]

In the first twenty-six months of operation, ninety-nine patients were admitted. Of these, fifty-eight were cured, eleven were relieved, four withdrew, three were declared incurable, nine died, and fourteen remained in the hospital. Mental cases were excluded from these highly commendable figures because most of those admitted were chronic cases with little or no prospect of relief. From these figures Franklin argued that, if the contributions of a limited number of contributors could do so much good, a more widespread charitable investment could not fail to do more good. His optimism was justified. In the first five five-year periods of operation, admissions advanced progressively from 399 in 1753–57 to 688 in 1758–62; to 1552 in 1763–67; to 1936 in 1768–72; and to 2031 in 1773–77.[10]

The cornerstone for the building, as originally planned, was laid on May 28, 1755, and patients were admitted to its first section in December 1756. The completed structure (still in use) consisted of a central administration area, two wings of wards two stories high, and a basement. It was completed in 1805.

Around 1788 a distinguished Frenchman, M. de War-ville, visited the Pennsylvania Hospital and wrote subsequently:

> I have seen the hospitals of France, both at Paris and in the provinces; I have known none of them but the one at Besançon that can compare to this at Philadelphia. Every sick and every poor person has his bed well furnished, but without curtains, as it should be. Every room is lighted by windows placed opposite, which produce plenty of light.
>
> Blacks are here mingled with the whites and lodged in the same apartments. This to me seemed a balm to my soul. I saw a negro woman spinning with activity by the side of her bed. She seemed to expect a word of consolation from the director; she obtained it, and it seemed to be heaven to her to hear it. On our return from the hospital we drank a bottle of cider. Compare this frugal repast to the sumptuous feasts given by the superintendents of the poor of London—by those humane inspectors who assemble to consult on making repairs to the amount of six shillings and order a dinner for six guineas! You never find among the Quakers these robberies upon indulgence, these infinite treasons against beneficence. . . .
>
> The hospital is fine, elegant and well kept. I observed the bust of Franklin in the library and was told this honor was rendered to him as one of the principal

founders of the institution. Each one of the lunatics (about fifteen) has a cell, with a bed, a table and a convenient window fitted with grates. Stoves are fixed to the walls to warm the cells in winter. . . . I observed that none of the [lunatics] were naked or indecent—a thing very common with us. . . .[11]

BENJAMIN RUSH

The contributions to medicine made by Benjamin Rush (1745–1813) included work with the mentally ill. His *Medical Inquiries and Observations upon the Diseases of the Mind,* published in Philadelphia in 1812, was the first American textbook on psychiatry. By 1835 it had run through five editions. It was based on almost thirty years' observation at the Pennsylvania Hospital, where Rush was in charge of mental patients.

On November 11, 1789, six years after Rush joined the staff, he wrote the board of managers:

> Under the conviction that the patients afflicted by Madness, should be the first objects of the care of a physician of the Pennsylvania Hospital, I have attempted to relieve them, but I am Sorry to add that my attempts which at first promised some Improvement were soon afterwards rendered Abortive by the Cells of the hospital.
>
> These apartments are damp in Winter & too warm in Summer. They are moreover so constituted, as not to admit readily of a change of air; hence the smell of them is both offensive and unwholesome. . . .[12]

This letter has peculiar significance. There have been suggestions that Rush's work was not original, that it was based on the work of Philippe Pinel (1755–1826) of the Paris School of Hygiene and the work of William Tuke (1732–1822), the English businessman who in 1794 founded the Quaker York Retreat for the insane. It was Pinel and Tuke's aim to replace prevailing medical and lay practices with a humanitarian approach. They "emphasized psychological factors. They believed that insanity could be cured and based their therapeutics on kindness and the consideration of each patient's physical and emotional needs. The ideal regimen included placing the patient in a mental hospital where he would receive considerate treatment, occupational therapy, entertainment, mild exercise, good food, and comfortable lodgings." [13]

Pinel wrote a treatise on insanity that was published in Paris in 1791 but did not appear in an English translation until 1806; the first detailed description of the York Retreat was published in 1813. Rush may have been influenced by what he heard and read from abroad; he may even have read Pinel's treatise before he completed his book on diseases of the mind; but Rush had been at work on the problem since 1783, and his inquiries and observations cannot be dismissed as wholly derivative.

As early as the 1770s Rush's medical philosophy involved a belief that good health depended on the social, political, and economic environment as well as on physical factors. His crusade for reform in the treatment of the insane evolved from this philosophy. While he held moral treatment secondary to medical treatment, he at the same time considered psychological approaches important in the treatment of all disease.

Breaking with tradition, he demanded that mental illness be freed from moral stigma, that the insane be handled with kindness, and that, in cases of religious melancholia, the patient be treated with medicine rather than preaching and moralizing. However, he remained firmly committed to such eighteenth-century practices as bloodletting, purging, heavy dosing with emetics, physical restraint, chastisement, and shock therapy—cold showers and stimulation of terror. In short, while advocating a humanitarian approach and "moral treatment," Rush continued to hold the view that insanity was fundamentally somatic, a pathological brain condition producing psychological symptoms. Rush believed that all disease involved tension in the blood vessels (to be relieved by bloodletting) and that in mental disorders the abnormal condition of the blood vessels localized in the brain.

As an alternative to shock therapy, Rush invented a tranquilizing chair that, by holding the patient upright and immobile, slowed the movement of the blood to the brain and, by directing it elsewhere, relieved tension.

Rush urged his mental patients to write their thoughts, experiences, recollections, and secrets on paper. He believed that when patients saw what they had written down they would be shocked into rejecting their morbid ideas. This was hardly anticipation of the Freudian theory of the subconscious, but he was moving in the right direction.

Rush recognized the paramount importance of the doctor-patient relationship. Discussion, he saw, mitigated the undesirable effects of repressed emotions and inspired the patient with a hope of recovery. He classified as possible emotional disorders many antisocial actions considered sinful—suicide, impulse to murder, compulsive stealing, habitual lying, drunkenness. Despite his basically medical approach, Rush held with Pinel that insanity did not always involve disorder of

66

the intellect. Some insane persons reasoned well but became "the involuntary vehicle of vicious actions, through the instrumentality of their passions." Rush called this condition "mental derangement." [14]

In the field of mental illness Rush produced more effect on medical thought than any other American. Those who have called him the Father of American Psychiatry have done so with justification.

THE NEW YORK HOSPITAL

On May 16, 1769, Dr. Samuel Bard (1716–1799) delivered a "Discourse upon the Duties of a Physician" to the first graduating class of King's College School of Medicine,

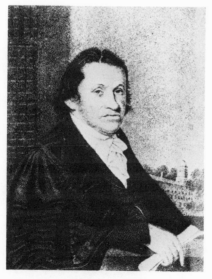

SAMUEL BARD

of which he was professor of the practice of medicine. Toward the conclusion of the discourse he called to his hearers' attention the unhappy state of the poor man struck down by disease and his helpless family. The budding doctors would find themselves treating such patients under the difficult and deplorable conditions existing in their homes, because there was no public hospital in which these miserable objects of charity might be cared for.

The benefits of such a hospital, he felt, should not be confined to the poor but should extend to the safety and welfare of the whole community. Nor, in his opinion, was the scheme for a public hospital impractical. It had for some time past engaged the attention of many charitable and benevolent individuals, particularly in medicine and religion, and it was now time to recommend it to the serious consideration of the public.[15]

On November 3, 1769, in an address delivered at King's College, Dr. Peter Middleton (d. 1781) said:

> The necessity and usefulness of a public infirmary has been so warmly and pathetically set forth in a discourse delivered by Dr. Samuel Bard . . . that his Excellency Sir Henry Moore immediately set on foot a subscription for that purpose, to which himself and most of the gentlemen liberally contributed. His Excellency also recommended it in the most pressing manner to the Assembly of the Province as an object worthy of their attention.[16]

Two years were to elapse before funds, voted and collected, were sufficient to warrant the purchase of a site. Five acres were acquired, and construction of the central building was begun in July 1773. Plans for the building had been obtained by Dr. John Jones (1729–1791), professor of surgery at King's College School of Medicine, during a trip to Europe in 1772. Dr. Jones was hopeful that the hospital would "have fewer objections to its plan, than any Hospital hitherto constructed;—the principal wards, which are to contain no more than eight beds, are thirty six feet in length, twenty four wide, and eighteen high;—they are all well ventilated, not only from the opposite disposition of the windows, but by proper openings in the side walls, and the doors open into a long passage or gallery, thoroughly ventilated from north to south." [17]

In 1775, when the buildings were close to completion, they were almost totally destroyed by fire. Owing to the War of Independence and the subsequent derangement of city affairs, rebuilding was not completed and the hospital formally opened until January 1791, twenty years after it had been chartered. In the interim part of it was used as an infirmary and part for dissections.

During the next century the hospital earned a reputation equal to that of any other institution of its kind. In an address delivered in 1855, Dr. Joseph M. Smith, professor of theory and practice of physic and clinical medicine at the College of Physicians and Surgeons of New York, praised the staff of the hospital in these words:

> There has been no case admitted into the house warranting and requiring an operation, however formidable, which has not here found a surgeon qualified by his knowledge, his eye, heart, and hand, for its performance. Operations of which there were few or no precidents, and

so unpromising in their results as scarcely to justify their performance or repetition, have been executed with a skill that elevated the operator to the level of those enjoying the highest European reputation.[18]

Part II

---∽⚬∾---

THE DEVELOPMENT OF
MEDICAL EDUCATION

---∽⚬∾---

⚾(6)⚾

Dissection and Anatomy

Down through the ages men interested in science have had to fight for the right to dissect bodies in order to learn and teach anatomy. Antagonists of dissection maintained their position on both religious and political grounds. When advocates of dissection did win a victory, its effect was apt to be local rather than universal.

In the British Isles, the earliest reference to dissection dates from 1505, when the magistrates of Edinburgh, in a charter granted to the city's Guild of Surgeons and Barbers, made provision for the body of an executed criminal to be dissected annually. In 1540 the English Parliament followed suit, providing "That the said masters or governors of the mystery and commalty of barbers and surgeons of London and their successors yearly for ever . . . shall and may have and take without contradiction four persons condemned . . . and put to death for felony . . . and to make incisions in said dead bodies . . . for further and better knowledge, instruction, insights, learning, and experience in the science and faculty of surgery." [1] In 1564 this privilege was extended to the College of Physicians.

The practice of permitting a judge to add dissection to the death penalty for murder was clearly recognized in the colonies which were governed by English statutory and common law. As early as 1641, *The Body of Liberties* (or code of laws) adopted by the Massachusetts Bay Colony provided that the body of an executed man might not remain unburied for twelve hours "unless it be in the case of Anatomie."

According to John Winthrop in his *History of New England,* the first autopsy in the colonies was undertaken in September 1639, two years before the promulgation of the code, when the body of a boy who had been ill treated by his master was examined. "After the boy gate a bruise on his head, so as there appeared a fracture in his skull, being dissected after his death." [2]

On February 23, 1643, a jury of twelve men rendered this verdict in the case of an Indian boy: "We find that this Indian (named Edward) came by his death by a bullett shot by John Dandy, which bullett entered the epigastrium near the navell on the right side, obliquely descending & piercing the gutts, glancing on the last vertebra of the back, and was lodged in the side of the Ano." The technical language of the report would indicate that the autopsy must have been performed by a medical man.[3]

Several authorities consider the first "Anatomie" in America to have been performed by Giles Firmin, Jr., sometime prior to 1647, which was referred to earlier in John Eliot's let-

ter to Thomas Shepherd. Involved may be a distinction between an autopsy or postmortem and a dissection for educational purposes. Firmin's dissection was probably made at
Ipswich, perhaps "on a body secured by robbing a grave. Like-
lier it was on the body of an executed murderer, a procedure
permissible under the common law and the code of 1641." [4]

Dr. Oliver Wendell Holmes offered this fanciful recon-
struction of the Firmin dissection:

> Of the making of that anatomy in which my first
> predecessor in the branch I teach did read very well, we
> can know nothing. The body of some poor wretch who
> had swung from the gallows was probably conveyed by
> night to some lonely dwelling at the outskirts of the vil-
> lage, and there, by the light of flaring torches, hastily dis-
> sected by hands that trembled over the unwonted task.
> And ever and anon the master turned to his book, as he
> laid bare the mysteries of the hidden organs; to his pre-
> cious Vesalius, it might be, or his figures repeated in the
> multifarious volume of Ambroise Paré; to the Aldine oc-
> tavo in which Fallopius recorded his fresh observations;
> or that giant folio of Spigelius, just issued from the press
> of Amsterdam, in which lovely ladies display their viscera
> with a coquettish grace implying that it is rather a plea-
> sure than otherwise to show the lace-like omentum, and
> hold up their appendices epiploicae as if they were say-
> ing "these are our jewels." [5]

LECTURERS IN PRACTICAL ANATOMY

There are accounts of some autopsies involving dissection
in the century following John Eliot's plea on behalf of "young
students of Physic." In 1674 John Josselyn wrote of a "young

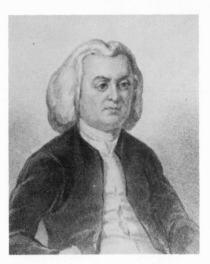

THOMAS CADWALADER

maid that was troubled with a sore picking at her heart" whose "friends desirous to discover the cause of the distemper of her heart, had her opened, and found two crooked bones growing upon the top of her heart, which as she bowed her body to the right or left side would job their points into one and the same place, till they wore a hole quite through." The same year the records of Roxbury Church report on John Bridge whose "body was opened. He had sundry small holes in his stomach & bowels, & one hole in his stomach yt a man's fist might passe through." In 1676, in a complaint against Giles Cory, an examination was made of the body of Jacob Goodale by a "Jury . . . among which was Dr. Zorobbabel Endicot; who found the man bruised to Death, and having clodders of Blood about his Heart." Two years later a surgeon reported: "Search the Body of one called Edward Boyle; I made Incision upon the parte of his Body which was most suspitious which was upon the Temporall Muscle: I layd the Bones Beare; wee could nott find any fracture in the least neither was the flesh in any wise corrupted or putrified." [6]

In 1691 came the celebrated autopsy of Governor Slaughter of New York. The circumstances under which the governor died suggested poisoning, but an examination by six doctors led by Dr. Johannes Kerbyle revealed that he "died of a defect in his blood and lungs occasioned by some glutinous tough humor in the blood, which stopped the passage thereof and occasioned its settling in the lungs." [7]

However, between 1647 and 1750, records "of human dissection in colonial New England were rare. There were no medical colleges and no medical journals, and such events would not be likely to be published in any of the few newspapers . . . because of the public aversion to the procedure." [8]

Dissection for educational purposes took a step forward when Dr. Thomas Cadwalader (1708–1799) of Philadelphia returned to America around 1730 after studying abroad. The son of John Cadwalader, who had emigrated from Wales in 1689, Thomas attended the Friends Publick School and, at the age of eighteen, was apprenticed for two years to his uncle, Dr. Evan Jones. He completed his medical education at the University of Rheims and in London, where he studied under William Cheselden (1688–1752).

After Cadwalader's return from Europe he became "so proficient in dissection . . . that students and physicians alike urged him to give a public course of lectures on the cadaver." The impression that the demonstration made upon William Shippen, Sr. (1712–1801), was largely responsible for his decision to send his son, William Shippen, Jr. (1736–1808), to England for his medical education. This decision led to the first scholastic teaching of anatomy in the American colonies. While nothing more is known of Cadwalader's anatomical dissections, he utilized this skill in the performance of autopsies, described in his celebrated work, *Essay on the West-India Dry-Gripes,* printed by Benjamin Franklin in 1745.[9] To appreciate the full significance of Cadwalader's contribution in the field of anatomy and dissection one must realize that medicine in the colonies in the first half of the eighteenth century was at a low level.

By mid-century things were beginning to improve. In 1750 in New York City, Dr. John Bard (1716–1799), father of the more famous Samuel Bard and Dr. Peter Middleton "injected and dissected" the body of an executed criminal, "for the instruction of young men then engaged in the study of medicine." [10]

On January 27, 1752, the *New York Weekly Postboy* carried what was almost certainly the earliest printed announcement in the colonies for a series of lectures on anatomy. Thomas Wood, Surgeon, of New Brunswick, New Jersey, was offering a

> COURSE of OSTEOLOGY and MYOLOGY [in which] all the human BONES will be separately examined, and the Connections and Dependencies on each other demonstrated; and all the MUSCLES of the human BODY dissected; the Origin, Insertion, and Use of each plainly shown. . . .

Subject to proper encouragement of the original course, Mr. Wood proposed a further course in

> ANGIOLOGY and NEUROLOGY . . . performing

all the OPERATIONS of SURGERY, on a dead body. . . .[11]

There is no evidence that Mr. Wood's courses were ever given, but it is quite definite that William Hunter (1729–1777) delivered a series of lectures on anatomy and comparative anatomy in Newport, Rhode Island, between 1754 and 1756. Hunter, a relative of the famous brother-anatomists, William Hunter (1718–1783) and John Hunter (1728–1793), was educated at Edinburgh, where he studied under Alexander Monro (1697–1767), or Monro Primus, the founder of the Monro medical dynasty that flourished in Edinburgh for 126 years. After more study at Leyden, he settled in Rhode Island in 1752.

It was in 1758 that William Shippen, Sr., sent his son to England to study anatomy under John Hunter and obstetrics under William Hunter, William Smellie (1697–1763), and Colin Mackenzie (d. 1775). Young Shippen became well acquainted with the celebrated Quaker physician, John Fothergill (1712–1780). Dr. Fothergill was particularly interested in the Quaker Pennsylvania Hospital that had opened its doors in 1752. He impressed Shippen and John Morgan (1735–1789), another American who was studying in England, with the desirability of establishing a medical school in the colonies, and it may have been this interest that prompted Fothergill in 1762 to make a gift to the Pennsylvania Hospital of eighteen crayon anatomical drawings, made in 1755 by J. Van Riemsdyck, and three gypsum casts of pregnancies.

Shippen, after finishing his studies under Alexander Monro (1733–1817), or Monro Secundus, obtained his degree from Edinburgh and returned to Philadelphia in May

1762. The *Pennsylvania Gazette* for the following November 11 carried a letter by Shippen announcing a course of anatomical lectures:

> The necessity and public utility of such a course in this growing country, and the method to be pursued therein will be more particularly explained in an Introductory Lecture, to be delivered the 16th instant, at six o'clock in the evening at the State House. . . . The lectures will be given at his father's house in Fourth Street. Tickets for the course to be had of the Doctor at five pistoles each; and any gentleman who may incline to see the subject prepared for the lectures and to learn the art of dissecting, injecting, etc. is to pay five pistoles more.[12]

The initial course attracted only ten students but in subsequent years enrollment ran as high as two hundred. The lectures continued without interruption until 1777.

In 1763, a year after Shippen started his lectures, Samuel Clossy (fl. 1760), a graduate of Trinity College, Dublin, lectured on anatomy as part of a course in "natural philosophy" at King's College (now Columbia University), New York. In 1768 the Medical School of King's College came into being with Clossy as professor of anatomy.

Sometime between 1760 and 1770 organized anatomical instruction was introduced into Baltimore by a Prussian, Charles F. Wiesenthal (1726–1789), who arrived there in 1755 and came to be regarded as the father of its medical profession.

In 1773 the *Providence Gazette, and Country Journal* for

April 24 (and some subsequent issues) carried a half-column advertisement by Daniel Hewes, a practitioner of medicine and setter of bones, in which is described "the wired skeleton prepared from an executed negro" and in which an invitation is extended "to see the Frame of Bones." [13]

In 1770 Abraham Chovet (1704–1790), an English anatomist, was forced by a slave insurrection to flee from Jamaica. He settled with his family in Philadelphia. The author of *A Syllabus or Index of the Parts that Enter into the Composition of the Human Body,* published in London in 1732, Chovet had been a demonstrator to the barber-surgeons of London in 1734. He brought to Philadelphia a collection of wax models and dried and injected specimens. Late in 1774 he inaugurated a course of lectures which "were so well attended that, in 1778, he erected an amphitheater on Water Street in Philadelphia." [14] John Adams saw the Chovet anatomical collection and wrote in his diary on October 14, 1774:

> Went in the morning to see Dr. Chovet and his skeletons and wax works—most admirable, exquisite representations of the whole animal economy. Four complete skeletons; a leg with all the nerves, veins and arteries injected with wax, two complete bodies in wax, full grown; waxen representations of all the muscles, tendons, &c., of the head, brain, heart, lungs, liver, stomach, &c. This exhibition is much more exquisite than that of Dr. Shippen at the hospital [presumably the Fothergill gift]. The Doctor reads lectures for two half joes a course, which takes up four months. These wax-works are all of the Doctor's own hands. [15]

Massachusetts lagged well behind Philadelphia and New York in providing lectures in anatomy and formal medical education. The first public lecture on anatomy was not given in Boston until shortly before the Revolution. The lecturer was Boston-born John Jeffries (1744–1819). After graduating from Harvard College in 1759, Jeffries studied under the celebrated James Lloyd (1726–1810) in Boston; he began to practice in 1766. Soon realizing a need for further study, he went abroad, obtained his M.D. degree from the University of Aberdeen in 1769, and then returned home. Jeffries served with the British army throughout the Revolutionary War. In 1779 he moved his family to England, where he became interested in balloon flights. He made two ascents, the second of which involved crossing the English Channel. He was the first to study scientifically the composition of the upper air and, in 1786, published a book on aeronautics.[16] (In 1940 the Institute of Aeronautical Science created the John Jeffries Award to go each year to the physician making the greatest contribution to aviation in the field of medicine.)

In 1780 John Warren (1753–1815) gave so successful a course of anatomical lectures and dissections that the Boston Medical Society voted that it be repeated. When Harvard Medical School came into being in 1782, he was the first professor of anatomy and surgery.

THE GRAVE ROBBERS

It was a principle of English common law that a dead human being was not property. Therefore "grave robbing," as commonly applied to the seventeenth- and eighteenth-century practice of taking bodies from the ground, was something of a misnomer when reference was to the corpse. The shroud or other funeral garments could be "stolen" "for the property thereof remains in the executor or whoever was in charge of the funeral." Except for this, England had no law related to grave robbing until 1788, when it was "determined that stealing dead bodies, though for the improvement of the science of anatomy, is an indictable offense as a misdemeanor." [17]

In seventeenth-century America grave-robbing—a term more acceptable than the "body snatching" of the vulgar or the "resurrection" of the elegant physician—was not seemingly a severe enough problem to warrant legislation against it. *The Body of Liberties* (1641) made no mention of disinterment of human bodies. Nor did the Connecticut code of 1659 or the New Hampshire code of 1679. The only legal source of bodies for dissection was at the discretion of judges who might order that the body of a convicted murderer be delivered to a physician. Executions for murder were rare in New England, and dissection as an additional punishment even rarer.

Physicians needed human bodies not only to increase their own knowledge but also properly to prepare apprentices and students for the practice of surgery. There probably "was grave robbing by physicians or their agents . . . in excess of what the public suspected." Before 1760 "dissections were seldom performed . . . except by stealth." [18]

For obvious reasons little is known of the activities of the grave robbers, but as often as not the procurers were students. In 1771, or possibly a dozen years earlier, Harvard undergraduates founded an anatomical society known as the Spunks or Spunkers. The date of inception turns on whether the organizer was Joseph Warren (1741–1775), or his brother John Warren. Speaking of the Spunkers' activities, John Warren wrote: "Brutes were dissected and demonstrations on the bones of human skeletons were delivered by the members." Most members of the Spunker Club "were religious and respectable enough not to pillage the churchyards, limiting themselves to the corpses of friendless derelicts and criminals." If the body of an executed murderer was not assigned to a physician for dissection, the club members would go into action. The game was a dangerous one. The students might be beaten (or even killed) by friends of the deceased, by rival hijackers, or the guards whose duty it was to dispose of the body, but to the Spunkers it was an adventure.[19]

On one occasion no less than three groups were intent on obtaining the body of a criminal. A friend of the deceased named Stillman had sworn to keep the body from a group of doctors (John Clark, John Jeffries, James Lloyd, and Benjamin Church) who were after it, and the Spunkers were also in the race. One of them, William Eustis, recorded their attempt:

> . . . as soon as the body of Levi Ames was pronounced dead by Dr. Jeffries, it was delivered by the Sheriff to a person who carried it in a cart to the water side, where it was received into a boat filled with about twelve of Stillman's crew, who rowed it over to Dorchester Point. . . . When we saw the boat land at Dorchester Point, we had a consultation, and Norwood, David, one Allen and myself took a chais and rode round to the Point, Spunker's like, but the many obstacles we had to encounter made it eleven o'clock before we reached the Point, where we searched and searched and rid, hunted and waded; but alas, in vain! There was no corpse to be found. . . . [We] have since heard that Stillman's gang rowed him back from the Point up to the town, and after laying him

out in mode and figure, buried him—God knows where! Clark & Co. went to the Point to look for him, but were disappointed as well as we.[20]

Sometimes procurement was by the master rather than the student. In the eighteenth and nineteenth centuries the "first professor of anatomy in almost every medical school in . . . America had to face charges, usually verbal but sometimes delivered by armed mobs, that he engaged in grave-robbing to get materials for classroom dissections." William Shippen, Jr., was no exception. In a notice that appeared in the *Pennsylvania Gazette* of January 11, 1770, he denied "sundry wicked and malicious Reports of my taking up Bodies from the several Burying-grounds in this Place; . . . I never have had and . . . I never will have, directly or indirectly, one Subject from the Burying-grounds belonging to any Denominations of Christians whatever." To meet the insinuation "that Subjects might have been brought from these Burial Places by my Pupils, without my Knowledge, I have added an Affidavit of Joseph Harrison, Student of Medicine, who has lived in my Father's House ever since I began my anatomical Lectures, and who has had an Opportunity of knowing where every Body was obtained, that ever I dissected in America." Harrison swore before the mayor and one of the aldermen that to his knowledge "there never was . . . any dead Body taken from any of the aforesaid Burying-grounds to be dissected by any other Person whatsoever, and . . . no such Thing could have been done by any of the Students of Anatomy, without his Knowledge." However, as Shippen once admitted, bodies may have been taken from potter's field.[21]

It was inevitable, of course, that direct procurement by

physicians and students would give way to purchase of bodies from "professional" grave robbers, and that this would finally lead to murder as the alternative means of providing bodies for dissection. The best-known cases of such murder for profit were those of Burke and Hare in England, who killed sixteen victims between February 12 and November 1, 1828. In America, though grave-robbing was prevalent, there has been only one recorded instance. In 1887 a Baltimore woman who had come down in the world was living with a man named Perry who worked in the dissecting laboratory at Maryland University. Perry hired John Thomas Ross to kill the woman for fifteen dollars, intending to sell the body to the medical school for a larger sum. Ross was convicted and executed, but Perry went free.

THE NEW YORK DOCTORS' RIOT

No one factor causes a riot, but in the case of the New York Doctors' Riot of 1788, Richard Bayley (1745–1811) seems to have been a major contributor.

During the Revolutionary War, Dr. Bayley served as a surgeon in the British army, in charge of a hospital at Newport, Rhode Island, for a time. In 1787 he started lecturing on surgery (with his son-in-law lecturing on anatomy) in some unused rooms at New York Hospital. Objection was promptly raised by some of his contemporaries, who claimed that at Newport he had initiated the practice "of cutting up his patients, and performing cruel experiments upon the sick soldiery." [22]

Nevertheless his classes went forward. The zeal with which his students were robbing graves to furnish anatomical material drove the Negroes and slaves to petition the common council on February 4, 1788:

> MOST HUMBLY SHEWETH—That it hath lately been the constant Practice of a Number of Young Gentlemen in this City who called themselves Students of Physick, to repair to the Burying Ground assigned for the Use of your Petitioners, and under cover of the Night, and in the most wanton Sallies of Excess, to dig up the Bodies of the deceased friends & relatives of your Petitioners, carrying them away and without respect to Age or Sex, mangle their flesh out of a wanton Curiosity and then expose it to Beasts and Birds.
>
> That your Petitioners are well aware of the Necessity of Physicians & Surgeons consulting dead Subjects for the Benefit of Mankind, and far from presupposing it an injury to the Deceased, in particular Circumstances and conducted with that decency and propriety which the Solemnity of such Occasion requires Your Petitioners most humbly pray your Honors to take their case into Consideration, and adopt such Measures as may seem meet to prevent similar Abuses in the future.[23]

There followed an exchange of letters in the *Daily Advertiser* in which a "Student of Physic" defended grave-robbing as essential to the advance of medicine. At about the same time a shocking notice appeared in the same paper offering a reward for the apprehension of offenders who had robbed a grave in Trinity Church Yard. (On April 26 Isaac Gano, a medical student, and George Swinney were indicted for this act.) Under-

standably the public was already keyed up when the events occurred that led to the Doctors' Riot of April 13–15, 1788.

An eyewitness of the scene was Colonel William Heth of
the Army of Virginia, who wrote to the governor of Virginia:

> . . . We have been in a state of great tumult for a day
> or two past—The causes of which, as well as I can digest
> them from various accounts, are as follows. The Young
> students of Physic, have for some time past, been loudly
> complained of, for their very frequent and wanton tres-
> passes in the burial grounds of this City. The Corpse of a
> Young gentleman from the West Indias, was lately taken
> up—the grave left open, & the funeral clothing scat-
> tered about. A very handsome & much esteemed young
> lady, of good connections, was also, recently carryd off.
> These—with various other acts of a similar kind—
> inflamed the minds of people exceedingly, and the young
> members of the faculty, as well as the Mansions of the
> dead, have been closely watched. On Sunday last, as some
> people were strolling by the hospital they discovered *a*
> *something* hanging up at one of the windows, which ex-
> cited their curiosity, and making use of a stick to satisfy
> their curiosity, part of a man's arm or leg tumbled out
> upon them. The cry of barbarity &c was soon spread—
> the young sons of Galen fled in every direction—one
> took refuge up a chimney—the mob raisd—and the
> Hospital apartments were ransacked. In the Anatomy
> room, were found three fresh bodies—one, boiling in a
> kettle, and two others cuting up—with certain parts of
> the two sex's hanging up in a most brutal position. These
> circumstances, together with the wanton & apparent inhu-

man complexion of the room, exasperated the Mob beyond all bounds—to the total destruction of every anatomy in the hospital, one of which, was of so much value
& utility, that it is justly esteemed a great public loss having been prepared in a way, which costs much time & attention, and requires great Skill to accomplish.[24]

There were other versions of what set off the riot. According to one, it was a group of young children playing in the rear
of the hospital who saw the human limb hung out to dry. In
another, a young surgeon, in the process of dissecting a cadaver, waved its arm at a small boy who had climbed a ladder
resting against a hospital window.

The mob, having ransacked the hospital, widened its
search for bodies to the residences of the doctors, even destroying the home of Sir John Temple in the mistaken belief that he
was "Surgeon" Temple. The following day, Monday, the mob
resumed its attack. According to Colonel Heth:

> Not a man of the Profession thought himself safe. An
> innocent Person got beat & abused, for being *only dressed
> in black.* Two, of the young tribe were unfortunate
> enough to fall into their hands. But the Mayor obtain
> them, upon a promise of sending to gaol—a measure,
> to which in their rage, they submitted—not reflecting,
> that *sending them to gaol,* would secure them from their
> violence & resentment. And therefore, as soon as they
> found themselves defeated in their furious intentions, re-
> specting their captives they repair to the gaol, & com-
> menc'd their attack (with all the intemperence & folly,
> which ever marks the conduct of People assembled in that

way)—vainly endeavouring to break in—when they could do nothing more than break windows &c which they will be tax'd to repair. The militia were orderd out —small parties were sent to disperse them, but they instantly disarmd these detachments, & broke their guns to pieces, & made them scamper to save their lives. The evening advanced a pace; . . . about dark . . . the Adjutant Genl of the Militia . . . led up in good order, about 150 men—(tho' not more than half with fire arms). . . . This body were not long before the gaol before the bricks & stones from the Mob, provoked several to fire. . . . Three of the mob were killd on the spot & one has since died of his wounds, & several were wounded. One of them was bayoneted on attempting to force into a window of the Prison, which he saw filld with armd Men— a proof, of the astonishing lengths to which popular rage will sometimes carry Men. . . .

Yesterday [Tuesday], the Militia turn'd out again, made a respectable appearance, & paraded about exceedingly—both *Horse & foot*—but it must be observd, *that the enemy were not to be heard of.* In truth, numbers who were *in the Mob on Monday evening*— turn'd out *yesterday to support government.*[25]

THE RESURRECTION WARS

On the one hand, patients wanted their physicians to be thoroughly acquainted with anatomy. On the other hand, ignorance, superstition, and religious prejudice were driving these same patients to demand the enactment of laws restrictive of dissection as a means of learning anatomy.

At the close of 1839 a woman died at Columbus (Ohio)

State Hospital and was buried in potter's field. When her son arrived to transfer her remains to a Marietta cemetery, her body was missing from the grave. This precipitated a "resurrection war" against Worthington Reformed Medical College, whose faculty and students had on a number of prior occasions been accused of resurrecting bodies from Columbus and Delaware cemeteries. Learning that a mob of irate citizens was headed in their direction, the faculty and students prepared to defend the college, rifles in hand.

The defense cannot have been very effective. The mob searched the house and office of Dr. Thomas V. Morrow, president and professor of anatomy and surgery. While the house was clean, the attackers found the dead body of a Negro in a corn shock behind it. Gaining admittance to the college building after threatening to break down the doors, they found on a dissection table the missing body that had incited the attack.

In 1831 the Ohio General Assembly had enacted a statute providing for a fine not to exceed $1000 and/or imprisonment of up to thirty days on convicting for wantonly exhuming a corpse from any cemetery or burial ground. As a consequence of the Worthington riot, the Ohio House of Representatives introduced a bill that would have increased the prison term to from one to three years. Thirty physicians attacked this bill through a notice in several newspapers. They decried this "act of the House . . . as an insult, directed against the members of an honorable profession," reminding "the lower branch of the Legislature . . . that there is a law giving the power to impose heavy penalties upon Physicians for mal-practice—and that there is a Medical Society at Cincinnati, whose interests will become seriously affected, should the bill under consideration, pass the Senate." The bill failed to pass the Senate.[26]

In 1852 investigation of a small shanty on the outskirts of Cincinnati revealed that it was a workshop for preparing human skeletons. The disconnected parts of about twenty bodies, some destitute of flesh, others as they were in life, offered a gruesome picture. When an infuriated mob descended on the place, the proprietor and another man made their escape in a horse-drawn vehicle. It was their good fortune to be arrested for fast driving by two police officers. Even then, on the way to jail, the mob attempted to seize the prisoners with a mind to hanging them on the spot. The officers, while severely beaten, managed to get them to jail. It was subsequently learned that the bodies had been legally procured and that the skeletons were being prepared for scientific purposes.

The newspapers did not always help the situation. The following editorial appeared in the *Zanesville* (Ohio) *Daily Courier* for November 18, 1878:

> In all parts of the country are established medical colleges. In fact a second class city is not thought to be complete unless a medical college is established within its limits. Here collect ignorant professors to lecture to still more ignorant pupils. Surgery! Not one in a hundred knows anything about surgery. But bodies must be secured to make the brainless youths believe the brainless professors know something about surgery. These brainless youths, who will soon be turned out to prey, like a set of harpies, upon the people, must be taught, however, to make sport over the remains of some body, which has been stolen from where relatives and friends have tenderly placed it. It is a most disgraceful thing that people are preyed on by ignorant blockheads who sail under the name of physicians.

LEGISLATION

Laws passed in New York after the Doctors' Riot of 1788 and in Connecticut after a less violent riot in 1824 eased the situation slightly in those states. Massachusetts, in 1829, was the first to approach the problem logically.

On February 4 the Counsellors of the Massachusetts Medical Society appointed a committee of three, including John C. Warren (1778–1856), "to prepare a petition to the legislatures, to modify existing laws, which now operate to prohibit the procuring of subjects for anatomical dissection." At the annual meeting of the society on June 3 the committee was enlarged to nine members. The committee reported on October 7. Their findings were published in an *Address to the Community on the Necessity of Legalizing the Study of Anatomy.* Their opening statement put the matter succinctly:

> It is a truth sufficiently mortifying to the practitioners of the healing art, and disastrous to the community, that while all other pursuits of science are encouraged and facilitated in this Commonwealth, and throughout New England, that alone, which has for its object a knowledge of the structure of man, with a view to heal the diseases to which he is subject, is not only not provided for, but virtually disgraced and condemned.[27]

The problems of the surgeon were presented: "In all surgical cases, the hand of the operator is paralyzed, if not guided by a knowledge of the parts in which the operation is going forward." It then cited a number of situations in which the difference between success and failure rested on the degree of the practitioner's anatomical knowledge.[28]

The address asked the reader to concede that anatomical knowledge was necessary to medical men yet

> . . . the impediments to the indispensable pursuit are multiplying, and the power of the healing art to promote the health and happiness of the community must be more and more diminished as these impediments increase. . . . In the preamble to that celebrated law of the Old Colony of Massachusetts, passed within twenty years of the date of the first charter, providing for the support of common schools, the necessity of this enactment is stated in these remarkable words,—"to the end that *learning* be not *buried in the graves of our forefathers."* The wisdom of *our* forefathers is now manifest in the general diffusion of common learning, and yet *we,* their descendants, have been willing to suffer a department of knowledge no less necessary to the well-being of society than common learning, to be burdened with oppressive and unnecessary restrictions, and in a fair way to be buried in the tombs of our fathers. . . . Is it not time for our well-intentioned editors, our legislators and magistrates, to break off the shackles of prejudice and superstition from the community under their influence, and to give them those liberal views that are becoming the philosophic and philanthropic spirit of the age? [29]

On January 6, 1831, a select committee of the Massachusetts House of Representatives reported:

> The subject . . . is beset with difficulties even in approximating a satisfactory, practical result. On the one

side are health, the safety of the limbs and lives of a whole community; on the other are encountered those strong prejudices, powerful associations, and earliest impressions of awe and reverence, for the repose of the dead, which are too strong to be conquered, too delightful to be despised, and too solemn and hallowed to be effaced.

The committee then set itself to consider and report on the rise and progress of anatomical science; the indispensable importance of both branches of the healing art—medicine and surgery ("We next propose to show, that the study and knowledge of Anatomy are essential to the safe and successful practice of Medicine."); the interest, first of society at large and then of the medical profession, in modification of the laws of the Commonwealth; the provisions, character, and effect of existing laws ("We have no direct law in this Commonwealth upon the subject of Anatomical Dissections."); and the "Provisions that have been made in France and other enlightened countries for the promotion of Anatomical Science." [30]

The committee found that anatomy was an important science of essential interest to all classes of the population, that dissection for anatomic purposes was deserving of public encouragement, and that existing laws should be changed and the study of anatomy legalized. The committee's proposals, which were essentially embodied in the act, altered an 1815 statute, designed to protect the sepulchres of the dead, that gave the right to dispose of the bodies of executed criminals to the court. Now the right to dispose of certain bodies, including those of executed criminals, would be vested in proper municipal authorities. The effect was twofold. It would gradually disabuse the public mind of "that association [of dissection with capital convictions] which now, above all others, makes it odious." It would create a broader base by authorizing the municipal authorities "to deliver to any physician . . . such dead bodies as may be required to be buried at public expense and which shall not be claimed . . . within twenty-four hours from and after death," for executed criminals represented only a fraction of bodies that might have to be buried at public expense. While the act increased the severity of penalties for grave-robbing or knowingly accepting the fruits of such activity, Section 4 provided:

> That from and after the passing of this Act, it shall be lawful for any physician duly licensed according to the laws of this Commonwealth, or for any Medical Student under the authority of such physician, to have in his possession, to use and employ human dead bodies, or parts thereof, for purposes of anatomical inquiry or instruction.[31]

Pennsylvania did not adopt a statewide anatomy law until 1883. Its passage was prompted by the discovery late in 1882 that an organized gang of grave robbers was operating in Philadelphia. The movement for legislation was led by Senator William James McKnight (1836–1918), who, twenty-five years earlier as a young physician, had taken part in a grave robbery.

In 1867 the legislature, in a feeble effort to combat grave-robbing, had authorized authorities in Philadelphia and Allegheny counties to deliver to physicians, surgeons, and particularly medical schools bodies that were otherwise to be buried at public expense. Unfortunately there just were not enough bodies to meet the demand.

Over the next fifteen years it was suspected that grave

robbers were active. Then in the winter of 1881–1882 Louis N. Megargee, editor of the *Philadelphia Press,* and four colleagues posing as doctors made contact with the organized gang. They learned that doctors, graveyard superintendents, and undertakers were involved. By December 1882 the investigators were ready to act. Jefferson Medical College, of which McKnight was an alumnus, was seriously involved. He recognized that the time had come to face the problem.

On February 28, 1883, a bill that would provide ample subjects for dissection was offered for adoption to the state senators. There was considerable opposition. McKnight argued that laboring men would be the beneficiaries rather than the victims of the proposed statute: if more doctors could be trained, they would be available to treat the injured in mines, lumber camps, pineries, and on the farms. "Humanity . . . should first be shown to the living. We must legislate for [them], not the dead," he said in conclusion. When the favorable vote (later confirmed in the lower house) was in, a Dauphin County judge who was visiting the senate chamber told McKnight: "I was violently and bitterly opposed to this law, but since I have heard your remarks I am just as violently in favor of it." [32]

The states, with local variations, continued to provide the bodies of those who would otherwise be interred at public expense. In 1869 Maine enacted a law, unique in its day, providing that if a person requested or consented before his death that his body be used to advance anatomical science, it might be so used if no kindred objected. This pioneer approach has spread across the nation, and it is quite common today for scientifically oriented individuals and humanitarians to will their bodies for anatomic dissection, usually to a university medical school.

❧(7)❧

The Early
Medical Schools

When the conditions prevailing in the colonies are considered, it is quite remarkable that two medical schools should have been established there before the Revolution. Not only was the supply of competent teachers limited, but the student body that might have been assembled in any one of the provincial capitals was correspondingly small. Since travel between the provinces was difficult and fraught with danger, it was almost as easy to go abroad for a medical education.[1]

Would-be doctors who did not attend European medical schools were trained under the apprentice method, which was not without its advantages. "At a time when in Paris and most European universities medicine was taught purely theoretically, without any concrete bedside illustration, in America [under the apprentice method] it was learned in daily contact with patients."[2]

Nevertheless a craving for broader knowledge on the part of young men bent upon medicine demanded that the gap between apprenticeships and medical school be filled, and this was at least partially achieved through the lecture series undertaken by a number of intelligent doctors—among them Thomas Cadwalader, William Hunter, Samuel Clossy, and Abraham Chovet, as we have seen. Besides the anatomical lectures begun in 1762, William B. Shippen, Jr., initiated a course of lectures in 1765 on midwifery. The twenty lectures, open to both sexes, were designed to train obstetrical physicians as well as midwives. They covered, among other topics, the anatomy of the pelvis and the reproductive organs, physiology of pregnancy, the management of normal and complicated labors, and the diseases of women and children. These were "the first systematic teaching of medical subjects at anything approaching an academic level in the American colonies." [3]

THE SCHOOL OF MEDICINE, UNIVERSITY OF PENNSYLVANIA

Shippen, in his first lecture on anatomy, had discussed the need for education in all branches of medicine. There is no record of what he had in mind, and it is just possible that he was whistling in the dark, for he was never a good planner and organizer. Perhaps he was waiting for John Morgan, who had promised to join him in getting a college program under way.

Morgan returned to Philadelphia in 1765 "to see whether, after fourteen years' devotion to medicine, I can get my living without turning apothecary or practicing surgery." He brought with him a well-considered plan, approved by the Hunters, Fothergill, and others with whom he had studied abroad, for a faculty of medicine in the College of Philadel-

99

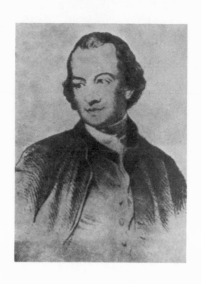

JOHN MORGAN

phia, which had been founded in 1740. His plan was looked on favorably by Thomas Penn, proprietor of the Province of Pennsylvania. Morgan was considered an "enterprising young man who would make Shippen a good assistant in organizing a school of medicine," but he "deftly and ruthlessly prepared to take the lead himself." [4]

At a special meeting on May 3, 1765, the trustees of the college, having "duly weighed" Thomas Penn's written recommendation and Dr. Morgan's proposal, "entertaining a high sense of Dr. Morgan's abilities, and the honors paid to him by different learned bodies and societies in Europe, . . . unanimously appointed him Professor of the Theory and Practice of Physic in this College." [5]

It was an obvious next step to have the new professor speak at the commencement, held on May 30–31. Morgan began by defining medicine and the various subjects that must be studied. These included anatomy, the firm foundation of all knowledge of the human body, in health or illness, and the basis for diagnosis and treatment, including surgery; the study of drugs and botany, "branches of science [from which] we derive our knowledge of that part of natural history, which more immediately relates to the health giving arts"; the "theory of physic," covering physiology and pathology; and the *practice* of medicine, wherein one learns the diseases themselves and how to diagnose and treat them.[6]

Morgan considered medical apprenticeship inadequate. It was physically impossible, he said, for a busy practitioner thoroughly to instruct his students in all branches of medicine, and they were left to pick up information during patient rounds or by reading indiscriminately whatever might be in the preceptor's library. "A contracted view of Medicine naturally confines a man to a very narrow circle, and limits him to a few partial indications in the cure of diseases. He soon gets through his little stock of knowledge; he repeats over and over his round of prescriptions, the same almost in every case; and, although he is continually embarrassed, has the vanity to believe that, from the few maxims he had adopted, he has within himself all the principles of medical knowledge, and that he has exhausted all the resources of art. This is a notion subversive of all improvement." [7]

While speaking of the advantages that would stem from the establishment of a medical school, particularly in Philadelphia, he mentioned that Dr. Shippen, Jr., had espoused a plan for medical lectures, "but I do not learn that he has recommended at all a collegiate undertaking of this kind." Then, as a sop, he suggested that, if there was to be a professor of anatomy, Shippen should fill the chair.[8]

Shippen seemed to take the slight lying down, but in September, in making application for the chair of anatomy, he struck back on two counts: "The instituting of medical schools in this country has been a favorite object of my attention for seven years past, and it is three years since I proposed the expediency and practicability of teaching medicine in all its branches in this city. . . . I should long since have sought the patronage of the trustees of this College, but waited to be joined by Dr. Morgan, to whom I first communicated my plan in England, and who promised to unite with me in every scheme we might think necessary for the execution of so important a point." [9] His "revenge" was not limited to this wrist-slapping. As we shall see, its full impact was felt when, during the Revolutionary War, he exercised his political influence to ruin his rival.

When the school opened its doors in the fall of 1765 it boasted a faculty of two—Professor of the Theory and Practice of Physic Morgan and Professor of Anatomy and Surgery Shippen. There could be no pretense that a complete medical curriculum was being offered. In fact, an announcement in the *Pennsylvania Gazette* for September 26 promised only "that lectures on two of the most important branches of medical knowledge would be helpful to young men [that is, apprentices] who were attending the practice of the physicians and surgeons of the Pennsylvania Hospital." Seemingly these young men did not beat a path to the college door. [10]

The situation gradually improved. In the fall of 1766 Dr. Thomas Bond, who had been influential in establishing the Pennsylvania Hospital, proposed to the hospital managers that he deliver a series of clinical lectures covering the treatment of acute and chronic diseases. Bond was a trustee of the college, and his lectures remained part of the school's curriculum from 1767 until his death in 1784, but he was never given the title of professor, nor did he receive an appointment to the faculty —probably because "he was not on friendly terms with Morgan." [11]

Students seeking admission to the medical school were found to be lacking in training regarded as fundamental. Consequently, in 1766, at the request of the medical trustees, the Reverend Dr. William Smith, provost of the College of Philadelphia, initiated a course of free lectures designed to give medical students an opportunity "of completing themselves in the Languages and any parts of the Mathematics at their leisure hours." It had been Morgan's view from the start that certain premedical educational standards be set, and a code was drawn up in May 1767, requiring "that such students as have not taken a degree in any College shall, before admission to a Degree in Physic, satisfy the Trustees and Professors of the College, concerning their knowledge of the Latin Tongue, and in such branches of Mathematics, Natural and Experimental Philosophy, as shall be judged requisite to a Medical Education." [12]

It was not until early in 1768 that a third professor was added to the roster. This was Adam Kuhn (1741–1817), who filled the chair of materia medica and botany. The following year Benjamin Rush was appointed professor of chemistry. (Rush had attended the first classes taught by Shippen and Morgan in 1765 and then gone to Edinburgh, where he obtained his M.D. degree.) If a faculty of four professors plus one clinical lecturer (Bond) seems scant, it must be borne in mind that renowned Edinburgh could then only boast seven professors and a lecturer in surgery.

In May 1767 requirements for medical degrees were established, and on June 21 the degree of bachelor of medicine (M.B.) was conferred on the first ten candidates. This degree could be *advanced* to an M.D. degree after an interval of time (three years at the College of Philadelphia) and evidence (by examination or preparation of a thesis) of satisfactory professional progress. By the turn of the century this two-step process had been abandoned (except by Harvard and Dartmouth) and the M.D. degree was granted on completion of the course of study. While this change was taking place, there were both "advanced" and "initial" M.D.s.

In November 1779 the College of Philadelphia became the University of the State of Pennsylvania; in January 1792 it was merged with the University of Pennsylvania. By the end of 1800 the medical school under its three names had conferred ninety-six M.B. degrees out of a national total of 149, sixteen of nineteen advanced M.D. degrees, and eighty-six of 108 initial M.D. degrees.

"The University of Pennsylvania School of Medicine was eminently successful in the performance of its mission as the first and foremost medical school in the English colonies of America and the United States. More than six thousand graduate physicians had gone from the institution by the close of the academic year of 1850–51. Probably another fifteen thousand attended lectures but did not remain to qualify for the degree. . . . Being a direct descendant of the University of Edinburgh, the University of Pennsylvania in turn became the progenitor of a group of schools which sprang up throughout the country during the first and second quarters of the [nineteenth] century." [13]

THE MEDICAL DEPARTMENT OF
KING'S COLLEGE, NEW YORK

On November 20, 1767, Dr. John Morgan wrote to a friend in London:

> I have twenty pupils this year at about five guineas each. Next year we shall confer the degree of Bachelor of Physic on several of them, and that of doctor three years after. New York has copied us and has six Professors, three of whom you know, to wit: [Samuel] Bard, Professor of Physic; [John V. B.] Tennant, of Midwifery; and [James] Smith, in chemistry; besides whom are Dr. [John] Jones, Professor of Surgery; [Peter] Middleton, of Physiology; and [Samuel] Clossy, of Anatomy. Time will show in what light we are to consider the rivalship; for my part, I do not seem to be under great apprehension.[14]

The touchy Morgan must have been annoyed when, three years later, despite the fact that King's had begun operations two years after Philadelphia, it conferred its first (advanced) M.D. degree on a 1769 baccalaureate in medicine, Robert Tucker—this was a year ahead of the school first in the field. The following year the M.D. was awarded to Samuel Kissam. These were the only M.D. degrees (with twelve M.B. degrees) conferred by King's prior to the Revolutionary War, when the school closed down for the duration. The standards of the new school in the first year compared favorably with those of the College of Philadelphia, then in its third year.[15]

After the war King's College was reorganized and took the name of Columbia College, but its medical department was not reactivated. The hiatus between the King's College closing and the Columbia revival was filled by private instruction, and among these preceptors Dr. Nicholas Romayne (1756–1817) was possibly the most popular. Certainly his Edinburgh degree and postgraduate work at several continental schools led him to rate himself highly and to depreciate the efforts of less well-trained colleagues. In 1792, observing "the negligence of Columbia's medical faculty to promote formal training," Romayne obtained authority "to establish a College of Physicians and Surgeons" in New York State.[16]

Columbia, faced with the possibility of losing its medical department, asked the regents of the University of New York to give it another chance. Romayne's charter was revoked, and a new faculty of physic was organized under the leadership of Samuel Bard, the only member of the original faculty returned to service.

Bard's ability notwithstanding, the next twenty-one years were bleak. Bard and his five professors cannot have been severely taxed by an average attendance of under forty-five students annually. The same period saw an average of just under two (initial) M.D. degrees conferred annually, with no graduates at all in five of the years. The scholastic standards set up in 1792 were no advance on those initiated in 1767. The M.B. degree was no longer given, and with no established requirements of preliminary education the doctorate level was regrettably low.[17]

Romayne, meanwhile, as the first president of the New

York Medical Society in 1806, had again obtained a charter (1807) and had established the College of Physicians and Surgeons. In 1813 the Columbia medical department was merged with the new school. After a major reorganization in the late 1820s the College of Physicians and Surgeons was placed on the firm foundation that has kept it in an outstanding position to the present day.

THE HARVARD MEDICAL INSTITUTION

Strictly speaking, the third college to establish a medical department was Virginia's William and Mary. The department was chartered in 1779, but beyond the fact that Dr. James McClurg (1745–1823) was appointed professor of anatomy and medicine and held the chair for three years (after which it was mysteriously left vacant), little is known. The department conferred a single M.D. degree (honorary) in 1782. Consequently Harvard (with a medical school chartered in 1783) is rated number three.

Harvard was founded in 1636. Eleven years later President Henry Dunster petitioned the New England Confederation for funds to purchase books "especially in law, phisicke, Philosophy, and Mathematickes" to advance scholarship in "all professions." [18] This suggests an early effort toward at least some instruction in medicine, but about a hundred and twenty-five years were to pass before a concerted move was made. In 1770 Dr. Ezekiel Hershey (1709–1770) of Hingham, Massachusetts, described by President Quincy of Harvard as "among the most beloved and honored of the distinguished men of that period," bequeathed the college one thousand pounds for the establishment and maintenance of a

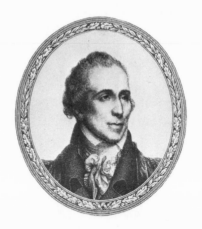

JOHN WARREN

chair in anatomy and surgery. Another dozen years elapsed before the Harvard Medical Institution began operations.[19]

Meantime there had been a move in the Boston area, initiated prior to the Revolutionary War by Joseph Warren, to improve the system of apprenticeships by offering organized courses in various fields of medicine. John Warren's series of anatomical lectures with dissections, begun in 1780, was the first to be offered in Massachusetts. Originally intended to elevate the standards of the doctors under his direction at the military hospital in Boston, where he was senior surgeon, they were repeated on an open basis in 1781 and 1782. The lectures had the approval of the Boston Medical Society (organized in 1780), and in 1782 the society strongly recommended Dr. Warren to Harvard College.

The Harvard Corporation, intent on establishing a medical institution, invited Warren to submit a plan. His plan was adopted on September 19, 1782. In November, John Warren, who incidentally had no medical degree, was appointed professor of surgery and anatomy. A month later Dr. Benjamin Waterhouse (1754–1846), who in 1800 would introduce vaccination into America, was selected to fill the chair of theory and practice of physic. It had been part of the plan that either Warren or Waterhouse would lecture on chemistry and pharmacology, but in May 1783 Aaron Dexter (1750–1829) was made professor of chemistry and materia medica. It was said of Dexter, as recorded by Dr. Oliver Wendell Holmes, a member of the class of 1829, that in the conduct of an experiment in which a powder touched with a drop of fluid was supposed to burst into brilliant flame, nothing happened. "Gentlemen," said Dexter with a serene smile, "the experiment has failed; but the principle, gentlemen,—the principle remains as firm as the everlasting hills." [20]

On September 18, 1783, Boston's *Continental Journal and Weekly Advertiser* carried an announcement by the University at Cambridge of the opening of the Medical Institution. The first lecture series was attended by some twenty students "and also by those members of the Senior Class of the University who obtained the consent of their parents." [21]

By the turn of the century, apart from honorary degrees, Harvard had conferred only twenty-nine M.B. degrees and one (advanced) M.D. degree (in 1795). Thirty earned degrees in eighteen years suggest "a rather feeble accomplishment for a college-attached school several days' journey from its nearest competitor." [22]

The school continued to stagnate until 1810. This was partly due to a scarcity of anatomical and clinical material, partly to inadequate facilities, and, possibly largely, to tense relations existing between Warren and Waterhouse. Like their earlier counterparts in Philadelphia, John Morgan and William Shippen, they periodically accused each other of deceit, double-dealing, lying, and slander.

In 1810 the school was moved from Cambridge to Boston, where there were better facilities and greater opportunity for practical experience. In making this move, the Harvard Medical School exchanged the status of a country school for that of a city school to which students might be expected to travel "from every part of the country," to the end that it might become "what it ultimately should be, The Medical School of New England." [23]

The Harvard Medical School's association with its parent university and its high admission standards kept it in the top rank, not only in New England but throughout the growing country.

THE MEDICAL DEPARTMENT OF DARTMOUTH COLLEGE

The medical department of Dartmouth College, chartered in 1797, ranks fourth on the eighteenth-century roster of important schools.

Nathan Smith (1762–1829) grew up in the Connecticut Valley and the shadow of the Green Mountains at a time when both were harried by Indians and Britishers, but he managed enough education to qualify as a schoolmaster. At twenty-one his ambition took a new direction when he was called upon to assist Dr. Josiah Goodhue of Ludlow, Vermont, in a leg amputation at the thigh. Smith was so impressed by the surgeon's skill that he asked Goodhue to take him on as a pupil. A review of Smith's educational credentials found him deficient in preliminary training. He went to work with a will and within a year had mastered sufficient Latin and natural philosophy to satisfy his preceptor. In 1787 he finished his apprenticeship and began practicing in Cornish, New Hampshire. Two years later he recognized that he needed more training and enrolled at Harvard's Medical Institution. He resumed practice in 1790, possessor of the seventh M.B. degree conferred by that school.

Smith was not to remain just another practitioner of medicine. Three medical schools in the entire country seemed insufficient. It was time, he decided, for a fourth.

Dartmouth College had been founded in Hanover, New Hampshire, by the Reverend Eleazar Wheelock (1711–1779) in 1770, and twenty-five years later was highly regarded as an educational institution. In 1796 Smith, backed by John Wheelock, who had succeeded his father to the presidency, presented to the trustees a plan for the establishment of a medical school. The trustees approved the plan in principle but, probably for lack of funds and possibly because Smith had had no training beyond his bachelor's degree, postponed final action for a year. Smith spent the interim studying in London and Edinburgh. In the fall of 1797, although the trustees had still not acted, he returned with books and apparatus for the new school, and he delivered a series of lectures on anatomy, surgery, chemistry, and the theory and practice of physic. In August 1798 the trustees instituted the plan originally proposed by Smith. Under it he became professor of all medical subjects.

Smith's only assistant from 1801 to 1810 was a former student, Lyman Spaulding (1775–1821). In 1810, because of ill health due to overwork, Smith had Cyrus Perkins (Dartmouth M.B., 1802; M.D., 1810) appointed professor of anatomy and surgery. Smith resigned his professorship in 1814.

The president and the college authorities in general were excited by the success of the medical school. On one occasion in 1810, Wheelock, fresh from Dr. Smith's lecture room, gave thanks in these words during evening prayers in the old chapel: "Oh, Lord! we thank Thee for the Oxygen gas, we thank Thee for the Hydrogen gas; and for all the gasses. We thank Thee for the Cerebrum; we thank Thee for the Cerebellum, and for the Medulla Oblongata." [24]

Its rural location and limited faculty kept the school from turning out many graduates in its formative years, but after 1812, with a more representative faculty, the medical department began to grow more rapidly. Dartmouth remained essentially a country school but attracted some excellent men to its faculty.

TRANSYLVANIA UNIVERSITY'S MEDICAL DEPARTMENT

In 1783 the Virginia General Assembly chartered the Transylvania Seminary, located in what is now Lexington, Kentucky. In 1784 the Kentucky General Assembly gave a charter to the Kentucky Academy. In December 1798 these two schools merged to become Transylvania University.

The trustees of the new institution met early in 1799 and established a medical department. On October 16 Dr. Samuel Brown (1769–1830) was made professor of chemistry, anatomy, and surgery. A month later he was joined by Dr. Frederick Ridgely (1754–1824), who became professor of materia medica, midwifery, and the practice of physic. Dr. Brown was authorized to spend $500 for books and apparatus, a considerable sum for a beginning school. This would indicate that the trustees were serious in their intention to establish a medical school and faculty, but there is little evidence that the medical department truly functioned prior to 1816–17. Thereafter, for thirty years, this first midwestern medical school reigned supreme. Its reputation faded at mid-century when the medical department of the University of Louisville and the Kentucky School of Medicine were opened.

{(8)}

Medicine and War

The relationship between medicine and war is meaningful only in terms of what medical knowledge can be acquired and what medical advances made as the result of participation of doctors in military activities.

In America medical men have served in a military capacity since early colonial times. Among the first to merit recognition was Gershom Bulkeley (c.1635–1713). Born in Concord, Massachusetts, he was graduated from Harvard in 1655. After studying for the ministry, and possibly studying medicine at the same time, he accepted a call to New London, Connecticut, in 1661. Five years later he moved on to Wethersfield. This post he resigned early in 1667, probably because his voice was weak.[1]

Thereafter he devoted himself to medicine. While there is no record of earlier medical activities, he must have had considerable experience and success because in October 1675, during the prosecution of King Philip's War, the English Court appointed him "chyrurgion to the army" and made him a member of the colony's Council of War. Between January and May 1676 he accompanied three expeditions against the Indians. During the second he was wounded in the thigh, seemingly not too seriously.

On May 13, the Court, "being informed that sundry wounded men are come to Mr. Buckly, desired Mr. Buckly to take the care and trouble of dressing the s^d wounded soldiers till God bless his endeavours with a cure." [2]

On January 2, 1677, the Council returned him "hearty thanks . . . for his good service to the country, this present war [and did] order the Treasurer to pay unto him the sume of thirty pounds as an acknowledgement of his good service to the country, besides the sattisfying of those that have supplyed his place in the ministry." [3] After his death in 1713 Bulkeley was eulogized by a grateful public.

THE FRENCH AND INDIAN WARS

The war that broke out in Europe between England and France in the early 1740s had its repercussions in the New World. New Hampshire proposed an expedition against Louisburg at the extreme east of Cape Breton Island. Massachusetts rejected the plan as "bold and hopeless." New York and Pennsylvania held back, although the latter subsequently advanced £4000 to defray expenses. Connecticut, however, responded keenly, adding four hundred men to New Hampshire's contingent of five hundred. In addition, she sent her sloop, *The Defence*, with one hundred men for sea service.

The Louisburg expedition produced several medical men of subsequent stature. Matthew Thornton (1714–1803), surgeon to the New Hampshire Division, who would affix the final signature to the Declaration of Independence, held the rank of colonel at the outbreak of the Revolution and earned the reputation of a great patriot. Alexander Wolcott (b. 1711), son of Major-General Roger Wolcott, second-in-command of the Connecticut forces, was appointed physician and surgeon's mate to the expedition. He later "distinguished himself . . . by his excellence in the classics and . . . by the energy with which he delved into the mysteries of the healing art." The post of surgeon went to Norman Morrison (1706–1761). Born in Scotland and educated at Edinburgh, he settled in Hartford, Connecticut, in 1733. He was the first Connecticut doctor to encourage the separation of medicine and pharmacy, and was "a thorough and diligent scholar for he possessed a valuable library and inspired his pupils, many of them distinguished, with a taste for reading. Because of his influence as a medical teacher and his superior eminence and judgment as a physician he enjoyed a large consultation practice." [4]

Participants in the war that ended with the victory on the Plains of Abraham in 1763 were John Cochran (1730–1807) and James Craik (1730–1814). The former, a surgeon's mate on duty with the British, would become "Physician and Surgeon of the Middle Department of the Continental Army" and, in 1781, "Medical Director of the Army." Craik, who came to the colonies in 1755 in the army of General Edward Braddock, later served as "Assistant Medical Director of the Continental Army." He was physician to George Washington at the time of his death.

The conquest of Canada was perhaps "the first circumstance which materially improved the condition of medicine in [New York] State. The English army employed for that purpose, left Europe, accompanied by a highly respectable medical staff, most of whom landed in the city of New York, and continued some years in the neighboring territories, affording to many young Americans opportunities of attending the military hospitals, and receiving such professional instruction as gave them afterward consideration with the public. . . . In this manner a new order of medical men was introduced into the Community." [5]

Nonetheless, the outbreak of the Revolutionary War in 1775 found the American colonists unprepared. There was a "lack of well-trained physicians and surgeons and the supplies and equipment needed to set up temporary hospitals for the care of sick soldiers and casuals of battle. Some . . . military officers and a few doctors had had experience . . . in the wars fought . . . between English and French armed forces. The British Army had a well-developed medical and hospital service. It was logical that this should be the pattern on which the early American military hospital system was planned." [6]

THE REVOLUTIONARY WAR

On July 17, 1775, the Colonial Congress, meeting in Philadelphia, passed an act for the establishment of a military hospital, thereby, in effect, creating the Medical Department of the United States Army. Prior to this, the Colonial Militia lacked an organized medical arm, and care of the military sick and wounded was in the hands of surgeons recruited locally as necessity dictated.

Numerous physicians and surgeons were active in the cause of independence. Dr. Joseph Warren and Dr. Benjamin Church (1734–1776) were prominent members of the Committee of Public Safety of Massachusetts and the Massachusetts Provincial Congress. In 1774–75 twenty-two physicians were members of this congress, nearly all of whom served as surgeons during the war. Of the over four hundred casualties at Bunker Hill, eleven were surgeons or surgeon's mates. [7]

Among these casualties was Joseph Warren. Despite holding the rank of major-general in the Massachusetts Militia, he insisted, in order to gain experience, on serving as a volunteer in

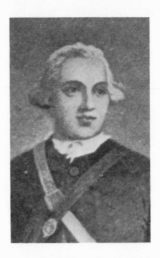

JOSEPH WARREN

the ranks. It is generally agreed that he was killed late in the day among those who were covering the retreat.

The ability of the volunteer medics varied greatly. Of the nearly twelve hundred physicians involved in the war, there were probably not more than a hundred with medical degrees. Many of the older men had served as regimental surgeons or assistants in the war of 1754–1763, and, for the Continental Army that assembled around Boston in 1775, surgeons and assistants were often selected on the basis of personal friendship or political influence. Consequently physicians were in positions of trust beyond their capacity and experience. This "contributed to the general confusions and friction that characterized the medical service during the first years of the struggle." [8]

THE MEDICAL DEPARTMENT OF THE ARMY

As there was no advance plan for care of the casualties of Bunker Hill, the wounded were carried to one side and their wounds dressed hastily. Later they were housed in deserted residences impressed for use as temporary hospitals or in barns and sheds euphemistically styled "regimental hospitals." This description derived from the fact that the doctors serving with the hurriedly assembled troops did so on a regimental basis, bringing with them their own few medicines and surgical instruments. Recognizing the inadequacy of these "hospitals," the Massachusetts Provincial Council decided to provide "better equipped units" under the direction of their own appointees in four strategically placed houses. The regimental surgeons were quick to protest that these facilities were no better than their own, and they were in no mood to transfer their patients to them.

One of the first undertakings of George Washington after he became commander-in-chief was an inspection of camps, fortifications, and hospitals. Afterward he wrote the Continental Congress at Philadelphia that an army medical department must be organized. The Congress took action on July 17, 1775, providing for the appointment of a "Director-general and chief surgeon," four surgeons, one apothecary, twenty mates, one clerk, two storekeepers, one nurse to every ten sick, and occasional laborers. The directorship proved a quagmire for a succession of competent practitioners, educators, and organizers.

The first victim was Dr. Benjamin Church. A leading physician and tried patriot, he stood high in the councils of the revolutionaries. He seemed eminently suited to iron out the differences that had arisen between regimental military surgeons and the fledgling government, but he was faced with a situation beyond his control when Congress failed to bring the regimental surgeons under the Medical Department. The result was two services competing for strictly limited supplies, and accusations were hurled back and forth between the two sides. Word of these difficulties reached General Washington. While he supported

Church's organizational approach, he ordered an official inquiry into the functions of the hospital department in relation to the regiments, stating his personal conclusion that there was "either unpardonable abuse on one side, or an inexcusable neglect on the other." [9]

Preliminary hearings were held without delay, but a final hearing never took place because, in the interim, Church was arrested for engaging in treasonous correspondence with the enemy.

> A letter, in cipher, addressed to a British officer in Boston (then within the enemy's lines), had been intercepted. The messenger, who turned out to be Church's mistress, had steadfastly refused to disclose the identity of the writer. Under "threat and persuasion" she had finally broken down and named Dr. Church as its author. Church was immediately apprehended. He did not deny having written the letter, but he assured his interrogators that it contained nothing criminal. When deciphered it was found to be a queerly garbled, apparently innocuous document. Church's papers, which had been seized at the time of his arrest, contained, as far as could be seen, nothing incriminating. However, there was a strong suspicion that a confidant of Church's had had access to them prior to seizure.[10]

A Council of War, presided over by the commander-in-chief, found Church guilty. The army and the country were shocked; Washington, in reporting the outcome to the Congress, considered it a "painful though necessary duty." In further proceedings before the Massachusetts House of Representatives, Church maintained in his own defense that "he had attempted to contact the British for the purpose of bringing about a termination of hostilities," but the House found him guilty of attempting to carry on a "highly criminal and dangerous" correspondence with the enemy. Sentenced to solitary confinement, he was released after a year (for reasons of health) and given permission to leave the country. The ship on which he sailed for the West Indies was lost at sea, and he was never again heard of.[11]

Dr. Church was succeeded by Dr. John Morgan of Philadelphia in October 1775. Army morale was at its lowest. Supplies of food and clothing were meager. Malnutrition was common. The army was ravaged by smallpox, typhus, cholera, rheumatism, pneumonia, and dysentery, to which inadequate sanitation in the camps and putrid drinking water contributed.

Morgan was further plagued by petty politics and professional jealousy. Not the least of the harassment came from the regimental surgeons for whom Congress had not seen fit to provide supplies. Morgan backed the surgeons in petitioning Congress for supplies, but Congress, while reacting favorably, attached so much paper work and so many restrictions on regimental hospitals that the field surgeons in their resentment sought to undermine the director-general. In this they were abetted by Dr. William Shippen, Jr.

Boston was evacuated by the British in March 1776. During the summer and fall Morgan traveled back and forth between Boston and Baltimore, laboring to supply various divisions of the general hospital. He appeared to be all places at once, picking sites for new hospitals, supervising the evacuation of patients and the removal of supplies when the enemy's advance threatened existing sites. Meanwhile Shippen spent most of his time in Philadelphia, ingratiating himself with Congress.

The regimental surgeons were continuing their attacks on

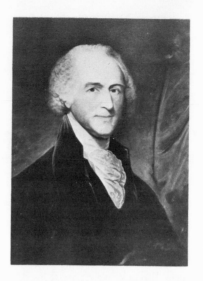

WILLIAM SHIPPEN, JR.

Morgan with such vehemence that General Washington became
convinced that they were aiming to break up the Medical Department. He so informed Congress, recommending that the regimental surgeons be required to accept the director-general as their superior. Congress not only ignored Washington's advice but
further undermined Morgan's authority by creating an independent medical department, headed by Shippen, for the army of
New Jersey. Over this department the director-general would exercise no authority. Morgan regarded this step as a demotion.

Shippen's father and his brothers-in-law, Richard Henry
and Francis Lightfoot, were members of Congress. Shippen let
his "friends in Congress" know that "neglect and inequity in the
medical department" had been responsible for the death of many
more "brave Americans" than had been the "sword of the
enemy." [12] On January 9, 1777, Morgan was dismissed with neither an explanation nor a hearing.

He immediately requested an investigation of his steward-ship, but it was not until June 12, 1779, that a congressional committee appointed to hear him declared that ". . . Dr. John Morgan hath in the most satisfactory manner vindicated his conduct in every respect. . . ." [13] The reprieve came too late. Morgan, a broken man, retired more and more from public life and died a decade later at the age of fifty-four.

Not surprisingly, William Shippen, Jr., was the next director-general. A reorganization of the department placed the regimental surgeons within his jurisdiction. Two months after his appointment the following appeared in the *Pennsylvania Evening Post* for June 5, 1777:

> None but gentlemen of the best education and well qualified are employed as Senior Physicians; Surgeons; and the Eastern and Northern Departments are filled with gentlemen of the first characters in these countries; and the public may depend on it that the greatest exertions of skill and industry shall be constantly made, and no cost spared to make the sick and wounded soldierly, comfortable, and happy. W. Shippen, Jun., Director-General of the American Hospitals. [14]

Despite this promising beginning, the new director fared little better than his predecessors.

Among the doctors appointed by Congress to serve under Shippen was Benjamin Rush. This capable, young, ambitious physician had signed the Declaration of Independence and now, just over the threshold of his thirties, was a member of Congress and chairman of its medical committee.

A number of army medical men had deplored Congress's

treatment of Morgan, and they greeted Shippen's appointment with critical skepticism. Rush, who sympathized with Morgan, led this opposition. Nor was Shippen helped by the lowered morale that followed the battle of Valley Forge in the winter of 1777–78. Shippen, preferring the comforts of his headquarters, did not circulate among the hospitals under his direction, as Morgan had.

Rush, who had seen duty in the military hospitals in the late summer of 1777, was convinced that radical administrative reorganization was necessary. He also believed that Shippen was incompetent, negligent in the performance of his duties, not above filing misleading reports as to the number of sick and dead, and was possibly speculating in hospital stores.

Rush sent a letter to General Washington in which he detailed the abuses he had seen in the hospitals and offered suggestions for rectifying them. No direct attack on the director-general was involved, but Congress, to which Washington turned over the letter, called both Shippen and Rush before an investigating committee. A court-martial proceeding ordered against Shippen in the spring of 1780 ended in acquittal on most counts on the grounds that the charges were not clearly proved, but the court found that Shippen had speculated in hospital supplies, conduct it considered "highly improper, and justly reprehensible." [15] Congress dismissed Shippen from his post, but when the department was reorganized in the fall Shippen was reappointed to the directorship, seemingly a face-saving gesture engineered by his friends in Congress, for on January 3, 1781, he resigned "voluntarily." Unlike Church and Morgan, he went on to enjoy a long and honorable life.

Shippen was succeeded on January 17, 1781, by his former deputy, Dr. John Cochran, whom General Washington had highly recommended to Congress four years earlier. Cochran served through the remainder of the war without meeting the fate of his predecessors, though his task was no easier. He took over at a time when the department was near disintegration for lack of funds. There was no money for hospital upkeep or the salaries of army surgeons, many of whom, Cochran told Congress, "had not received a shilling in nearly two years." One physician, appealing to a civilian friend for help, wrote: "Joe and myself have spent all our money, and fear, unless we can borrow, we shall starve; do pray prevent it by sending us cash. You may depend upon it, no Surgeons of the army can lend us a shilling." [16]

After the war President Washington named Cochran Commissioner of Loans for the State of New York, basing the appointment on "a cheerful recollection of his past services." [17] Cochran held this post until a stroke forced him into retirement. He died at Schenectady, New York, at the age of seventy-seven.

DOCTORS AT THE FRONT

The Medical Department was organized by trial and error. There were limited supplies, sometimes none at all. Following heavy battles, surgeons had to use razor blades instead of scalpels. Overcrowded barracks, insufficient food and clothing, lack of sanitation, and polluted water encouraged epidemics of virulent diseases and produced a high mortality rate. There were, however, bright moments, such as the occasion when five hundred troops were inoculated with smallpox, of whom only four died.[18]

In face of adversity and at great personal risk, since proportionately more army doctors met their death than did officers of the line, the medical men of the Revolution carried on. "Some may have been but fairly good doctors, some may not have been worthy of the trust placed in them, but the vast majority served their country faithfully, according to their lights." [19]

These army doctors "constituted the backbone of American medicine and surgery. . . . They could pull teeth, set a horse or human fracture, excise a tumor if it presented, evacuate an abscess, probe and remove a ball, and remove by Caesarean section a baby after the mother had expired." The dental reference is an oblique one to the fact that, when George Washington was suffering unmercifully from aching teeth, Major Charles Gilman, M.D., suggested that he "wash out his mouth with rum and then be given an ample dose of Tincture of Opium, to give him some much needed sleep." As for obstetrics, Colonel Nathaniel Scudder, M.D. (1733–1781), like Gilman a commander of line troops as well as a medical officer, was at the head of his regiment at the battle of Monmouth when a harassed civilian asked for help for his wife, who was ready to deliver. Scudder, an obstetrician in the days when midwives dominated the field, decided that his professional duty to medicine outweighed his duty to the army. He accompanied the man to his home. When he had completed his mission he "found he was within British lines, and so, from an attic window, watched the tides of battle flow back and forth. Finally, when the British were pushed from the field, Colonel Scudder, M.D., descended through a trap door from his undignified observation perch, met his men, and led them forward." [20]

Charles Gilman had quite accidentally discovered the disinfecting properties of alcohol. By his own account, "At the battle of Haarlem' Heights, I received a crease wound in the back of the hand. Painful, it would not heal and exuded laudable pus. In camp at Newburgh, I spilled—quite accidentally—for I had had too much rum, some upon the member. I covered it, and in two days I noticed no odor. I removed the cover and the wound was healing. Thereafter, all wounds were soaked in rum clothes before covering." [21]

In September 1783 Congress authorized the commander-in-chief "to grant furloughs to all of the medical staff whose services were no longer needed." This was tantamount to disbandment of the Medical Department. Nine months later the "Commanding Officer [was] directed to discharge the troops now in the service of the United States, except twenty-five privates to guard the stores at Fort Pitt; and fifty-five to guard the stores at West Point, and other magazines; with a proportionate number of officers; no officer to remain in service above the rank of Captain, and those privates to be retained who were enlisted on the best terms." [22] The practice of post-bellum economizing had been initiated. The Medical Department of the Army was not fully revived until 1818.

THE MILITARY JOURNAL OF JAMES THACHER

John Adams, writing in 1824, said of *A military journal* by James Thacher (1754–1844) that it was "the most natural, simple, and faithful narration of facts that I have seen in any history of that period [the American Revolutionary War]." [23]

Thacher at twenty-one was fresh from an apprenticeship under Abner Hershey, the leading physician of Barnstable, Massachusetts. He became a surgeon's mate to John Warren, who was one year older but already senior surgeon at the provincial military hospital in Cambridge.

Thacher was to become a prolific writer and produce a diversity of works: *The American new dispensatory . . .* (1810); *Observations on hydrophobia . . .* (1812); *American modern practice . . .* (1817); *The American orchardist . . .* (1822); *A*

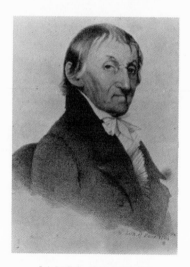

JAMES THACHER

military journal . . . (1823); *American medical biography . . .* (1828); *A practical treatise on the management of bees . . .* (1829); *An essay on demonology, ghosts and apparitions, and popular superstitions . . .* (1831); and *History of the town of Plymouth . . .* (1832).

An observant man with such broad interests must inevitably triumph over the mere physician. Consequently *A military journal* is not, as might have been expected from a doctor, primarily devoted to medical aspects of the war. References to medical performance and the problems of medicine are scattered through the journal and seem largely incidental.

Thacher's entry for March 29, 1776, states: "One of our soldiers found a human skeleton in complete preparation, left by a British surgeon [at the evacuation of Boston], which I have received as an acceptable present." In May, with smallpox in many parts of Boston, Thacher was inoculated by his friend Dr. John Homans, "though contrary to general orders." But July 3 saw or-

ders given "to inoculate for the small pox, all the soldiers and inhabitants in town, as a general infection of this terrible disease is
apprehended. Dr. Townsend and myself are now constantly engaged in this business." [24]

April 1777 found Thacher at the Ticonderoga general hospital as surgeon's mate to his friend, senior surgeon David Townsend. They were taking care of "about eighty soldiers laboring
under various diseases, and eight or ten that had been cruelly
wounded by savages who had been skulking in the woods in the
vicinity." He was still there in July. On the 5th he noted with as-
tonishment that "the enemy have taken possession of an eminence called *Sugar-loaf Hill*, or *Mount Defiance*, which, from its
height and proximity, completely overlooks and commands all
our works at Ticonderoga and Mount Independence. . . . The
situation of our garrison is viewed as critical and alarming. . . .
[About midnight] I was urgently called from sleep, and informed that our army was in motion. . . . It was enjoined on me
immediately to collect the sick and wounded, and as much of the
hospital stores as possible, and assist in embarking them on board
the batteaux and boats . . . [for] our voyage up the South bay to
Skeensboro', about thirty miles. . . . At three o'clock in the afternoon we reached our destined port . . . unsuspicious of danger;
but, behold! Burgoyne himself was at our heels. . . . The officers
of our guard now attempted to rally the men and form them in
battle array; but this was found impossible. . . . I perceived our
officers scampering for their baggage; I ran to the batteau, seized
my chest, carried it a short distance, took from it a few articles,
and instantly followed in the train of our retreating party."

In a skirmish with the British and Indians on the 7th, a
"surgeon with a wounded captain and twelve or fifteen privates,
were taken and brought into our fort. The surgeon informed me

that he was in possession of books, &c. taken from my chest at Skeensboro', and, singular to relate, some of the British prisoners . . . had in their pockets . . . *private letters* which I had received from a friend in Massachusetts, and which were now returned to me."

The next day a move was begun to Fort Edward on the Hudson River where, Thacher reported on the 25th, "the sick soldiers under my care at this place have been accommodated in barracks and tents. I have now received orders to accompany them to the hospital at Albany, [down river] about fifty-five miles." The hospital at Albany, a city of about three hundred houses, was erected "during the last French war . . . on an eminence overlooking the city. . . . It contains forty wards, capable of accommodating five hundred patients." By September 21 the Albany hospital was admitting a considerable number of officers and soldiers wounded in the battle of Saratoga. "Several of these unfortunate but brave men have received wounds of a very formidable and dangerous nature, and many of them must be subjected to capital operations." Three weeks later Thacher "watched with the celebrated General [Benedict] Arnold, whose leg was badly fractured by a musket-ball. . . . He is very peevish and impatient under his misfortunes, and required all my attention during the night."

On August 7, 1778, Thacher, now on the east bank of the Hudson about two miles from West Point, noted that an "unusual number of patients have been brought into our hospital within a few days. Their diseases are putrid fever and dysentery; many of the cases appear so malignant, that it is feared they will baffle all the skill of the physician." A month later Major-General Israel Putnam arrived in the vicinity with his troops and "visited our hospital, and . . . observing a considerable number of men were infected with the *ground itch,* generated by lying on the ground, he inquired why they were not cured. I answered, 'Because we have no hog's-lard to make ointment.' 'Did you never,' says the general, 'cure the itch with tar and brimstone?' 'No. sir.' 'Then,' replied he, good-humoredly, 'you are not fit for a doctor.' "

In October, General Washington visited the hospital. His "arrival was scarcely announced, before he presented himself at our doors. . . . He appeared to take a deep interest in the situation of the sick and wounded soldiers, and inquired particularly as to their treatment and comfortable accommodations. Not being apprised of his intended visit . . . we were not entirely free from embarrassment, but we had the inexpressible satisfaction of receiving his excellency's approbation of our conduct, as respects the duties of our department."

The next two years saw Thacher constantly on the move. In October 1780 he was back in the West Point area, and March 1781 found him twenty miles down river at Crompond. Here, during a night foray, a man "named Hunt, received a dangerous wound through his shoulder and lungs, the air escaped from the wound at every breath. Dr. Eustis came to the lines, and dilated the wound in the breast, and as the patient is athletic and has not sustained a very copious loss of blood, he recommended repeated and liberal blood letting, observing that, in order to cure a wound through the lungs, you must bleed your patient to *death.* He eventually recovered, which is to be ascribed principally to the free use of the lancet and such abstemious living as to reduce him to the greatest extremity. . . . A gentleman volunteer, by name Requaw, received a dangerous wound, and was carried into the British lines. I was requested by his brother to visit him, under the sanction of a flag of truce, in company with Dr. White, who resides in this vicinity. This invitation I cheerfully accepted, and . . . we arrived before evening, and dressed the wounded man. . . . The next day we visited our patient again [and] paid the necessary attention."

In April, Thacher "received orders to return to the highlands near West Point, to inoculate the troops with small-pox. . . . The old practice of previous preparation by a course of mercury and low diet, has not been adopted on this occasion; a single dose of jalop and calomel, or of the extract of butternut, *juglans cinerea,* is in general administered previous to the appearance of the symptoms. . . . As the butternut-tree abounds in this country, we may obtain at very little expense a valuable domestic article of medicine."

A year later Thacher was again engaged in smallpox inoculation. On April 5, 1782, having "completed the inoculation of the soldiers, and attended them through the small-pox, and my professional duty being considerably diminished, I have obtained a furlough for forty-five days to visit my friends in Massachusetts."

After his return to camp the *journal* contains nothing more of medical interest. On December 25, Thacher wrote: "It is incumbent on me to express my unfeigned gratitude to the All-wise Author and Preserver of men, that he has been pleased to confer on me innumerable blessings, and preserved my life and health during a long period while exposed to the greatest hardships and imminent perils." And then on January 1, 1783: "This day I close my military career, and quit for ever the toils and vicissitudes incident to the storms of war. . . . I retire with honorable testimonials from very respectable authority of my punctuality and faithful performance of duty . . .

and with a heart fraught with grateful recollections of . . . my numerous companions and associates."

JAMES TILTON ON MILITARY HOSPITAL CONDITIONS

Born in what was to become the state of Delaware, James Tilton (1745–1822) trained under Dr. Ridgely of Dover and at the newly established medical school in Philadelphia. Here he was among the first group of graduates, obtaining his M.B. degree in 1768 (with a thesis on respiration) and his M.D. degree three years later (with a dissertation on dropsy). He established himself in practice in Dover, where he remained until 1776, when, combining "the characters of patriot and physician . . . he relinquished a lucrative practice, his friends and his home [and] entered as a surgeon the Delaware regiment, with $25 a month." [25]

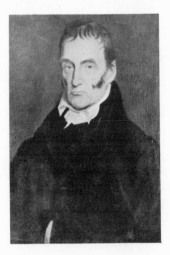

JAMES TILTON

133

He served at Wilmington through the winter of 1776–77. The following summer his "devotion to duty was recognized . . . by appointment as Hospital Surgeon . . . in charge of the hospital at Princeton." Here "he narrowly escaped with his life from an attack of hospital fever [typhus]. His sufferings from this disease must have been of a most distressing kind; and his recovery was almost a miracle. At one period of his disease eleven surgeons and mates, belonging to the hospital, gave him over, and only disputed how many days he should live. Providence ordered otherwise. To his friend . . . Dr. Rush, and the attention of a benevolent lady in the neighborhood he chiefly attributed his recovery, which was slow and painful." [26]

From 1777 to 1779 he undertook a survey of military hospitals in Pennsylvania, Rhode Island, and New Jersey, which later served as the basis of his *Economical Observations on Military Hospitals; and the Prevention and Cure of Diseases Incident to an Army,* published in 1813. This was doubtless a factor in his selection the same year as "Physician and Surgeon-General." [27]

"It would be shocking to humanity," Tilton wrote in *Economical Observations,* "to relate the history of our general hospital in the years 1777 and 1778, when it swallowed up at least one-half of our Army, owing to a fatal tendency in the system to throw all of the sick of the Army into a general hospital. . . . The sick and the wounded, flowing promiscuously into the hospital, it soon became infectious and was attended with great mortality." He observed "that tents in all cases are to be preferred to enclosed buildings." [28]

During the winter of 1779–80 he experimented with

"hospital huts," an idea he borrowed from Marshal Saxe, a German soldier of fortune in the service of the French, who wrote a book on the art of war, *Mes Rêveries* (1757). Tilton's "improvements exceeded his most sanguine calculations; they consisted in having an earthen floor, instead of wood, with a hole in the centre of the roof for the purpose of allowing the smoke to escape from the fire, which was made in the middle of the hut. So deep was his conviction of the absurdity and inhumanity of the existing hospital arrangements, that in the year '81 he determined to resign his situation in the army, unless they were radically changed." [29]

Reforms were instituted, and Tilton remained with the army. When it was disbanded he returned to his practice in Dover.

Benjamin Rush supported Tilton's concepts. In *Medical Inquiries and Observations,* Rush wrote: "It is proved, in innumerable instances, that sick men recover health sooner and better in sheds, huts, barns, exposed occasionally to wind, and sometimes to rain, than in the most superb hospitals of Europe." [30]

JOHN JONES ON WOUNDS AND FRACTURES

After Dr. Jones returned to King's College in 1775 from a trip to England, he wrote a manual of inestimable value to surgeons, civilian and military. While he had been abroad he had acquired considerable contemporary information on the treatment of wounds and fractures, which he added to his own experience as a surgeon during the French and Indian Wars.

In *Plain Concise Practical Remarks, on the Treatment of Wounds and Fractures,* Jones warned against the practice

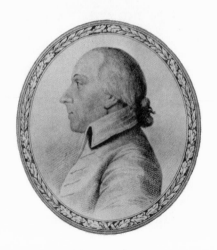

JOHN JONES

among wounded soldiers of resorting to stiff drinks to ease their pain while they were waiting for the surgeon's attention. The imbibing of alcohol, he said, caused dilation of blood vessels and led to fresh hemorrhaging.

In gunshot wounds, he noted, some physicians refrained from attempting to extract any ball or foreign body lying beyond finger's reach. Jones believed that any ball that could be felt under the skin should be removed by excision. A patient suffering from a large wound made by a cannon ball was to be given quinine, which Jones apparently regarded as a vasoconstrictor that would reduce hemorrhaging. "If the patient became constipated as a result of this treatment, a few grains of rhubarb helped to overcome this."

Superficial burns were to be treated with spirit of wine, deeper burns with linseed oil, and third-degree burns should be soaked twice daily until the dead tissue separated. Despite the fact that Jones generally distrusted ointments, which he categorized as salves and balsams peddled by quacks, he prescribed *unguentumum e stramonio* (prepared by boiling thorn apple leaves in fresh hog's lard) for severely burned surfaces.

Jones distinguished between the treatment of compound fractures by big city surgeons, working in dirty hospitals crowded with highly infectious putrid wounds and ulcers and treatment by country surgeons in the clean country air. The former frequently recommended amputation as a life-saving procedure; the latter avoided amputation wherever possible. In all cases, Jones favored a nourishing diet, warm alcoholic soaks, and the liberal use of Peruvian bark (quinine). In cases of skull fracture and trepanning, Jones cautioned the surgeon against being "in too great haste to cut." If he has patience, "he will frequently succeed in preserving the scalp and avoiding that deformity which a large scar and a loss of hair must inevitably produce." [31] A "good surgeon," Jones wrote, should "have firm steady hands, and be able to use both alike; a strong clear sight, and above all, a mind calm and intrepid, yet humane and compassionate, avoiding every appearance of terror and cruelty to his patients, amidst the most severe operations." [32]

ᡣᡰ

The extent to which the Revolutionary War contributed to the advance of medicine has long been a subject of debate. At one extreme is the opinion that although "some sound principles were enunciated, the record of the profession is not distinguished by originality or far-sighted progress." On the other hand there is the view that the "medical men of the American Revolution experienced some of their greatest days" by performing the seemingly impossible.[33]

The war was a great leveler. It brought together doctors

from the relatively isolated communities on an unprecedented scale to treat traumatic injuries in undreamed of numbers, to fight rampant epidemic disease, and to learn the rudiments of hygienics.

In addition, the war provided practical medical education which raised the general level of medical care.

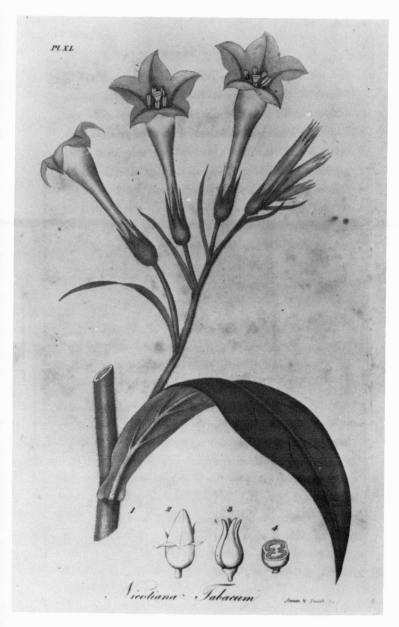

Tobacco, used by both Indians and colonists in a variety of medical treatments

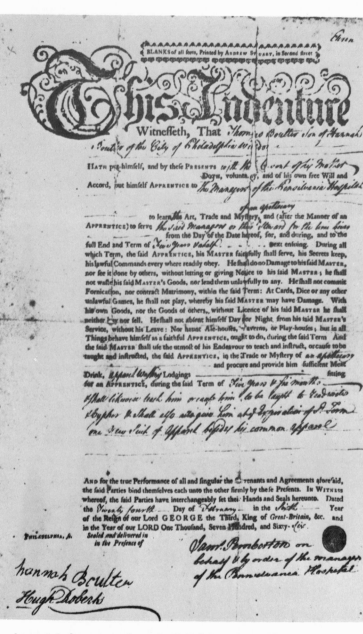

Apothecary's indenture, made out in Philadelphia in 1766

Admission card for the Pennsylvania Hospital, signed by Benjamin Rush, who also signed the Declaration of Independence

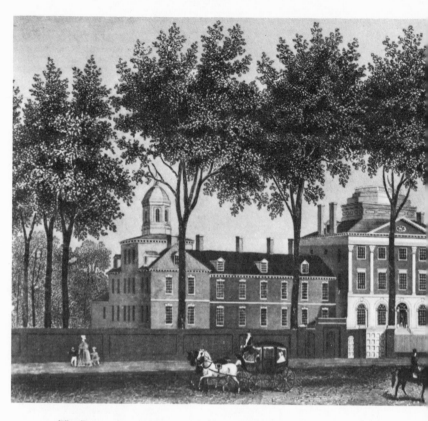

The Pennsylvania Hospital (about 1894); the oldest major hospital in the United States, it was founded in 1751

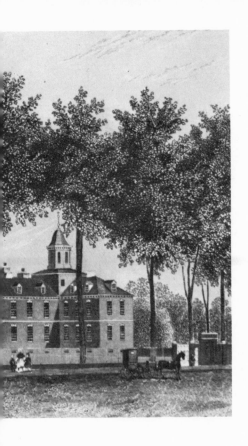

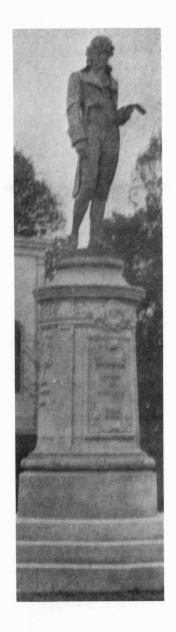

Statue of Benjamin Rush, physician, patriot, and humanitarian, erected in Washington, D.C., by the medical profession

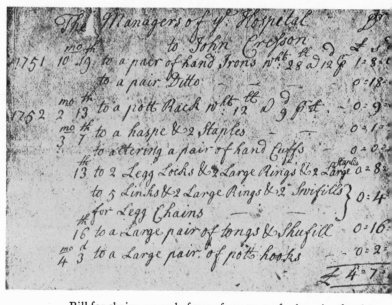

Bill for chains, an early form of treatment for lunatics, for the Pennsylvania Hospital

Jefferson Medical College, Philadelphia, founded in 1826; it has had many outstanding students and faculty members

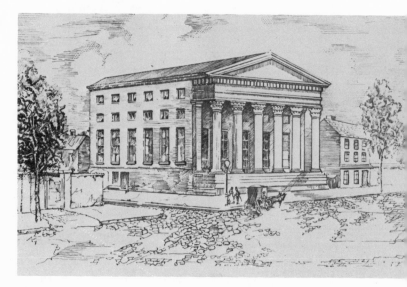

THE

INDIAN DOCTOR'S
DISPENSATORY,

BEING

FATHER SMITH'S ADVICE

RESPECTING

DISEASES AND THEIR CURE;

CONSISTING OF PRESCRIPTIONS FOR

MANY COMPLAINTS:

AND A DESCRIPTION OF MEDICINES,

SIMPLE AND COMPOUND,

SHOWING THEIR VIRTUES AND HOW TO APPLY THEM.

DESIGNED FOR THE BENEFIT OF HIS CHILDREN, HIS FRIENDS AND THE PUBLIC, BUT MORE ESPECIALLY THE CITIZENS OF THE WESTERN PARTS OF THE UNITED STATES OF AMERICA.

BY PETER SMITH,
OF THE MIAMI COUNTRY.

Men seldom have wit enough to prize and take care of their health until they lose it—And Doctors often know not how to get their bread deservedly, until they have no teeth to chew it.

CINCINNATI:
PRINTED BY BROWNE AND LOOKER,
FOR THE AUTHOR.
1813.

The Indian Doctor's Dispensatory, typical of the home remedy books which were the source of most of the medical care available on the frontier

A manuscript home remedy book; such collections were common, sometimes, as in this case, made by physicians and sometimes compiled by laymen

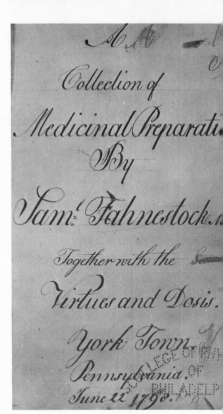

"Thomson's patent"—this "Certificate of Family Right" permitted members of a family to treat themselves by the Thomsonian System

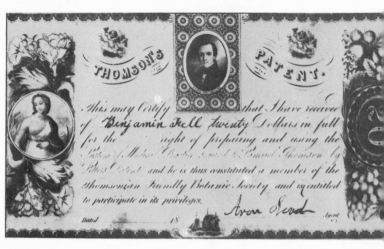

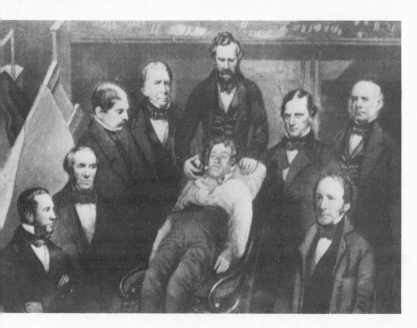

The first public demonstration of surgical anesthesia, October 16, 1846; left to right, around the patient, Gilbert Abbott, are H. J. Bigelow, A. A. Gould, J. Mason Warren, J. C. Warren, W. T. G. Morton, Samuel Parkman, George Hayward, and S. D. Townsend

Medal commemorating Ephraim McDowell, the backwoods doctor who was the first surgeon in the world to perform an ovariotomy successfully

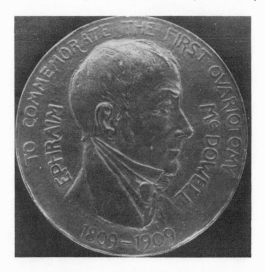

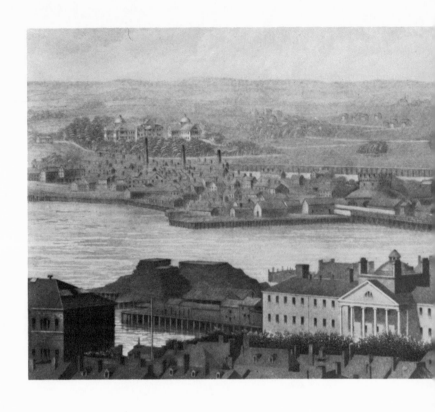

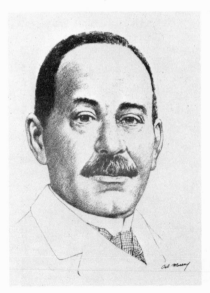

Daniel Hale Williams, courageous
physician, surgeon, and hospital
administrator

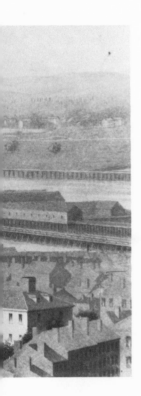

The Massachusetts General Hospital in about 1850, with the Charles River in the background (engraved from a daguerreotype taken from the top of the State House in Boston)

Harvey Cushing (right), internationally known neurosurgeon, with his protege Walter Dandy, also a major contributor to the field of neurosurgery

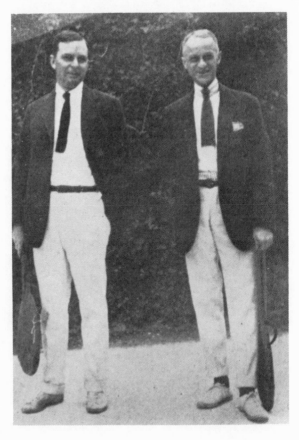

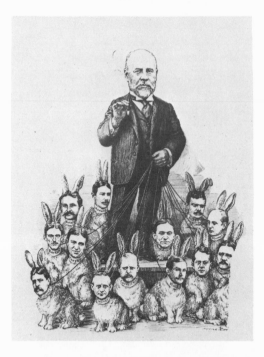

William H. Welch, pathologist, educator, and administrator, with some of his colleagues at Johns Hopkins
(CARTOON BY MAX BRÖDEL)

The Mayos (left to right): Charles H., William W., and William J.

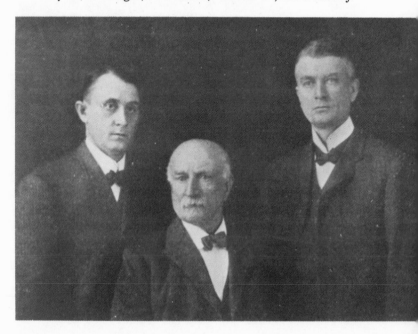

Part III

—⁂—

PROGRESS IN THE
NINETEENTH CENTURY

—⁂—

⁅(9)⁆

Medicine beyond the Alleghenies

FRONTIER DOCTORS

The close of the Revolutionary War saw the beginnings of a westward march through the mountains, and before the end of the century there were settlers in Kentucky, Tennessee, Ohio, Illinois, and Missouri. The number of doctors was not proportionate to the total flow. Throughout the eighteenth century the demand for medical care had exceeded the supply, especially in the rural areas into which a rapidly expanding population was moving. Physicians who settled in the country were likely to be poorly trained men who had not succeeded in the city. Rural dwellers perforce learned to physic, bleed, and sweat themselves, their families, and their slaves, relying on such manuals as *Every Man His Own Doctor* by John Tennent of Virginia, published in the 1730s. In Middle Tennessee, where for many years the only doctor was a horse doctor and settlers were dependent on their own administrations when they became ill, "men . . . exchanged prescriptions for rheumatism and fever as women exchanged recipes for bread and cake." [1]

The frontiersman and his family had to cope with the diseases and physical discomforts generated by their living conditions. As a consequence, the pioneer was "wan with fever, gaunt, and spindle-shanked. His wife was scrawny and peaked; their children were sick and fretful. . . . It was a hard-scrabble life. In the forests people existed in log huts with clapboard roofs, clay chimneys, and puncheon [roughly smoothed timber] floors on which they sat if a box or stool were not handy and slept if there were no pole-frame bed. . . . Fleas and bedbugs made nightly sallies from their nests in the cracks and chinks of frontier dwellings. . . . Pioneers settled close to streams when they could and were pestered by flies and gnats by day and mosquitoes by night. Malarial and typo-malarial fevers sapped their strength. Nobody suspected the role insects played in spreading them." [2]

The woman of the house, who did most of the doctoring, relied on a combination of home-made science, practical experience, and superstition. When all else failed she turned to Indian remedies, including herb and root concoctions, sweatings, rubbings, and ceremonial incantations. When the frontier physician appeared on the scene he too availed himself of Indian healing methods (usually eliminating the elements of superstition).

Of these early doctors Peter Smith (1753–1816) was a typical example. He was born in New Jersey and educated at Princeton. About 1780 he and his wife began wandering through the southern Atlantic states. Peter, an itinerant Baptist preacher, acquired medical knowledge from such physicians as he encountered. In 1794 he reached Cincinnati (by way of Tennessee and Kentucky) and settled at Duck Creek. Here he preached frequently, engaged in farming, and practiced medicine, styling himself an Indian doctor because of the extensiveness with which he employed herb and root remedies. In 1813 he published *The Indian Doctor's Dispensatory,* a compendium of frontier medical practices, with emphasis on botanicals.

The doctor most needed in the hinterland was, of course, the surgeon. The early frontier was the land of the ax and the rifle, the scalping knife, and the bite of the grizzly bear. If a surgeon was not available, it was a case for hunting-knife surgery performed by a companion, with whisky the anesthetic. There were even cases of auto-surgery. "Pegleg" Smith, as he came to be known, was trapping beaver when an Indian bullet smashed his leg. "He should have died because there was no companion to help him, but he wrapped a tourniquet of buckskin thongs around his thigh and amputated with a hunting knife. He clamped off the bleeding arteries with a bullet mold. He whittled himself a leg of hickory." [3]

The pioneers, who were quite proficient in the management of gunshot wounds, had also to deal with cases of scalping. The procedure involved taking a pegging awl and thickly perforating the naked area so that granulation would occur and form a covering to the denuded skull before its investing fibrous membrane should die and exfoliate. A somewhat unique case presented itself when a bear took almost all of Captain Jedediah Smith's head in its huge mouth, causing a wound extending from close to his left eye to his right ear. James Clyman, a young member of the party, agreed to undertake "surgery," but only after asking Captain Smith, whose head was bleeding freely, for guidance. The leader of the expedition told him to get out a needle and thread and sew up his wounds. "I got a pair of scissors and cut off his hair and then began my first job of dressing wounds," Clyman reported subsequently. When the young doctor had finished, Smith mounted his horse and rode to camp.[4]

Few frontier doctors were much better equipped than Clyman. Surgical instruments necessary for the treatment of gunshot wounds were rudimentary. At best, a physician might carry in his saddlebags a set of amputating instruments, a set of trephining instruments for penetrating the skull, a case of pocket instruments, and some crooked and straight needles. (It must be remembered that on July 3, 1776, there were only six sets of amputating instruments to be distributed among fifteen regiments of Washington's army.) Some early physicians carried a scalpel or incision knife for dilating wounds and a pair of forceps for extracting bullets.

The general practitioner "who rode west . . . slept on the ground when he could to aboid flea-infested cabins and inns, where a dozen men were customarily lodged in a room with three or four in each bed. He crunched through winter forests on snowshoes, forded swollen rivers on his horse in the spring, and rode sweating down the hot trails of summer. Often the only drugstore in hundreds of miles was in his saddlebag. He pounded his own drugs, made tinctures and infusions, and put up prescriptions with the aid of horn balances and a china mortar.

"At the end of a long and wearisome ride, the doctor set broken limbs, bound up wounds and injuries, delivered babies, fought smallpox, pneumonia, and dyphtheria. His cures were blunt. He slit the throat of a child choking with dyphtheria and opened the windpipe. He kept the aperture from closing with fishhooks. A frontier doctor's cures were vigorous too. Seizing a patient sick with fever, the doctor opened a vein and drew blood until unconsciousness was near. The patient broke into perspiration. His fever and delirium vanished. The doctor next administered tartar as an emetic and followed it with a calomel purge. Finally he 'locked the bowels,' as the expression went, with opium. When the doctor paid a return visit, the patient usually declared himself 'well, if a little weak,' most likely to prevent additional treatment. The doctor was ingenious too. If a man broke his leg, he reduced the fracture and tied rough-hewn shingles on each side of the break. To keep the leg.pulled straight, he constructed a traction apparatus with a rope and a flatiron or a few horseshoes." [5]

In this medical wilderness, in the first quarter of the nineteenth century, several outstanding innovators emerged.

EPHRAIM McDOWELL, INNOVATOR IN GYNECOLOGY

Ephraim McDowell (1771–1830), was born in Rockbridge County, Virginia. When he was thirteen the family moved to Danville, Kentucky, where the 150 inhabitants made the senior McDowell their judge. Judge McDowell led the militia against the Indians, opposed the Aaron Burr faction that was conspiring with the Spanish to detach the west from the Union, and raised his son to be God-fearing, self-reliant, courageous, and enterprising. When Ephraim was nineteen he went to Staunton, Virginia, to become a pupil of Dr. Alexander Humphreys, an Edinburgh graduate. In 1793 young McDowell went on to Edinburgh, where he studied chemistry under

Joseph Black (1728–1799), anatomy under Monro *secundus*, medicine under James Gregory (1753–1821) at the university, and surgery under the lecturer John Bell (1763–1820). He left Edinburgh without a degree and returned to Danville, by then the capital of Kentucky with a population of about a thousand. He began to practice in 1795.

His practice covered hundreds of miles, and he made his calls on horseback, often riding through the trackless wilderness where Indians and wolves were plentiful. Because distances were so great, McDowell was frequently absent from home for a week or more. In addition to practicing medicine, he performed all the operations then known to surgery, unassisted; often a log cabin was his operating room. McDowell preferred to perform his major operations on Sundays because the thought of the congregations at services strengthened both him and his patient.

Late in 1809 Jane Todd Crawford, wife of a pioneer farmer, believed she was pregnant. She had already given birth to five children and knew the signs. Her body swelled as her time drew near, but she felt no stirring of life. She passed through her ninth and into her tenth month, but nothing happened. A local doctor was called in; then another. Neither knew what to do. They suggested sending for Dr. McDowell, sixty miles distant, who had the reputation of being a good surgeon.

When McDowell arrived on December 13 his examination revealed that the supposed pregnancy was a tumor. "There were no hospitals in that region, no professors whose counsel might be sought. Here everyone was thrown on his own resources. . . . McDowell came to the conclusion that nothing short of an operation, the removal of the tumor with a knife, would be of any use. It was an unheard-of-risk to take. No such operation had ever been carried out." [6]

McDowell told Mrs. Crawford that the procedure he proposed was experimental and that danger was involved. Realizing that she could not function as a pioneer's wife with such a growth in her body, she agreed to the operation. McDowell said she would have to come to Danville. Mrs. Crawford made the winter trip on horseback, since there was no other way, with the tumor resting on the pommel of her saddlebow. It was a slow journey and took several days.

The contemplated surgery was opposed by McDowell's friends and relatives. The minister pleaded, "If she must die, it is God's will. But Ephraim, you are doing the devil's work if you open her with a knife." [7] McDowell's doctor-nephew, Joseph Nash McDowell, stormed angrily out of the house but returned to help his uncle with the operation. "The day having arrived, and the patient being on the table, I marked with a pen the course of the incision to be made, desiring [my nephew] to make the external opening, which, in part, he did; I then took the knife and completed the operation." [8] The procedure, performed of course without anesthesia, took about twenty minutes. A 22½ pound ovarian tumor was removed. Five days later the patient was making her own bed. She lived another thirty-three years until the age of seventy-eight.

This first successful case was followed by two more cases in 1813 and 1816. (In all McDowell appears to have performed the operation thirteen times.)

In 1816 he wrote a simple, straightforward account of his successes and sent one copy to his former teacher and friend, John Bell of Edinburgh, and another to a famous Philadelphia physician, Philip Syng Physick (1768–1837). Bell, who was dying in Italy, never saw the letter, but it came into the hands of his pupil, John Lizars (1787–1860), who followed up McDowell's work and, in 1825, published his *Observations on Extraction of Diseased Ovaria*. Meantime, finding Physick's attitude wholly negative, McDowell's nephew William, who served as messenger, passed the letter on to Thomas C. James (1766–1835), professor of midwifery at the University of Pennsylvania and one of the editors of the *Eclectic Repertory and Analytical Review*. When McDowell's communication was published in an 1817 issue of the *Review,* the author was written off as a man from the backwoods telling tall stories. Two years later, when the *Review* published his account of two more cases, he began to be taken seriously.

The second American to perform an ovariotomy was Nathan Smith, the former professor of medicine at Dartmouth, in July 1821. There were a few cases undertaken by other doctors prior to 1835, but thereafter the procedure went into disuse until it was revived in 1853 by John Light Atlee (1799–1885), who performed seventy-eight ovariotomies (with sixty-four recoveries), and by his brother, Washington Lemuel Atlee (1808–1887), who undertook the procedure 387 times.

McDowell died in 1830 without "having dreamed that he had achieved immortality as the father of ovariotomy," [9] a title conferred on him in 1879 by Sir Spencer Wells (1818–1897). Thanks to followers on both sides of the Atlantic, the procedure that McDowell undertook in 1809 because there was seemingly no choice became one of the supporting pillars of the specialty of obstetrics and gynecology.

DANIEL DRAKE, "FATHER OF WESTERN MEDICINE"

Daniel Drake (1785–1852) was described as the "greatest physician of the West, and one of the most picturesque figures in American medicine. . . . [He] was the first after Hippocrates and Sydenham to do much for medical geography," and his position "in relation to the topography of disease" was unique.[10] This was eulogistic indeed for a man who was born in abject poverty and never saw the Atlantic Ocean.

When Daniel was three years old his father, Isaac, moved the family from New Jersey to Mayslick, Kentucky, a new settlement about seventy-five miles from Lexington, bringing nothing but two horses and the load of one wagon. The family fortune consisted of one dollar, the purchase price of a bushel of corn.

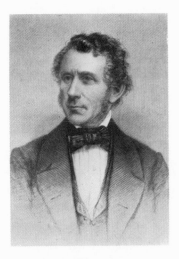

DANIEL DRAKE

There were no schools. Daniel helped with the farm work. Growing up in the woods, he developed an intimate relationship with nature in all its aspects. From time to time a wandering schoolmaster or preacher would settle in the area for a while and teach the children reading, writing, and arithmetic. From this background emerged a great but restless teacher and lecturer, who held almost a dozen professional chairs in half-a-dozen medical schools, established two medical schools (the Medical College of Ohio in 1821 and the Medical Department of Cincinnati College in 1835), and founded the *Western Journal of Medical and Physical Sciences* (1827–38), the most important medical periodical of its time. Drake was also a forceful writer with a clear style; the topics that interested him ranged from meteorological and climatic conditions, plant life, and geological formations to medical education and *Diseases of the Interior Valley of North America* (1850–54). He even found time for papers on the evils of city life, mesmerism, and moral defects in medical students.

When Daniel was fifteen it was decided that he should become a doctor. There has been some suggestion that young Drake would have preferred a business career, following in the footsteps of an uncle, a prosperous local storekeeper. This seems unlikely because the son of the same storekeeper, about six years Daniel's senior, was already studying medicine when Daniel was twelve or thirteen, and when John Drake came home for the holidays, his young cousin is said to have pored over his textbooks. Furthermore, while Isaac was an illiterate man who spent most of his life in dire poverty, he was determined that his children should better themselves. According to one story, in 1788 when Daniel was three, Isaac told Dr. William Goforth, who had also migrated from New Jersey to the wilds of Kentucky, that his son should be his pupil and become a doctor. If this was so, Daniel must have grown up with an understanding of what his calling would be.

By 1800 Goforth had moved to Cincinnati, where he would become the city's leading physician, and in December fifteen-year-old Daniel began a four-year apprenticeship. He mixed drugs, compounded salves, and accompanied his preceptor on his professional rounds. At the same time he went to school to learn Latin. He later wrote:

> My first assigned duties were to read Quincy's dispensatory and grind quicksilver into ungumentum mercuriale; the latter of which, from previous practice on a Kentucky handmill, I found much the easier of the two. But few of you have seen the genuine old doctor's shop of the last century, or regaled your olfactory nerves in the mingled odors which, like incense to the God of Physic, rose from brown paper bundles, bottles stopped with worm-eaten corks, and open jars of ointment, not a whit behind those of the apothecary in the days of Solomon; yet such a place is very well for a student. However idle, he will be always absorbing a little medicine, especially if he sleeps beneath the greasy counter. It was my allotted task to commit to memory Chesselden [sic] on the bones, and Innes on the muscles, without specimens of the former or plates of the latter; and afterwards to meander the currents of humoral pathology of Boerhaave and Vansweiten [sic]; without having studied the chemistry of Chaptal, the physiology of Haller or the materia medica of Cullen.[11]

The works of Benjamin Rush were forbidden—Goforth had no use for his therapy—but, in secret, Drake read everything by Rush he could lay his hands on. At the end of Drake's apprenticeship, Goforth took him into partnership. In his first year under this arrangement, Drake earned enough money to finance five months' schooling in Philadelphia. He set forth with a diploma from Goforth certifying that he had successfully completed his period of preparation—the first medical diploma conferred west of the Alleghenies. During his attendance at the university, he heard Rush and was enraptured by his lectures.

In 1815 Drake completed his medical education and received an M.D. degree from the University of Pennsylvania. Meantime, after attempting for a while to practice in the village where his parents lived, he returned to Cincinnati and in 1807 took over the practice of Dr. Goforth, who was moving to New Orleans.

Drake's career as a teacher and promoter of medical schools began in 1817 when he was appointed to the chair of materia medica at Transylvania University. From then on he moved from place to place in the cause of medical education, and apparently was "dissatisfied with every condition he met." [12]

His dissatisfaction sprang largely from the fact that, while he recognized that the growing nation needed physicians, he also recognized that they must be well grounded. Medical schools were springing up like mushrooms. Whenever two doctors got together they were apt to found a school, admit paying pupils, and deal out diplomas. The product of such schools was too often a bungling charlatan.

In his essays on medical education (1832), Drake directed

attention to inadequate preparation of students and often of teachers, to inadequate equipment and inadequate periods of training. Many schools offered only two sessions of four months each; Drake demanded four years' training, with practical demonstrations at the bedside. His voice was heard but not generally heeded, although he practically created decent medical teaching in Cincinnati.

For all his outspoken aggressiveness and belligerent attitude, Drake was essentially modest—the backwoods boy raised in a log cabin on the frontier. Asked by his friend and colleague, Samuel D. Gross (1805–1884), the greatest American surgeon of his time, why he did not go abroad where his fame would ensure his being received with respect and deference, he replied: "I don't care to be brought into contact with the great physicians on the other side of the Atlantic, men of university education, whose advantages were so much greater than my own. I think too much of my country to place myself in so awkward a position." [13]

WILLIAM BEAUMONT, PIONEER IN PHYSIOLOGY

William Beaumont (1775–1853) was not a product of the frontier but achieved fame there. He was, in fact, born in Lebanon, Connecticut, a member of a family that had emigrated from England in 1635. At the age of twenty-one, determined to see the world, he hitched a horse to a light sleigh, loaded aboard a barrel of cider, and, with $100 in his jeans, headed north. Impressed by Champlain, New York, near the Canadian border, he obtained the post of village schoolmaster and taught there for three years before deciding to study medicine. He crossed Lake Champlain to St. Albans, Vermont,

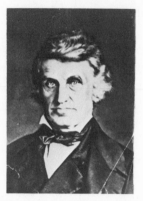

WILLIAM BEAUMONT

where he became apprenticed to Dr. Benjamin Chandler. On June 2, 1812, the Third Medical Society of the State of Vermont granted him a license to practice. The same month war was declared against England; in September, Beaumont joined the American army as a surgeon's mate and served until 1815. For four years he practiced medicine in Plattsburg, New York. Then the army was reorganized, and Joseph Lovell (1788–1836), the new Surgeon-General, remembered his comrade-in-arms of an earlier day and invited Beaumont to rejoin. Beaumont was immediately assigned to Fort Mackinac, a trading post on an island in the Straits between Lake Michigan and Lake Huron.

On June 6, 1822, a nineteen-year-old French-Canadian employee of the American Fur Company, Alexis St. Martin, was standing in front of the company store with a group of men when one of them accidentally discharged his shotgun. The full charge entered the left side of St. Martin's abdomen, causing an external wound the size of the palm of a man's hand. Beaumont was summoned promptly. He wrote in his account:

154

I saw him in 20 or 30 minutes after the accident, and, on examination, found a portion of the lung, as large as a turkey's egg, protruding through the external wound, lacerated and burnt; and immediately below this another protrusion, which, on further inspection, proved to be a portion of the stomach, lacerated through all its coats, and pouring out the food he had taken at breakfast, through an orifice large enough to admit my forefinger.

In attempting to return the protruded portion of the lung, I was prevented by a sharp point of the fractured rib, over which it had caught by its membranes; but, by raising it with my finger, and clipping off the point of the rib, I was able to return it into its proper cavity; though it could not be retained there on account of the incessant efforts to cough. The projecting portion of the stomach was nearly as large as that of the lung; and it passed through the lacerated diaphragm and the external wound, mingling the food with the bloody mucus blown from the lung.[14]

It seemed inevitable that the wound would prove fatal, but Beaumont, after putting back the lung and stomach, covered the wound with "a carbonated fermenting poultice, composed of flour, hot water, charcoal, and yeast," and by the next day the patient was not only alive but somewhat improved. After some months he was recovered except for a fistulous opening in the stomach.[15]

In April 1823 the Mackinac town authorities declared St. Martin an "infirm pauper" and proposed returning him to his birthplace in Canada. Beaumont, believing that the journey might well prove fatal, took him into his home, where he "nursed him, fed him, clothed him, lodged him and furnished him with every comfort and dressed his wounds daily and for the most part twice a day." [16]

It appears that it was 1825 before it occurred to Beaumont that the case offered an unusual opportunity for studying the gastric juices and the process of digestion. He carried out four experiments before St. Martin, who disliked the experiments and was of too little intelligence to appreciate their importance, ran off. It took Beaumont two years to locate him and another two years to get him back. Thereafter Beaumont continued his investigations. (St. Martin, incidentally, lived to be eighty-three.)

Beaumont, weak in chemistry, consulted Professor Robley Dunglison (1798–1869) of the University of Virginia and Professor Benjamin Silliman (1816–1885) of Yale, sending them samples of St. Martin's gastric juices. Dunglison offered valuable suggestions, and Silliman identified the free acid as chiefly hydrochloric acid. (In 1835 Theodor Schwann (1810–1882), the German physiologist, proved the other chemical substance to be pepsin.)

In 1833 Beaumont published his *Experiments and Observations on the Gastric Juice and the Physiology of Digestion.* He refuted the claim of the pioneer experimental physiologist, François Magendie (1783–1855) of France, that gastric secretion is continual; he showed that the gastric juice is secreted only when food is present and that mechanical irritation of the mucous membranes produces congestion but only a limited local secretion of gastric juice.

What is truly remarkable is that an army doctor in the primeval forests of Michigan realized, when an accident threw an experimental subject his way, this was a unique opportunity, and, at considerable personal sacrifice and hardship, pursued his research.

JOHN SAPPINGTON AND MALARIA

Born in Maryland, John Sappington (1776–1856) served an apprenticeship under his physician-father and joined him in practice after the family moved to Nashville, Tennessee. As a medical student at the University of Pennsylvania in 1814–15, he took issue with the practice of Benjamin Rush and other Philadelphia physicians of purging, inducing vomiting, and bloodletting in the treatment of fever. Sappington believed that such treatment served only to weaken the already weakened patient.

In 1819 Sappington established himself and his family in a log cabin at Arrow Rock, Saline County, Missouri. This area was part of the Louisiana Purchase acquired by Thomas Jefferson sixteen years earlier. At that time he was accused of having bought a vast amount of uninhabitable land; its eastern boundary was the Mississippi River, and the Mississippi River Valley was malaria-infested. A year after Sappington settled at Arrow Rock, two young French chemists, Pelletier and Caventou, isolated quinine from cinchona bark, which had been used as a fever fighter for several centuries. The first American quinine factory was established in Philadelphia in 1822.

Even as progressive a doctor as Daniel Drake hesitated to give up purgatives and the knife in the treatment of malaria. Henry Perrine (1797–1840), botanist and doctor, who practiced at Natchez, Mississippi, in the middle 1820s, while harboring reservations, used large doses of quinine at the first signs of malarial fever. An article by Perrine in the *Philadel-*

phia Journal of the Medical and Physical Sciences in 1826 was probably the first on the subject published in America.

Sappington had no reservations. He actively championed the use of quinine in the prevention and treatment of malarial fever. Quinine was his sole method of treatment as soon as it became available in 1823.

For a decade Sappington used quinine effectively but could do little at that time to change the attitudes of his fellow physicians. In 1832 he began the manufacture and sale of his "Anti-Fever Pills." These, at $1.50 for a box of twenty-four, were distributed by a regiment of drummers who traveled far and wide through the Mississippi Valley and into the Republic of Texas. Books and handbills as well as pills were distributed. The prescription for prevention was one pill three times daily. In ten years over a million boxes were sold. In 1844 Sappington published at Philadelphia his *Theory and Treatment of Fevers,* in which he presented in detail the method for preparing the "Anti-Fever Pills."

The malarial parasite was not uncovered until 1880 (a quarter of a century after Sappington's death). That the mosquito was the carrier was not proved until 1897. Sappington used and promoted quinine because it worked. And if proof was needed of the effectiveness of his bitter concoction of quinine sulphate, licorice, myrrh, and oil of sassafras, it was offered by the fact that his salesmen, who were themselves required to take three fever pills daily, marched through the areas where malaria was most prevalent without one of them contracting the disease. His successful program ultimately won many followers and became the recommended treatment.

⁅(10)⁆

The Phenomenon of Specialization

The distinction between medicine and surgery and pharmacy could not be maintained in colonial America. Doctors with M.D. degrees, "although educated abroad, were expected to practice just as other Americans did—including surgery and drug selling. . . ." [1]

In 1748 Dr. Adam Thomson (d. 1767), later famous in connection with inoculation, aroused professional resentment in Philadelphia by refusing to sell drugs. In the 1770s Dr. James McClurg, having returned to Virginia after considerable education abroad, attempted to limit his practice to medicine because of a nervous aversion to surgery. Despite the fact that the Virginia legislature had in 1736 ruled in favor of higher fees for doctors who possessed university degrees, he could not make a living.

When John Morgan returned to America in 1765, he brought with him a qualified apothecary and surgeon, David Leighton, to whom he proposed turning over all procedures not strictly related to the practice of medicine. Morgan considered that the limitations he placed on himself should be applied to others. He urged the separation of the practice of internal medicine from the practices of surgery and pharmacy. Pointing out that generals did not dig trenches, he stated: "No more then is a physician obliged, from his office, to handle a knife with a surgeon; to cull herbs with the botanist; to distill simples with the chymist; or compound drugs with the apothecary." [2]

The reaction of Philadelphia doctors was unfavorable. It was "perhaps fortunate that Morgan failed to convince his professional co-workers of the desirability of such a separation of function, for in America for the first time in history were abolished the barriers between physician and surgeon which had produced class distinctions and snobbishness in relegating surgery to an inferior role." [3] The concept of specialization did not take root in the United States until the middle of the nineteenth century. Even then it was an uphill battle. As late as 1869 the Committee on Specialties of the American Medical Association reported: "The chief objection brought against specialties is, that they operate unfairly toward the general practitioner, in implying that he is incompetent to properly treat certain classes of diseases, and narrowing his field of practice"; and in 1875 Abraham Jacobi (1830–1919), president of the New York State Medical Society and himself a pediatrician, could still point out that specialization tended "to degrade the general practitioner in the estimation of the public." [4]

The emergence of specialization was partly due to the natural human characteristic of doing what one is most capable of doing. As the colonial village advanced to a point where it could support more than one doctor, each tended to follow his own bent, so that, for example, one handled fever cases and the other delivered babies. Through the decades the work of the original doctor, who was a general practitioner in the fullest sense, was spread among the internist, the surgeon, the obstetrician, and the pediatrician.

Specialization was also the result of individual (sometimes collective discoveries) made by a doctor in pursuit of his professional activities. And as more and more knowledge became available, there developed an inevitable temptation for a physician to limit the acquisition of knowledge to a particular sphere of interest. The economic factor was also important since specialists usually enjoyed higher incomes than their generalist colleagues.

OBSTETRICS AND GYNECOLOGY

Obstetrics and gynecology involve the practice of both medicine and surgery. "One cannot draw any definite line between [them] for the two actually constitute one field dealing with reproduction and with the disorders and diseases of the reproductive tract. There is a single purpose and that is to preserve the function of reproduction where possible, at the same time preserving a woman's health in the face of damage or disease." [5]

James Marion Sims (*1813–1883*) is generally regarded as the founder of gynecology in the United States. McDowell contributed one important procedure, ovariotomy, but Sims was responsible for a number of innovations. "Probably the most

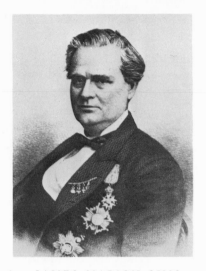

JAMES MARION SIMS

useful achievement in American surgery" was his "successful operation for vaginal fistula" in 1849.[6]

Sims was born in Lancaster County, South Carolina. His father, sheriff and tavern owner in a back-country village who rose to command a company in the War of 1812, wanted the best of education for his son. He was greatly disappointed when young Marion decided on medicine, describing that calling as "a profession for which I have the utmost contempt. There is no science in it. There is no honor to be achieved in it; no reputation to be made, and to think that *my* son should be going around from house to house through this country, with a box of pills in one hand and a squirt in the other, to ameliorate human suffering, is a thought I never supposed I should have to contemplate." [7]

Sims graduated from Jefferson Medical College in 1835 and settled in Mobile, Alabama. He quickly became known as a capable and inventive surgeon. Called upon in 1845 to examine a woman who had fallen off a horse and suffered a displacement of the uterus, Sims placed the patient in an unusual lateral position (the Sims posture or position), which afforded him a correct view of the vaginal canal:

> I saw everything, as no man had ever seen before. The fistula was as plain as the nose on a man's face. . . . I said at once, "Why can not these things be cured? It seems to me that there is nothing to do but to pare the edges of the fistula and bring it together nicely, introduce a catheter in the neck of the bladder and drain the urine off continually, and the case will be cured." [8]

These observations led him to invent a curved speculum for use in operating on fistulas between the bladder and the vagina (vesicovaginal fistulas). He also employed a special suture of silver wire (to avoid sepsis) and a catheter that would empty the bladder during healing without discomfort to the patient. Prior to 1852, when Sims published a paper in the *American Journal of the Medical Sciences* outlining several cures for vesicovaginal fistulas, many surgeons had tried unsuccessfully to treat this condition.

In 1853 Sims moved to New York, and two years later established the State Hospital for Women, which became the center of the best gynecological work of the day. In 1861 he developed a method for surgical removal of the neck of the uterus; in the same year he described the muscle spasm, "vaginismus." In 1878 he developed his operation for gallbladder disease.

Sims was rather an extraordinary man. In his day it was the practice of wealthy Southern planters regularly to employ prominent local physicians to take care of their plantations, including their slaves. In cases involving surgical intervention, permission of the master rather than the patient was required. On one occasion when Sims could not secure such permission he purchased a slave in order to operate on her.[9]

Oliver Wendell Holmes (1809–1896) was not only the first Brahmin of New England, he invented the term. Born in Cambridge in 1809 of a well-to-do family, in due course he undertook the study of law at Harvard but became sick of it. "I know not what the temple of the law may be to those who have entered it, but to me it seems very cold and cheerless about the threshold." The next year he entered medical school, "where he found the company of clammy corpses preferable to that of barristers." [10]

Holmes is remembered as a poet and an often witty man of letters. Consequently the importance of his place in the history of medicine is sometimes overlooked. The great Canadian physician Sir William Osler (1849–1919) described Holmes' contribution as having probably saved many more lives than had any other gynecologist.

It was on February 13, 1843, that Holmes read to the Boston Society for Medical Improvement a paper *On the Contagiousness of Puerperal Fever*. His paper was inspired by the death of a doctor who had cut his hand while performing an autopsy on a woman who had died of puerperal (childbed) fever and by the number of cases (which he had heard of or observed) where the disease seemed to have been conveyed by a victim to other individuals.

Holmes laid no claim to being first in the field. He had studied in France for over two years with side trips to England, Germany, and Italy. That puerperal fever was contagious and fatal had been noted by Hippocrates, by Paul-Jacques Malouin (1701–1778) of the Hôtel Dieu in Paris, France's leading hospital, and by Alexander Gordon (1752–1799) of Aberdeen. Charles White (1728–1813) of Manchester, England, had stressed the advantages of scrupulous cleanliness in such cases. What Holmes presented was, however, novel to his audience.

He suggested that, because the disease could be carried from patient to patient, physicians attending victims or making postmortem sections in cases of puerperal fever should avoid visiting women in childbed. If they could not, washing the hands in calcium chloride and a change of clothes after leaving the puerperal-fever case were the best available preventive measures.

The publication of Holmes' paper aroused the ire of prominent obstetricians. They were led by professors of obstetrics at the University of Pennsylvania and Jefferson Medical College, Hugh L. Hodge (1796–1873) and Charles D. Meigs (1792–1869). While Hodge opposed Holmes' views "in the most formal manner," Meigs committed the flagrant blunder of attacking the author's youth (he was then thirty-four), placing the article among "the jejeune and fizzenless dreamings of sophomore writers." [11] (It was Meigs, by the way, who would say, around 1850, arguing in favor of male midwifery, that "the first woman must have been assisted in labor by a man, for Eve could have had no other assistance than that of Adam.") [12] Holmes countered by describing his critics as "two professors, learned men both of them, skillful experts, but babies, as it seemed to me in their capacity of reasoning and arguing." [13]

In 1855 Holmes reiterated his views in *Puerperal Fever as a Private Pestilence*. The title derives from the final sentence in his earlier paper:

> Whatever indulgence may be granted to those who have heretofore been the ignorant causes of so much misery,

the time has come when the existence of a *private pestilence* in the sphere of a single physician should be looked upon not as a misfortune but a crime; and in the knowledge of such occurrences, the duties of the practitioner to his profession, should give way to his paramount obligations to society.[14]

Puerperal fever was a mere episode in his busy, varied life, but, having latched on to a brilliant and correct idea, he recognized a great opportunity to be of service to society and championed his cause with all the resources he could command.

Howard Atwood Kelly (1865–1943) was a recognized leader in American gynecology. A pioneer in the use of cocaine for local anesthesia (1881), he also devised many new operations and instruments, including the Kelly pad, the Kelly clamp, and the Kelly rectoscope. He served briefly (1888) as professor of gynecology at the University of Pennsylvania, then moved on in 1889 to Johns Hopkins University. His *Operative Gynecology* (1898) and *Medical Gynecology* (1908) are among the best American treatises of their time. Kelly's *Stereo-Clinic* (1910–13) is a photographic record of contemporary surgical procedures.

ANESTHESIA

The idea of alleviating the pain of surgery has tantalized man since earliest days. Homer mentioned the use of nepenthe for this purpose. Dioscorides in the second century A.D. recommended mandragora of the nightshade family. Indian hemp was used in the Middle Ages. Around the end of the first millennium, the soporific sponge was popular at the University of

Salerno. A few centuries later Gui de Chauliac described this as a sponge soaked in a mixture of opium, henbane, hemlock, lettuce, and mandragora dried in the sun. For use it was saturated with boiling water and its exhalations inhaled by the patient. These early practices died out.

Prior to the middle of the nineteenth century anesthesia was a matter of theory rather than practice. Hans von Gerssdorff (c. 1456–1517) probably reflected the attitude of his contemporaries when he wrote: "There has been much said and often written how you give a drink and make one sleep whom you wish to cut. I leave it alone. I have never used it or seen it even and at that I have cut off a hundred or two members." As late as 1839 Alfred Velpeau (1795–1867), the French author of an important treatise on surgical anatomy, declared: "To escape pain in surgical operations is a chimera which we cannot expect in our time." [15]

The work of the English chemist Humphry Davy (1778–1829) seems not to have made much impression. In 1799 he had observed: "As nitrous oxide in its extensive operation seems capable of destroying physical pain, it may probably be used with advantage during surgical operations in which no great effusion of blood takes place." [16]

By the early nineteenth century it was customary for surgeons to intoxicate their patients with alcohol or opium in cases requiring complete muscular relaxation—reduction of dislocations, ligations of large arteries, herniotomies, and so on. At the beginning of the 1840s the field was wide open for the development of effective anesthesia. Americans accepted the challenge.

The question of who was the first American doctor to introduce surgical anesthesia has been a matter of often violent controversy, with claims advanced on behalf of Crawford Williamson Long (1815–1878), Horace Wells (1815–1848), Charles Thomas Jackson (1805–1880), and William Thomas Green Morton (1819–1868). William E. Clark has been ignored in the debate, possibly because he was a student at Berkshire Medical College at the time. Clark may well have been the first individual to administer ether in America. The record shows that in January 1842 he did so to enable Dr. Elijah Pope to extract a patient's tooth.

It was in March of the same year that Dr. Long of Danielsville, Georgia, employed ether in the removal of a small cystic tumor from the back of a patient's neck. This experiment resulted from the fact that he had earlier been a witness to the "frolics" of some young men who had sniffed ether. Long had noticed that while stuporous they frequently injured themselves, as was confirmed subsequently by bruises on their bodies, without being aware that they had done so. Long used ether in other cases in 1842 and 1843.

If Long had communicated his findings, there could have been no grounds for dispute, but it was 1848 before he presented a paper on the subject to the Georgia State Medical Society and 1854 before, at the insistence of his friends, he entered his claim to be the discoverer of anesthesia.

The claim on behalf of Horace Wells, a dentist of Hartford, Connecticut, was a thin one. (He did not press it himself because, as a result of a patient's death under anesthesia, he retired from practice and then committed suicide.) Wells used nitrous oxide (laughing gas) not ether, which he had rejected after a superficial investigation. He first used anesthesia in 1844 and communicated his results to his friend and former partner, Dr. William Morton of Charlton, Massachusetts, who is generally acknowledged to be the first.

Charles T. Jackson, a Boston chemist of ability, was clearly psychotic. (He was in fact declared insane at the age of sixty-eight and died in an asylum seven years later.) He claimed that some years prior to Morton's demonstration of the anesthetic properties of ether he had deliberately rendered himself unconscious by inhaling ether and had informed Morton of this. He also claimed that he had suggested to Samuel B. Morse the essential features of the telegraph. There is no evidence to suggest that his claim against Morton was any more valid than his claim against Morse.

Morton's actual relationship to Jackson was that of pupil to preceptor. In 1844 Morton had undertaken the study of medicine (studies which he never completed owing to the distractions of the ether controversy), while continuing in the practice of dentistry. Dissatisfied with Wells' nitrous oxide, he asked Jackson to suggest a better anesthetic. Jackson proposed chloric ether, which Morton used with success in July 1844. Jackson then suggested sulphuric ether, with which, on September 30, 1846, Morton successfully extracted a deeply-rooted bicuspid.

Morton's next step was to persuade John Collins Warren, son of John Warren, to give his anesthetic a trial. On October 16, 1846, at the Massachusetts General Hospital, Dr. Warren removed a tumor from just below the jaw of an anesthetised patient. When the patient returned to consciousness, Warren exclaimed, "Gentlemen, this is no humbug." The next day George Hayward successfully removed a fatty tumor of the shoulder with Morton as anesthetist. On November 18, Henry

J. Bigelow (1818–1890) announced the discovery to the world in a paper in the *Boston Medical and Surgical Journal.* Since Warren and Bigelow enjoyed considerable reputation, ether anesthesia got off to a solid start.

As for the controversy, it boils down simply to a distinction between the first use and the first demonstration of its value. On this basis there is no question about Morton's primary position. Anesthesia "was a great technical achievement in improving the conditions faced by surgeons and at the same time was a milestone in the history of humanitarianism." [17]

SURGERY

It has been said that medicine had its beginnings in witchcraft and in religion, with the physician a priest who dispelled the evil spirits of disease, while "surgery sprang from injury and war. There were no mysteries about surgery. The surgeon was a warrior who displayed a special talent for binding the wounds of his companions. This distinction between the physician who was a priest, and the surgeon who was a 'dresser of wounds,' can be found in the Egyptian papyrus, in Homer and in the Bible. From the beginning, therefore, surgery has been more practical than medicine and the results of surgical treatment have been more immediate and apparent. The distinction has not always been complimentary to surgery. . . . Today, surgery is an applied science as well as a healing art." [18]

The American Civil War led to surgical progress far exceeding that achieved in earlier wars. As the use of surgical anesthesia broadened under military impetus, surgeons could accomplish feats never before attempted. An important tangential contribution was made by William Alexander Hammond

(1828–1900), who began a stormy and short-lived stint as Surgeon-General of the Army in April 1862. He promptly ordered that better records on the sick and wounded be maintained. He called for special reports on fractures, gunshot wounds, amputations, excisions, fevers, diarrheas and dysentery, scorbutic diseases, respiratory diseases, and other preventable diseases. Full reports on important cases and autopsies were required. This accumulation of data could not fail to promote knowledge and improve performance.

John Shaw Billings (*1838–1913*) may seem retrospectively to have only a remote connection with surgery. But it should be remembered that he began his career as an army surgeon and never abandoned his interest in surgery.

Born and raised on an Indiana farm, Billings early developed a thirst for knowledge. He learned Latin and Greek from an elderly clergyman, spent five years at Miami University, and graduated from Drake's Medical College of Ohio in 1860. Swept into the army, he served throughout the war, sometimes in hospitals, more often than not at the front, at Gettysburg and other bloody battles. In December 1864 he was ordered to the Surgeon-General's department in Washington. He remained there for thirty years.

Especially on the frontier where Billings grew up, books were scarce and acquired only at some sacrifice. When he arrived in Washington even the library of the Surgeon-General's office had only 1365 books. He decided to build this into a national library of medicine. With the blessing and, more important, the financial backing of Congress, Billings journeyed far and wide in search of books. By 1876 the library had grown to 40,000 volumes.

The next problem was a catalogue, which, Billings felt

should double as a bibliography of medicine. In 1876 he published a *Specimen Fasciculus* of an index catalogue of authors and subjects. In 1880, having been assisted by Robert Fletcher (1823–1912), originally from Bristol, England, he issued the first volume of the *Index Catalogue* of the library. This was the forerunner of the most comprehensive medical bibliography ever undertaken.

Close as books were to his heart, Billings was not exclusively a librarian and bibliographer. The army taught him many things, notably war surgery, military sanitation, the conduct of hospitals, and how to organize a project, whatever its nature.

In Washington he reorganized the Marine Hospital Service, which had been established by Congress in 1798 for "the relief of disabled seamen," doing away with abuses and preparing the department to assume increasing responsibilities. (In 1912 this would become the U.S. Public Health Service.)

Billings drew up the plans for the Johns Hopkins Hospital in Baltimore, begun in 1876. He was a pioneer believer in vital statistics, and since 1880 the population census has included medical data. He was also a prolific writer, and his *History of Surgery* is one of the best in English.

William Stewart Halsted (1852–1922) made many "contributions, not only to his craft but to the science of medicine in general, . . . fundamental in character and of enduring importance." [19]

In 1883 at the Chambers Street Hospital in New York City, one of six hospitals at which Halsted held a staff appointment, there was a steady flow of accident cases, many involving illumination gas poisoning. Halsted conceived the idea of what he called "refusion of blood." The procedure involved bleeding the patient, agitating the blood with air to remove carbon

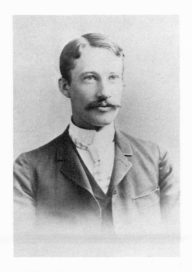

WILLIAM S. HALSTED

monoxide, and returning the blood by injection into an artery. His work had an important bearing on blood transfusion, then virtually unknown.

When in 1884 Carl Koller (1857–1944) of Vienna demonstrated the effectiveness of cocaine as a local anesthetic, Halsted recognized the importance of this discovery. He obtained a supply of cocaine and began recklessly experimenting on himself, his associates, and medical students. Halsted and three of his fellow experimenters became addicted. The three others died miserably; Halsted succeeded in "kicking the habit" and went on to be recognized as a pioneer in block (conduction) anesthesia and infiltration (local by injection) anesthesia, both important to surgery.

In 1889 he devised the supraclavicular operation for breast cancer; the same year, simultaneously with Edoardo Bassini (1844–1924) of Italy, he introduced the modern operation for hernia. Two years later he was the first successfully to ligate the large artery at the base of the neck that supplies blood to the arm. Halsted continued his experimental surgery into the twentieth century and made many advances.

Perhaps Halsted's greatest contribution to medicine was the lead he took in aseptic surgery. The antiseptic principle in the practice of surgery had been formulated in 1867 by London-born Joseph Lister (1827–1912) after two years of experimentation, based on the work of Louis Pasteur (1822–1895) in fermentation. Lister recognized that it was not exposure to air but exposure to germs in the air that produced suppuration. Lister's statement was poorly received. British medical men focused on the materials designed to keep the wound germ free—carbolic acid as the antiseptic agent and a covering of calico or lint—instead of on the actual principle. While senior surgeons in Glasgow, Edinburgh, London, and Dublin turned thumbs down on the sterilization procedure recommended, continental doctors were enthusiastic, especially in Germany, where Ernst von Bergmann (1836–1907) became Lister's devoted disciple. In 1886 von Bergmann devised a method of steam sterilization as an adjunct to the corrosive sublimate method.

Halsted read everything put forth by Lister, von Bergmann, and others. His "operating room was immaculate and he insisted on strict adherence to his rigid principles of asepsis from every member of the operating team. Sterilization was achieved by boiling or autoclaving, and the instruments were also immersed in a carbolic solution until needed. Caps and gowns were worn, but masks were not introduced until later. Hands were scrupulously cleansed, then immersed in bichloride of mercury solution in an effort to sterilize them, which Halsted admitted was virtually impossible."[20] In 1880–81 he introduced gutta-percha tissue in drainage; in 1890, rubber gloves.

He had considered rubber gloves as an added protective measure earlier than this, but, afraid they would cause a loss of manual dexterity and delicacy of touch, had ruled them out until in 1889, the nurse in charge of his operating room complained that the solution of mercuric chloride produced a dermatitis on her arms and hands. "As she was an unusually efficient woman," he wrote, "I gave the matter my consideration, and one day in New York requested the Goodyear Rubber Company to make, as an experiment, two pairs of thin rubber gloves with gauntlets." [21] For many years after gloves had been universally accepted in the operating room, Halsted continued to remove his glove to palpate the common bile duct.

On June 4, 1890, Halsted married the nurse in charge of his operating room, prompting John Miller Turpin Finney, a colleague on the Johns Hopkins Hospital staff, to remark of the rubber gloves incident: "Venus came to the aid of Aesculapius." [22]

Nicholas Senn (*1844–1908*) laid the groundwork, in a way, for a sub-specialty by his work in intestinal surgery. After graduating from the Chicago Medical School in 1868, he practiced in Milwaukee for some years, and then went abroad. He obtained an M.D. degree from the University of Munich in 1878. A decade later he accepted a surgical professorship at Rush Medical College in Chicago.

Senn made original contributions to the study of air embolism—obstruction of a blood vessel caused by the entrance of air into the bloodstream—(1885), to surgery of the pancreas (1886), to gunshot wounds, and to the formation of openings between portions of the intestines (which he closed with decalcified bone-plates). In 1888 he devised a method of detecting intestinal perforation by inflation with hydrogen gas. He was also the first to use X-rays in the treatment of leukemia (1903).

In another direction, he founded the Association of Military Surgeons of the United States in 1891. In the Spanish-American War he served as an army surgeon.

At his death he left his valuable collection of medical books to the Newberry Library (later transferred to the John Crerar Library) and made handsome bequests to Rush Medical College for the advancement of surgery.

NEUROLOGY

S. Weir Mitchell (1829–1914), neurologist, physiologist, novelist, and poet, holds a high place in both American and international medicine.

After graduating from Jefferson Medical College in 1850,

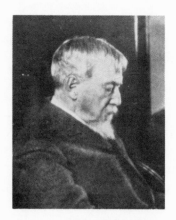

S. WEIR MITCHELL

Mitchell spent a year in Paris, where he was immensely impressed by the work of Claude Bernard (1813–1878), the great French physiologist. Between 1851 and 1863 Mitchell's investigations covered a wide range. His research extended from the formation of uric acid and blood crystals to the intercrossing of the nerves of the larynx of the turtle, the immunity of the pigeon to opium, and, perhaps the outstanding work of this period, a toxicological study of the venom of the rattlesnake. During the Civil War, Mitchell's work focused on the subject that would later be his central concern.

When William A. Hammond, with whom Mitchell had investigated arrow poisons in 1859, became Surgeon-General in April 1862, he created special military hospitals for diseases of the heart, lungs, and nervous system and placed Mitchell in charge of Turner's Lane Hospital in Philadelphia. Here Mitchell established a special ward for neurological patients. With George Reed Morehouse (1829–1905) and William W. Keen (1837–1932), he studied gunshot and other injuries of the peripheral nerves. A monograph was published by the three men in 1864, *Gunshot Wounds and Other Injuries of Nerves*. "Mitchell was the dynamic force behind the study. His analysis . . . [showed] his powers of observation and his genius for making sound physiological deductions." [23]

Mitchell and his colleagues found that, following the severance of an important nerve (especially when infection was involved), there was unusual sensitivity to pain or touch. Mitchell named this condition "causalgia." It was to be actively studied by succeeding generations for almost one hundred years, through World War II, when its incidence was frequent. They also produced clear-cut descriptions of primary and secondary shock. Discussing reflex paralysis, they wrote:

The majority of physicians will no doubt be disposed to attribute the chief share of the phenomena of shock . . . to the indirect influence exerted through and upon the heart. There are, however, certain facts, which duly considered, will, we think, lead us to suppose that in many cases the phenomena in question may be due to a temporary paralysis of the whole range of nerve centres, and that among these phenomena the cardiac feebleness may play a large part, and be itself induced by the state of the regulating nerve centres of the great circulatory organs. . . . But there do exist certain cases, more rare it is true, in which certain affections of the nerve centres, other than those of the heart, occur as a consequence of wounds.[24]

After the war Mitchell became a director and the moving spirit of the Philadelphia Orthopedic Hospital and Infirmary for Nervous Diseases. Here he did the clinical work that led to the publication in 1872 of *Injuries of Nerves and Their Consequences,* which includes the earliest description of ascending neuritis, clear accounts of the psychological problems of amputees, and many other data fundamental to neurology. Mitchell's style was both clear and enjoyable, and this assisted the early acceptance of his views.

Knowledge has been expanded to a degree that makes it impossible for an individual to be expert in all fields, and specialization has become an essential element in medical practice, but there is inherent in it an element of danger. For a number of perfectly logical and sensible reasons the specialist seeks to partition the patient's health-care problems, but a human being cannot be partitioned arbitrarily. The conscientious specialist should never forget that he is a physician first and a specialist second.

SPECIALTY MEDICAL SOCIETIES

The development of specialties brought in its train medical societies in special areas. The first was the Boston Phrenological Society, which survived for ten years, from 1832 to 1842. Because phrenology came to be exploited by quacks and charlatans, it was derided by scientists, and therefore seems like a strange candidate for the title of medical specialty, but at one time it was taken seriously. It was introduced by Franz Joseph Gall (1757–1828) of Vienna and his pupil Johann Caspar Spurzheim (1776–1832), who came to New York in August 1832 and died in Boston (probably of typhoid fever) a month before the Phrenological Society came into existence in December. Phrenology did not long survive in American medicine but in 1847, five years after the society's demise, Dr. John Collins Warren—of the Boston medical family—could still write: "The importance of phrenology is derived, according to my view, from the fact, that it leads to the development of the anatomy and physiology of the nervous system; and also the study of the forms of the crania enables us, in some measure, to understand the degree of intellectual power possessed by individuals." [25]

In 1837 William A. Alcott (1798–1859) and Sylvester Graham (1794–1851) of Boston formed the American Physiological Society to study personal hygiene and nutritional reform but they "damaged their cause by making up with enthusiasm what they lacked in knowledge." [26] The society survived for only three years.

A specialty society founded in Philadelphia in 1844 is

still active. The Association of Medical Superintendents of American Institutions for the Insane changed its name, in 1892, to the American Medico-Psychological Association and, in 1921, became the American Psychiatric Association. The Pathological Society of Philadelphia was also organized in 1844.

The real effort to establish national specialty societies came with the Civil War, which encouraged specialization in medicine. Aside from "the precursor of the American Psychiatric Association," there "was the American Ophthalmological Society, which in June, 1864, made its debut in New York." Ophthalmology as a full-blown specialty had not made its appearance until after 1859, although its antecedents "may be traced back to the earliest decades of the nineteenth century." [27]

After the eye came the ear. The American Otological Society was founded in 1868. By the end of the century, upward of twenty national specialty societies were functioning. Their purpose was twofold: the presentation, discussion, and publication of scientific information; and the public and professional relations of the group.

(11)

The Sectarians

The first quarter of the nineteenth century saw the emergence of a different type of specialist, one whose activity was limited not by an area of performance but by a method of treatment. These "specialists" have sometimes been called quacks and cultists. Undoubtedly some groups and individuals were deserving of condemnation, but others made an important contribution to American health, and it is to these sectarians that attention is directed here.

To a degree, their success represented a swing by the public away from the unpleasant and dangerous remedies of Benjamin Rush and his followers. European medicine, centered in post-revolutionary Paris, was marking time on the threshold of modern medicine, and its practitioners were also marking time. Their patients had become objects of research rather than human beings in need of help. While they investigated, they could only recommend that "nothing be done, and such nihilism seemed too negative to most [American] practitioners and doubtless also to their patients. Hence bleeding and purging were still common in the 1840s and even in the fifties. Homeopaths, in contrast, avoided the extremes of both nihilism and heroic practice." [1]

The sectarians were opposed by regular doctors, who for the most part would have none of them. Homeopaths and Thomsonians "became the modern medical sects. They founded their own schools and journals. . . ." [2]

Thomsonianism, a native product, appeared full grown on the American scene in 1813; homeopathy was imported in 1825; osteopathy, another American development, did not originate until 1874.

THE BOTANIC SYSTEM

Samuel Thomson (1769–1843), a native of New Hampshire, was entirely self-taught in medicine. There had been some attempt at an apprenticeship:

> Sometime during the year that I was sixteen years old, I heard my parents say, that as my mind was so much taken up with roots and herbs, they thought it best to send me to live with a Doctor Fuller . . . who was called a root doctor.

This "taking up" had occurred early:

> When I was between three and four years old, my father took me out with him to work. . . . I was very curious to know the names of all the herbs which I saw growing, and what they were good for; and . . . [I] was constantly making inquiries. . . . All the information I thus

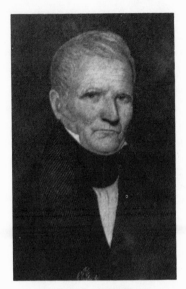

SAMUEL THOMSON

obtained, or by my own observation, I carefully laid up in
my memory and never forgot. . . . Some time . . . after I
was four years old . . . I discovered a plant which had a
singular branch and pods, . . . and I had the curiosity to
pick some of the pods and chew them; the taste and operation produced, was so remarkable, that I never forgot it.
I afterwards used to induce other boys to chew it, merely
by way of sport, to see them vomit. I tried this herb in
this way for nearly twenty years, without knowing any
things of its medicinal virtues. This plant [lobelia] is
what I have called the Emetic Herb, and is the most important article I have made use of in my practice.[3]

The stay with Dr. Fuller was brief. It was said that Samuel "had not learning enough." Since it was difficult for his

parents to spare him from the farm, he gave up hope of doing anything else.

When Samuel was nineteen he cut his ankle very badly. Its treatment illustrated "the Terrible Methods of Medical Practice, Domestic, Empirical, and Regular at that Date." [4] In dressing the wound his father drew

> a string through between the heel-cord and bone, and another between that and the skin; so that two thirds of the way round my ancle was hollow. [Dr. Cole was sent for and] ordered sweet appletree bark to be boiled, and the wound to be washed with it, which caused great pain, and made it worse, so that in eight days . . . the flesh on my leg and thigh were mostly gone and my life was despaired of. . . . [The doctor] did not know what to do; I told him there was one thing I had thought of. . . . I told him that if he could find some comfrey root, I would try a plaster made of that and turpentine. . . . The success which attended this experiment, and the natural turn of my mind to those things, I think was a principal cause of my continuing to practice the healing art at this time.[5]

Thomson moved into medicine first by treating his family (saving both his wife and daughter who were not expected to live) and then helping out his neighbors. Ultimately he began "to be sent for by people of this part of the country so much" that he was neglecting his farm and family. For the cases attended, he "received very little or nothing, not enough to compensate me for my time; and I found it to be my duty to give up practice altogether, or to make a business of it." [6] The outcome was Thomsonianism or the botanic system.

Thomson "adopted the dogma of Ionian and Greek sages, that heat, the calorific force of excitive energy, is the substance of life, and . . . that this primordial principle of life may also be its renovator and the restorer of health." [7] Thomson concluded that "all disease is the effect of one general cause, and may be removed by one general remedy." The general cause was "cold, or lessening the power of heat"; the remedy, to "increase the internal heat, remove all obstructions of the system, restore the digestive powers of the stomach, and produce a natural perspiration." [8] He used only two treatment aids: the botanicals, to which he had become attached at an early age, and external "steaming," a procedure developed to save his daughter.

In 1813 Thomson patented his system, began to advertise in newspapers and handbills, and issued a little booklet giving each purchaser the right to follow the system. Ten years later he was forced to take out a second patent because so many people had infringed his original one. Thomsonianism spread rapidly, especially in the southern and midwestern states.

In 1822 Thomson published two books, *New Guide to Health, or Botanic Family Physician* and *A Narrative of the Life and Medical Discoveries of Samuel Thomson*. In 1832 a follower, Dr. Thomas Hershey, began publishing the *Thomsonian Recorder*. The same year a national convention of delegates from the Friendly Botanic Societies, which Thomson had organized, met in Columbus, Ohio. States began to recognize the legal right of Thomsonians to practice within their borders, and infirmaries made their appearance throughout the United States. The Botanico-Medical College of Ohio (in Cincinnati) was chartered in 1838; a year later the Southern Botanico-Medical College was organized.

Unfortunately Thomson was dictatorial, jealous of his rights as founder of the system, and, because of his own lack of education, distrustful of educated men and educational institutions. In 1838 these traits led to a split of the Friendly Botanic Societies into two groups that became bitter rivals. Thomson continued to head the United States Thomsonian Society while Alva Curtis (1797–1881) organized the Independent Thomsonian Botanic Society, a group that numbered Thomson's sons among its members. What might be called pure Thomsonianism did not long survive the schism. Curtis's independent group was quick to join up with the Reformed System, later the Eclectic School, originated by Wooster Beach (1794–1859).

The use of plant remedies advocated by Samuel Thomson has not gone entirely into oblivion. "Secret remedies" that "contain only vegetable compounds" are still being advertised and "health food" stores are common.

Samuel Thomson was not an outright quack. It should be recalled that he faced a decision—"to give up practice altogether or to make a business of it." If his businesslike approach seemed beyond bounds to the regular physicians of the day, he was not willy-nilly a charlatan. The regular physicians had allowed a gap to form between heroic measures and none at all. The relatively pleasant and undemanding remedies of Thomson and his fellow sectarians filled that gap—for the benefit of the public.

LIKE CURES LIKE

If Thomson's status was open to question, that of Samuel Christian Frederick Hahnemann (1755–1843), the founder of homeopathy, was not. Born in Meissen, Germany, he became a medical student at the University of Leipzig, studied in

Vienna under Joseph von Quarin, the emperor's physician, and received his doctor's degree at Erlangen in 1779. In the final decade of the eighteenth century Hahnemann undertook a series of experiments, some made on his own person, which led to the formation of his system of homeopathy (from the Greek *homoios,* meaning "like" and *pathos,* "disease").

Hahnemann based his theories on three propositions: first, that like cures like (*similia similibus curantur*), a revival of the "doctrine of signatures" introduced by Paracelsus (1493–1541); second, that the effectiveness of drugs is heightened by the administration of infinitesimal doses; third, that most chronic diseases are the manifestation of suppressed psora (the common itch).

Paracelsus' doctrine of signatures assumed that God created plants in a form suggesting that organ upon which they acted. The sometimes "fanciful associative resemblance" might suggest "trefoil for heart disease, thistle for a stitch in the side, walnut shells for head injuries, bear's grease for baldness, topaz, the yellow celandine or turmeric for jaundice, powdered mummy for prolonging life, . . ." [9] Hahnemann differed from Paracelsus, however, in that he directed his medications against symptoms of disease rather than causes. Drugs producing certain symptoms in healthy persons would cure disease exhibiting these symptoms. Scarlet fever was, for example, associated with a sore throat; Hahnemann employed belladonna as a specific because it caused dryness of the throat if administered to a healthy person.

Hahnemann's second proposition was based on a belief in a spiritual power locked up in plants that was liberated by dilution. This being so, the active effect would increase with the dilution and be greater the smaller the dose.

As for the itch doctrine, Hahnemann called it "psora with

a view to giving it a general designation" ; he did not "regard it as *synonymous* with, or limited in its meaning to, *the* itch." However, he was "persuaded that not only are *the majority of the innumerable skin diseases* . . . but also almost all the pseudo-organizations, &c., &c., with few exceptions, merely the products of the multiform psora." [10]

Homeopathy was introduced into America by Hans Burch Gram (1786–1840), originally of Copenhagen, who settled in New York in 1825. He was "a mystic, a Swedenborgian, a man of spotless character, deeply convinced of the truth of Hahnemann's doctrine." [11]

Homeopathy fell on fertile ground. Conditions in American medical practice were chaotic. Therapeutic standards were low. Within a few decades homeopathy spread throughout the United States. When the regular medical practitioners tried to exclude the homeopaths from their institutions, the latter went ahead and established their own. In 1833 a Hahnemann Society was founded in Philadelphia, and two years later a homeopathic pharmacy was opened. In 1835 Dr. Constantine Hering started a homeopathic medical school in Allentown, Pennsylvania. Instruction was in German, and the institution did not survive. The Homeopathic Medical College of Philadelphia, chartered in 1848, became the Hahnemann Medical College in 1869. The Homeopathic Hospital of Philadelphia opened in 1874.

In New York City it was not until 1860 that the Homeopathic Medical College of the State of New York was chartered —an abortive attempt had been made in 1849. The Hahnemann Medical College of Chicago was also organized in 1860. In 1902 there were twenty-two homeopathic schools in the United States; a quarter of a century later they had fallen off to two.

Modern pharmacologists point out that Hahnemann's early experiments on himself and his friends must have involved a degree of self-delusion. They have also demonstrated that the effect of a drug is diminished, not increased, by dilution. Psora cannot be regarded as the basis of most ills. Hahnemann nonetheless played an important role. He protested the heroic measures of Rush and his followers. He advocated the use of few medicines in contrast with the complex therapeutics typical of his day. He introduced the small dose.

THE PERFECT MACHINE

"Osteopathy," said the founder of the discipline, Andrew Taylor Still (1828–1917), on his eightieth birthday, "deals with the body as a perfect machine, which, if kept in proper adjustment, nourished and cared for, will run smoothly into ripe and useful old age." [12] It was his belief that disease was caused

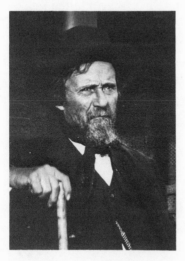

ANDREW TAYLOR STILL

by an abnormality someplace in the nerve divisions, with a resultant suspension, either temporary or permanent, of the blood either in the arteries or veins.

Still was born in Virginia. When he was six the family moved to Tennessee and, three years later, on to Missouri. It was here that he made his "first discovery in the science of Osteopathy":

> One day, when about ten years old, I suffered from a headache. I made a swing of my father's plow-line between two trees; but my head hurt too much to make swinging comfortable, so I let the rope down to about eight or ten inches of the ground and used the rope for a swinging pillow. Thus I lay stretched on my back, with my neck across the rope. Soon I became easy and went to sleep, got up in a little while with headache all gone. As I knew nothing of anatomy, I took no thought of how a rope could stop headache and the sick stomach which accompanied it. After that discovery I roped my neck whenever I felt these spells coming on. I followed that treatment for twenty years before the wedge of reason reached my brain, and I could see that I have suspended the action of the great occipital nerves, and given harmony to the flow of arterial blood to and through the veins, and ease was the effect.[13]

In 1844 the family moved to Kansas, where his father, a frontier physician and minister, had been appointed missionary to the Shawnee Indians. Here young Andrew was shocked not only by the extensiveness of disease (including such scourges, rarely encountered today, as cholera, smallpox, meningitis, and plague), but by the high mortality resulting from his father's lack of knowledge concerning the cause of disease and its treatment. Stimulated by frustration, Andrew determined to serve his fellow men with more efficient care than they were receiving.

Still's medical education, typical of the time, was largely by preceptorship. He did start on a course at the College of Physicians and Surgeons at Kansas City, only to have it interrupted by the Civil War. He enlisted at Fort Leavenworth in September 1861; he served with distinction and attained the rank of major. This experience seems to have amused him (at least in retrospect) for he wrote in his autobiography:

> During the hottest period of the fight a musket-ball passed through the lapels of my vest, carrying away a pair of gloves I had stuck in the bosom of it. Another minie-ball passed through the back of my coat just above the buttons, making an entry and exit about six inches apart. Had the rebels known how close they were shooting at Osteopathy, perhaps they would not have been so careless.

Back in the quiet of the frontier, surrounded by nature, he studied anatomy with more zest than he had at college. Recognizing that the greatest study of man is man, he pored over the skeleton until he was familiar with every bone in the human body. Then Indian after Indian was exhumed and dissected. At last he declared himself quite familiar with the bone structure. At the same time Still was not only farming but inventing aids to the "feeble right arm of man." His interest in machinery had developed as early as 1855. Nineteen years later he reached the conclusion that, while God had made the human body perfect and complete, it was subject to mechanical disorder.

Baldwin and Baker University at Baldwin, Kansas, had been founded in part through the generosity of Still's father and brothers. It seemed the proper place to introduce his new-found knowledge to the medical world. The university, however, declined to open its doors to him. Undaunted, he returned to Missouri to apply his ideas in medical practice.

During the winter of 1878–79 he was called to treat a patient whom he had doctored before. "I treated partly by drugs, as in other days, but also gave Osteopathic treatments. She got well." Thereafter he developed a large following and began to eliminate drugs from his practice.

There was a case of erysipelas that drugs had failed to cure. "I made a thorough examination of the great system of facial arteries and veins, treated her strictly by the teachings of Osteopathy, and she was well in thirty-six hours."

Four doctors had used four ounces of chloroform on a patient with a dislocated elbow and failed to reduce the bones. "I set it in about ten minutes without chloroform, and no machinery save my hands."

Still moved from disease entity to disease entity. "As nearly as I can remember," he wrote, "I had seventeen cases of flux [excessive drainage from the bowels] in a few days and cured all without drugs."

The American School of Osteopathy was established in Kirksville, Missouri, in 1892. By the turn of the century there were a dozen osteopathic schools spread across the country. In 1896 Vermont led the states in licensing osteopathic physicians. The American Association for the Advancement of Osteopathy (now the American Osteopathic Association) was founded in 1897.

There is a general impression that, in the course of the years, osteopathy has departed from Dr. Still's original precepts. Osteopathic physicians employ drugs to a marked degree and engage in surgical operations. The four-year curriculum of their medical schools closely parallels that of regular medical schools, with the addition of manipulative therapy. "At no time did Dr. Still believe that his word was the final one. At no time did he attempt to establish restrictive scientific dogma. . . . Dr. Still did not seek to destroy medicine. He sought to *contribute to it.* He was trained in and practiced the methodologies of the day. They were the best that were known, and he was *not* satisfied. . . . Still organized the first osteopathic college in order to 'improve' or, if you will, reform medicine on a basic biologic foundation." [14]

In the 1960s a movement to erase the difference between doctors of medicine and doctors of osteopathy got under way. In California a D.O. was automatically converted into an M.D. In the eastern United States osteopathic physicians generally held out against merger. Not only were they proud of their heritage, but they were afraid that in such a merger the prime objective of their philosophy of medicine—keeping the perfect machine in proper adjustment—might be eclipsed.

ᴄᴫᴐ

The distinguishing mark of the sectarians was a basic belief in the gospel of one cause, one cure. However, by the time of Thomson and his followers, Hahnemann and the homeopaths, and Still and the osteopaths, medical science was advancing to the point where things seemed too complex for single, simple solutions. Regular medicine tried to consign the sectarians to outer darkness, but the sects retained their appeal. They, after all, preached simple doctrines "within the comprehension of every one not born an idiot." [15]

§(12)§

Reforms in Medical Practice and Education

THE MEDICAL SOCIETIES

The first "medical society" of which a record survives was sponsored in 1735 by Dr. William Douglass (1692–1725), the only doctor in Boston possessing an M.D. degree. On February 18, 1736, Douglass wrote to Cadwalader Colden of New York: "We have lately in Boston formed a medical society. . . . We design from time to time to publish some short pieces; there is now ready for the press number one [of *Medical Memoirs*]. . . ." [1] This volume never reached the press; nor did the society survive. The last known contemporary reference dates from 1744.

A dubious claim to the honor of founding the country's second "medical society" goes to a group of physicians who, in 1739, met in New Haven, Connecticut, elected a chairman, remained in session for two days, and then, unable to agree on a program, adjourned *sine die*. Claims to second place have been made on behalf of Benjamin Franklin's American Philosophical Society and of New York's Weekly Society of Gentlemen. One of Franklin's reasons for sponsoring his society was to discuss the new methods of curing and preventing diseases. He intended that a physician be included in the membership and, when the society was formed a year later, Dr. Thomas Bond was indeed a member, but in this form the society existed only a year and could hardly be rated a medical society. The claim of the New York Gentlemen seems to have been based on the fact that in 1749 Dr. John Bard delivered a medical essay at one of its meetings.

In 1755 the "Faculty of Physic" in Charleston, South Carolina, under the leadership of John Moultrie (1729–1798), formed a society primarily concerned with the "better support of the Dignity, the Privileges, and Emoluments of their Humane Art." The emphasis on fees raised a furor in the press that the society did not survive.[2]

In 1763 Connecticut physicians attempted to organize societies in Norwich and New London. Another effort was sponsored by Dr. Cotton Tufts (1731–1815) in rural Weymouth, Massachusetts. He invited a number of physicians to meet with him at "Gardners Tavern on Boston Neck at the hour of two p.m. precisely on the third Monday in March, 1765," to consider regulations for a society that he had drawn up. The meeting took place and another was set for three months later, but it is doubtful "that the out-of-Boston physicians who associated themselves with this venture ever carried the organization beyond this introductory stage."[3]

In 1766 Dr. John Morgan organized the Philadelphia

Medical Society, which would three years later, through mergers, become a part of the American Philosophical Society.

The "early attempts to form medical societies, although almost inevitably abortive, intimate the motives that gave rise to them and that were to become increasingly strong as the colonies continued to grow. Although before the middle of the eighteenth century there was in each of the important colonial centers a nucleus of European-trained physicians, the early pioneer standards of medical practice necessarily continued to flourish—and more menacingly as populations increased out of proportion to the number of ethical, well-trained physicians. . . . In 1753, it was being said of the medical situation in New York: 'That place boasts the honor of above forty gentlemen of the faculty, and far the greater part of them are mere pretenders to a profession of which they are entirely ignorant.' In the absence of effective laws regulating the practice of medicine, . . . the medical society afforded the reputable physicians their only means of professional communication, their only hope of controlling the forces working against their professional interests." [4]

The New Jersey Medical Society (subsequently the Medical Society of New Jersey) was the earliest attempt "to establish a provincewide organization of the profession to form a program embracing all the matters then of highest concern to the profession: regulation of practice; educational standards for apprentices; fee schedules; and a code of ethics. Although its meetings were suspended during the Revolution, and its postwar course was bedeviled for some years by a rebellious member's organization of a rival society, the Medical Society of New Jersey survived all obstacles and remains the oldest medical society in the United States." [5] It came into being at a meeting at Duff's Tavern in New Brunswick on Wednesday, July 23, 1766. "Every gentleman of the profession of the province" was invited to the meeting but only sixteen appeared. These charter members adopted an "instrument of association" and elected Robert McKean of Perth Amboy their first president.[6]

One of the first efforts of the society was to establish a fee scale. Disputes over bills caused so much friction between doctors and patients that colonial legislatures had provided what they considered fair codes of charges. By the 1760s, however, practitioners were prepared to regulate themselves. The scale drawn up by the New Jersey society was typical of those subsequently put into effect by other societies.

At this time medical education was almost entirely in the hands of preceptors. In 1767 the New Jersey society ruled that no "student be taken as apprentice unless he has competent knowledge of Latin and some initiation in Greek. No member shall take an apprentice for less than four years, the fee to be one hundred pounds a year." [7]

The first law providing for the examination of prospective practitioners was passed in New York City in 1760. The New Jersey society, rounding out its program, persuaded the provincial legislature in 1772 to pass a comprehensive provincial licensing law, under which no person might practice as a physician or surgeon in New Jersey until he had been examined, approved, and given a testimonial by two judges of the supreme court of the colony (with such professional advice as they might deem desirable). Anyone practicing without a testimonial would be fined five pounds for each offense, one half of which would go to the informer. The law stipulated that all

197

medical bills were to be written out in English, and that any-one staging a show for the sale of drugs or medicines of any kind would be fined twenty pounds for each appearance.

Other state legislatures began to promulgate similar regulations for examining and licensing practitioners. By the beginning of the nineteenth century the establishment of standards and the certification of doctors was firmly in the hands of the societies. It was an easy step for the leaders in such societies to conclude that they were qualified to conduct training schools for physicians.

On March 12, 1807, a medical school to be operated by the Medical Society of the County of New York was chartered; on December 18 the College of Medicine of Maryland was incorporated under the auspices of the state medical society. Previously medical schools had been established as separate departments of existing colleges or universities, a relationship that tended to raise the standards of the medical degree conferred. Now society-affiliated institutions, called "proprietary" medical colleges, sprang up everywhere. An increase in the supply of doctors was urgent, but the products of these schools proved no answer. The elimination of two features standard in the programs of university-affiliated medical departments—a long general education and a long lecture term—attracted many students, but the schools failed to train them adequately.

A few doctors, aware that something must be done, attempted in 1835 and 1839 to call a meeting of representatives of the profession and the medical schools to create a national organization, but these efforts failed. Conditions grew steadily worse.

In 1845 the Medical Society of the State of New York was faced with a demand for a national convention to correct abuses in medical education, presented by Nathan Smith Davis (1817–1904) of Broome County and Alexander Thompson (1809–1869) of Cayuga County. Among the corrections they contemplated were a longer annual course of instruction (six months instead of four), sequence and grading in the curriculum, separation of the licensing power from the teaching function, and a fair standard of preliminary education.

On February 6, 1845, after considerable procrastination, the society passed a resolution introduced by Dr. Davis that earnestly recommended that "delegates from medical societies and colleges in the whole Union . . . convene in the city of New York, on the first Tuesday in May, in the year 1846, for the purpose of [taking] some concerted action." [8] When, thanks to the efforts of Dr. Davis, the national convention met at the time and place stated there were almost a hundred delegates representing sixteen states.

The program presented to the convention proposed the creation of a national medical association, the adoption of uniform, higher requirements for an M.D. degree by all medical schools, suitable preliminary education for prospective medical students, and a standard code of ethics to be maintained by the medical profession throughout the United States.

The convention reassembled at Philadelphia on May 5, 1847, with nearly two hundred delegates representing over forty medical societies and twenty-eight colleges in twenty-two states and the District of Columbia. The convention's first order of business was to resolve itself into the first session of the American Medical Association.

On the question of higher educational standards, it was decided that premedical training should include what amounted to a liberal education in the arts and sciences; that medical-college entrance should require a certificate of completion of training from the student's preceptor; and that the M.D. degree should entail three years of study, including two lecture sessions of six months each, three months devoted to dissection, and at least one session of hospital attendance.

The committee on the licensing of physicians reiterated the abuse-potential of schools that were both teaching agency and licensing authority and proposed that examining and licensing boards be established on a statewide basis. The matter was referred to the Committee on Medical Education for report at the next meeting of the association.

Under its constitution, the purpose of the association was declared to be

> for cultivating and advancing medical knowledge, for elevating the standards of medical education, for promoting the usefulness, honour, and interests of the Medical Profession; for enlightening and directing public opinion in regard to the duties, responsibilities and requirements of medical men, for exciting and encouraging emulation and concert of action in the profession, and facilitating and fostering friendly intercourse between those engaged in it.[9]

Nathaniel Chapman (1780–1853) was elected the first president of the American Medical Association. His exceptional qualifications included graduation from the medical department of the University of Pennsylvania followed by three years' study abroad, mostly in Edinburgh; practice in Philadelphia beginning in 1804; professor of materia medica at the University of Pennsylvania from 1813 to 1816, when he moved up to professor of the theory and practice of medicine, a chair he graced until 1850; original editor of the *Philadelphia Journal of Medical and Physical Sciences* (first published in 1820 by Mathew Carey), which in 1828 became *The American Journal of the Medical Sciences.*

While the 1847 meeting firmly established the American Medical Association, progress was slow. There was no legal authority by which its recommendations, resolutions, and proposed reforms could be enforced, and the proprietary schools were resistant.

In 1852 it was ruled that no medical school might send delegates to association meetings unless it had a faculty of six and gave a sixteen-week course of instruction annually on anatomy, materia medica, medicine, surgery, midwifery, and chemistry. Candidates for graduation were required to be twenty-one, to have studied three full years—two under an acceptable practitioner—and to have attended full courses of lectures in two different years—one at least at the institution granting the diploma. Under examination candidates had to show qualification for practice.

In 1873 a Judicial Council was created to rule on all matters ethical and judicial.

The association has grown into a formidable institution that exerts great power on matters medical. It "has never lowered its standards or forsaken its code of ethics." [10]

ADVANCES IN MEDICAL EDUCATION

Medical schools proliferated in the nineteenth century. Between 1802 and 1876 sixty-two regular medical schools (plus eleven homeopathic and four eclectic schools) came into reasonably stable existence. Many others started up, only to collapse in the matter of a few weeks, months, or years.

The advance was, of course, progressive. This is well illustrated by medical-school attendance and number of graduates at various times in the century: 650 students and 100 graduates in 1810; 2500 and 800 in 1840; 5000 and 1700 in 1860; 6500 and 2000 in 1870; 12,000 and 3200 in 1880; 16,500 and 5000 in 1890; and 25,000 and 5200 in 1900.[11]

Although the numbers of students and graduates showed a steady growth the total picture was not as bright as it might seem. Most of these students and graduates were both white and male.

Blacks had little opportunity even to apply for medical school and almost no chance of being accepted. One of the early outstanding black medical graduates, Daniel Hale Williams (1856–1931), was born in Holidaysburg, Pennsylvania. After overcoming many difficulties he obtained his M.D. degree from the Chicago Medical College of Northwestern University in 1883. Dr. Williams began practice in Chicago and was later instrumental in founding Provident Hospital, which is still serving the city's South Side.

On July 10, 1893, a young man was brought into Provident near death from a stab wound in the chest. Dr. Williams had sufficient knowledge and courage to open the man's chest, but he was then presented with an inch-and-a-quarter wound in the pericardium, the membrane that covers the heart. Though surgeons of the day considered the heart off limits, Dr. Williams sewed up the vibrating wound, and the young man eventually recovered completely. Before Dr. Williams' death he had raised the major hospital for members of his race, Freedmen's Hospital in Washington, D.C., out of the depths, and vastly improved the possibilities for medical care and medical education for his people.[12]

Women were in only a slightly better situation. The first woman to obtain the M.D. degree in the United States was Elizabeth Blackwell (1821–1910), who graduated from the Geneva College of Medicine in upstate New York in 1849. Her admittance to the school had been accidental, and it took many years of hard work by Dr. Blackwell, her sister Emily, and many others (men as well as women), before women had any real opportunity of obtaining a medical education.[13]

THE FLEXNER REPORT

In November 1908 the trustees of the Carnegie Foundation for the Advancement of Teaching authorized a study designed "to ascertain the facts concerning medical education and the medical schools themselves at the present time." [14] The assignment fell to Abraham Flexner (1866–1959), an em-

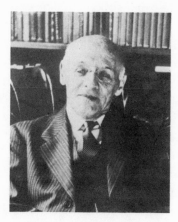

ABRAHAM FLEXNER

inent surveyor in the field of education. Flexner's report threw a brilliant light on the appalling conditions in many of the schools; but it was "more than a merciless piece of criticism; it offered a number of creative suggestions." [15] It had "not only a large influence upon the professional opinion, but especially a large influence on universities and upon public opinion." [16] Certainly the publicity arising out of discussion of the report in the news media "largely closed the gap between private knowledge of departures from accepted standards and public acceptance of those standards." [17]

Some reforms in medical education had already been started, as we have seen. Nathan Smith Davis in 1859 went to Chicago to found the medical department of Lind University, where he initiated the program that he had recommended to the New York State Medical Society. (This became the Chicago Medical College in 1864 and joined Northwestern in 1869.) The new institution "was organized for the express purpose of testing the practicability . . . of a thoroughly graded and consecutive system of instruction." The subjects in the curriculum divided into junior and senior groups, and new matriculates were required to follow this graded plan.[18]

Since 1858 the faculty of Harvard Medical School had *advised* students "to divide their studies into three groups in successive sessions." Charles Eliot, when he became president of Harvard in 1869, was ready to make the graded curriculum requisite. He invited the medical departments of Columbia and Pennsylvania to join with him. They declined. Members of the faculty of the Harvard Medical School were divided on the question. In his 1870 annual report President Eliot stated: "The course of professional instruction should be a progressive one covering three years." In 1871 a graded curriculum of three sessions was put into effect.[19] In 1901 the Harvard Medical School adopted an academic degree as a requirement of admission.

In 1869 the first university hospital, at the University of Michigan, was opened—an important element in turning out capable physicians. Laboratory instruction was introduced in 1878 by Dr. Francis Delafield (1841–1915) at the College of Physicians of New York, and by William H. Welch (1850–1934), who opened the pathological laboratory at Bellevue Hospital Medical College.

While the reform movement was gaining strength during the last half of the nineteenth century, it was as yet too feeble and disorganized to halt the multiplication of medical schools. There were disgraceful conditions in many schools, and unsatisfactory standards in all but a few.

The Association of American Medical Colleges, which had been formed in 1876, was totally inactive from 1883 through 1889, and when it resumed operation in 1890, having "learned by sad experience that attempting to raise educational standards rapidly resulted only in disagreement and loss of unity between the member colleges, the Association's moves toward higher standards were this time more carefully considered." [20]

Flexner's solution was to "reduce the number and increase the output of medical schools." Ideally, he wrote, "a medical school is . . . a university department; it is most favorably located in a large city, where the problem of procuring clinical material, at once abundant and various, practically solves itself. Hence those universities that have been located in cities can most advantageously develop medical schools." The problems of universities not so placed were not insurmountable, but Flexner did not approve of the establishment of remote medical departments as a solution. "As we need many universities and but few medical schools, a long-distance connection is justified only where there is no local university qualified to assume responsibility." Since "students tend to study medicine in their own states certainly in their own sections . . . arrangements ought to be made . . . to provide the requisite facilities within each of the characteristic state groups." [21]

Flexner was severely critical of the way medical schools had been "established regardless of need, regardless of the proximity of competent universities, regardless of favoring local conditions. An expression of surprise at finding an irrelevant and superfluous school usually elicits the reply that the town, being a 'gateway' or a 'center,' must of course harbor a 'medical college.' It is not always easy to distinguish 'gateway' or 'center': a center appears to be a town possessing, or within easy reach of, say 50,000 persons; a gateway is a town with at least two railway stations. The same place may be both—in which event the argument is presumably irrefragable. . . . The argument, so dear to local pride, can best be refuted by being pursued to its logical conclusion. For there are still forty-eight towns in the United States with over 50,000 population each, and no medical schools: we are threatened with forty-eight new schools at once, if the contention is correct. The truth is that the fundamental though of course not sole consideration is the university, provided its resources are adequate; and we have fortunately enough strong universities, properly distributed, to satisfy every present need without serious sacrifice of sound principle." [22]

THE IDEAL MEDICAL SCHOOL

Evident in Flexner's report was the influence of the Johns Hopkins Medical School. He wrote in his autobiography:

> Having finished my preliminary reading, I went to Baltimore—how fortunate for me that I was a Hopkins graduate—where I talked at length with . . . [those] who knew what a medical school ought to be for they had created one. . . . I became thus intimately acquainted with a small but ideal medical school, embodying in a novel way, adapted to American conditions, the best features of medical education in England, France and Germany.[23]

The Johns Hopkins University had been made possible by a legacy from Johns Hopkins, a Baltimore merchant. The establishment of a hospital for the poor of Baltimore and of a medical school as part of the university was stipulated in the bequest. The university opened in 1876, the hospital in 1889, and the medical school in 1893.

The first president of the university was Daniel Coit Gilman (1831–1908). "In the whole history of education" there has been no "other institution whose influence was so far-reaching and revolutionary." Its medical school was the first "in America of genuine university type, with something approaching adequate endowment, well-equipped laboratories conducted by modern teachers, devoting themselves unreservedly to medical investigation and instruction, and with its own hospital in which the training of physicians and the healing of the sick harmoniously combine to the infinite advantage of both. . . . It has finally cleared up the problem of standards and ideals; and its graduates have gone forth in small bands to found new establishments or to reconstruct old ones." [24]

Johns Hopkins University was different from the start—a research center on the European model where faculty and students could unite in the investigation of scientific problems. The hospital and the medical school, when they were opened, were also research-oriented. Sir William Osler was physician-in-chief, William H. Welch was in charge of pathology, William S. Halsted of surgery, and Howard A. Kelly of gynecology. These men stressed actual work in the wards, clinics, dispensaries, laboratories, and dead-house as the foundations of the curriculum. "They were splendid times, those first years at the Johns Hopkins. Everything was new—there was no shackling tradition. Everyone was young, and filled with an enthusiasm for his enterprise which carried all before it." [25]

The Johns Hopkins Medical School was a positive step toward the reorganization of medical education. It provided a model for university-affiliated medical schools and, at the same time, drove out of business a number of "commercial" medical schools that could not afford the laboratories, dissection rooms, clinics, and hospitals that were now obviously indispensable to practical instruction; nor could they provide the opportunity to study allied sciences.

"By 1930 nearly all medical schools required an arts degree for admission and provided a three- or four-year graded curriculum, improved hospital facilities and clinical instruction. In addition, boards [of examiners] in some thirty states insisted—in cooperation with the American Hospital Association (founded in 1898)—that candidates take a year's internship as well as a recognized degree. . . . As a result of these trends the ratings of medical schools rose rapidly. . . ." [26]

As Professor Welch has said:

> It is obviously impossible to impart the entire contents of medical and surgical science to the student. You cannot even impart the contents of any single subject in the curriculum. The most you can expect is to give to the student a fair knowledge of the principles of the fundamental subjects in medicine, and the power to use the instruments and the methods of his profession; the right attitude toward his patients and toward his fellow-members in the profession; above all, to put him in the position to carry on his education, because his education is only begun in the medical school.[27]

Undoubtedly there has been improvement in the selection and education of medical students and in the end product, but the end product can only be as good as the potential of the raw material, the quality of the teachers developing it, and the scientific curiosity of the fledgling doctor.

Part IV

THE PROBLEMS OF
PUBLIC HEALTH

§(13)§

The Smallpox Epidemics

The origins of smallpox, a deadly and terrifying disease that has plagued most of the world for centuries, are lost in the mists of time. By the beginning of the eighteenth century epidemics of smallpox were common in major British cities. Physicians were rarely called in because the infection was considered a children's disease, comparable to teething and worms. Many children died but relatively few adults, because most adults had survived childhood exposure and developed immunity.

It was another matter in the colonies, where outbreaks of smallpox were spasmodic. Few achieved immunity. When an epidemic did strike, adult cases were common, which "led to the popular colonial misconception that smallpox was peculiarly fatal to Americans. In actuality the death rate in the colony was, if anything, slightly lower than that in England. Because of its irregular appearance in the colonies, the disorder was far more dreaded than in England: even the rumor of a smallpox epidemic caused consternation among the colonists. In London, where the annual number of deaths from smallpox rarely was under a thousand, the disease was a familiar evil." [1] Bad as smallpox seemed among the American whites, it was worse for the Indians. It was not unusual for from half to almost a complete tribe to be wiped out during an epidemic.

While Samuel Fuller has been credited with serving the colonists during a smallpox epidemic in 1621, smallpox probably did not reach America until 1630, when it was brought in by the considerable number of settlers led to New England by John Winthrop. Thomas Hutchinson, an eighteenth-century historian and the last royal governor before the Revolutionary War, placed the first major epidemic in 1633, "when the small pox made terrible havoc among the Indians of Massachusetts [who] were destitute of every thing proper for comfort and relief, and died in greater proportion than is known among the English. However, John Sagamore of Winesimet, and James of Lynn, with almost all their people, died of the distemper." [2] This epidemic was responsible for the deaths of Samuel Fuller and about twenty other residents of Plymouth.

There were limited outbreaks of smallpox in 1638 and 1639. A general epidemic in 1648–49, while largely sparing Boston, hit outlying communities quite severely. Almost twenty years elapsed before the major epidemic of 1666, which resulted in forty or fifty deaths in Boston.

In the Dutch colony of New Netherlands "a most malignant epidemic of smallpox, which was of a virulent character, spread . . . with great rapidity" in 1633. [3]

The first recorded epidemic in Virginia occurred in 1667. When a sailor with smallpox landed at Accomack, he was placed in isolation but escaped to an Indian town and infected two tribes. The health officer promptly instructed all families affected with smallpox to allow no member "to go forth their doors until their full cleansing, that is to say, thirtie dayes after their receiving the sd smallpox, least the sd disease shoulde spread by infection." [4] Smallpox was prevalent in Jamestown in 1696.

In 1675, when a few cases appeared in New England, Increase Mather wrote: "The Ld. hath lifted up his hand agt. Boston in yt ye smallpox hath bin in ye harbor." [5] Two years later the disease struck Boston with full force. Brought by British ships to Charlestown in the summer of 1677, the epidemic took 500 to 700 lives in eighteen months. Across the river in Boston a peak was reached in September 1678 when thirty individuals died in one day and 150 in a four-week period. It was during this epidemic that Thomas Thacher produced his broadside, *The Brief Rule.*

THE BRIEF RULE

The first accurate description of smallpox was written in Arabic by a Persian medical authority, Abu-Bakr Muhammad ibn-Zakarīyā al Rāzi, or Rhazes (850–923). Thacher may have had a translation of this work on hand, and much in Rhazes' clear account found its way into the *Brief Rule,* but it was "more likely that recourse was to the account in *Observationes Medicae* by Thomas Sydenham (1624–1689), published in 1676." [6]

The *Brief Rule* begins: "The *small Pox* (whose nature and cure the Measels follow) is a disease of the blood, endeavouring to recover a new form and state." Then, in twenty-nine numbered paragraphs, Thacher describes how the disease manifests itself and why and how it runs its course. Progress, he says, may be retarded by ill-advised therapy that interferes with the natural progress of the disease, and he advises against "too much Clothes, too hot a room, hot *Cordials . . . bloodletting, Clysters, Vomits, purges, or cooling medicines. . . .*"

A proper diet, he continues, will include "small Beer only warm'd with a Tost . . . thin *water-gruel,* or *water pottage* made only of Indian Flour and water, instead of *Oat-meal* [and] *boild App'es.*" He enumerates "Signs discovering the Assault at first," "Signs warning of the probable Event," "signs [that] are hopeful," "signs [that] are doubtful," and finally "Deadly Signs."

He concludes:

> *These things have I written* Candid Reader, *not to inform the Learned* Physician *that hath much more cause to understand what pertains to this disease than I, but to give some light to those that have not such advantages, leaving the difficulty of this disease to the* Physitians *Art, Wisdome, and Faithfulness: for the right managing of them in the whole Course of the disease tends both to the* Patients *safety, and the* Physitians *desired Success in his Administration: For in vain is the* Physitians *Art imployed if they are not under a* Regular Regiment. *I am, though no* Physician, *yet a well wisher to the sick: And therefore intreating the Lord to turn our hearts, and stay his hand, I am* A Friend, Reader to thy Welfare, *Thomas Thacher.*[7]

In Massachusetts the next major epidemic broke out in October 1689 and continued through the following summer. Smallpox appeared in Portsmouth and Greenland, New Hampshire, but seems then to have run its course, for the following February 23 the colonists held a thanksgiving.

An outbreak in New York City in 1689 led to the issuance on October 16 of this proclamation:

> William Lynes Master of ye ship Anne & Catherine arriving here from Nevis with a parcell of negroes whereof some have ye small pocks Ordered that all which are sound in Body may be landed cleaning themselves sufficiently & those which are sick to be Landed a Mile or thereabouts from the City & to Permit none to come to them but ye doctors Chirurgeons & attenders.[8]

New York was hit again early in 1702, and Boston in the summer. In December, Cotton Mather, three of whose children were brought down by the infection, wrote in his diary: "More than four-score people were in this Black Month of *December,* carried from this Town to their long Home." [9]

THE BEGINNINGS OF INOCULATION

It had long been known that certain diseases, including smallpox, occur only once during the lifetime of an individual, and that the deliberate introduction of a mild form of the disease by inoculation might prevent a severe attack.

According to Dhanwantari, the earliest known Hindu physician (fl. c. 1500 B.C.), inoculation involved taking "the fluid of the pock on the udder of the cow or on the arm between the shoulder and elbow of a human subject on the point of a lancet, and lance with it the arms between the shoulders and elbows until the blood appears. Then, mixing this fluid with the blood, the fever of the smallpox will be produced." [10]

Smallpox inoculation is considered to have been introduced into Europe from Asia and Africa by way of Turkey and Greece. In 1715, in "An Essay on External Remedies," Peter Kennedy (fl. 1710) wrote of a method

> of giving or ingrafting the Small Pox practised in the *Peloponnesus* (now called the *Morea*), and, at the present time, is very much used both in *Turkey* and *Persia,* where they give it in order to prevent its more dismal effects by the early knowledge of its coming, as also probably to prevent their being troubled with it a second time. This method of the *Persians* is to use the *Pock* and matter dried into powder, the which they take inwardly; but the common way now used in *Turkey,* and more particularly at *Constantinople,* is thus: they first take a *fresh and kindly Pock* from some one ill of this distemper, and having made *scarifications* upon the forehead, wrists, and legs, or extremities, the matter of the Pock is laid upon the foresaid incision, being bound on there for eight to ten days together; at the end of which time the usual symptoms begin to appear, and the distemper comes forward as if naturally taken ill, though in a more kindly manner and not near the number of *Pox.*[11]

In the early eighteenth century two Italian physicians practicing in Constantinople, Emanuel Timoni (fl. 1714) and Giacomo Pylarini (1659–1718), noted the local use of inoculation and recommended it. The *Philosophical Transactions of the Royal Society* for 1714–16 carried two separate accounts of the Turkish procedure by the Italian physicians.[12] Cotton Mather must have heard about inoculation before he read the Timoni-Pylarini contributions to the *Transactions,* for on July 12, 1716, he wrote to Dr. Woodward of the Royal Society:

> Enquiring of my Negro-man *Onesimus,* who is a pretty Intelligent Fellow, Whether he had ever had y^e *Small-Pox;* he answered, both *Yes,* and *No;* and then told me, that he had undergone an Operation, which had given him something of y^e *Small-Pox,* & would forever praeserve him from it; adding, That it was often used among y^e *Guramantese* [an African tribe], & whoever had ye Courage to use it, was forever free from ye fear of the Contagion. He described ye Operation to me, and shew'd me in his Arm ye Scar, which it had left upon him; and his Description of it, made it the same, that afterwards I found related unto you by your *Timonius.* . . .
>
> [Why is] no more . . . done to bring this operation, into experiment & into Fashion in *England?* . . . For my own part, if I should live to see y^e *Small-Pox* again enter o^r City, I would immediately procure a Consult of o^r Physicians, to Introduce a Practice, which may be of so very happy a Tendency.[13]

In April 1721 Boston was invaded for the sixth time by smallpox. On June 6 Mather circulated a letter, most of which subsequently appeared in Boston newspapers, addressed to the physicians of Boston. It contained abstracts of the Timoni-Pylarini articles and concluded with a request that the physicians "consider this new and yet untried method for the prevention of smallpox, and if they thought it wise to employ inoculation, he begged them to do so." [14]

Led by Dr. William Douglass, the physicians were almost unanimous in rejecting Cotton Mather's proposal. Douglass argued that deliberately infecting people with smallpox could only result in more deaths, and the more people infected with smallpox the more the dread disease would spread. In face of contemporary knowledge these objections had a certain validity.

Douglass persuaded Lawrence Dal 'Honde, a Boston physician who had formerly been in the French army, to make a deposition showing the uselessness of inoculation. The latter stated that about twenty-five years earlier he was

> at Cremona, in Italy, . . . where . . . thirteen soldiers [were inoculated, of whom] four died; six recovered with abundance of trouble and care. . . . On the other three, the operation had no effect.
>   . . . At the battle of Almanza in Spain, the smallpox being in the army, two Muscovite soldiers had the operation performed upon them; one recovered, but the other received no impression, but six weeks thereafter was seized with a frenzy, and swelled all over his body. They, not calling to mind that the operation had been performed on him, believed that he had been poisoned.[15]

The deposition, made on July 22, 1721, came too late to prevent the introduction of inoculation into Boston.

ZABDIEL BOYLSTON

Zabdiel Boylston's grandfather, Thomas Boylston, had come to the colony at the age of twenty. He settled at Watertown, Massachusetts, in 1635. His son, also Thomas (1645–1695), was the earliest physician and surgeon in Muddy River, a part of Boston that became the town of Brookline in 1705. Of the twelve children born to Thomas's wife, Mary Gardner of Muddy River, the sixth was Zabdiel (1679–1766).

Zabdiel received his medical education from his father and Dr. John Cutler, a prominent Boston physician. He quickly built a fine practice in Boston and gained some reputation, but he attracted no special attention until 1721.

Boylston was an early believer in enlightenment of the public. Early in 1721, "aided and abetted by the Reverend Cotton Mather, [he] introduced public education of the layman on medical affairs, thus laying the foundation for all the Sunday afternoon public lectures and the popular books on health and hygiene that were to come later." [16]

On June 24, 1721, Mather wrote to Boylston:

> . . . I design it, as a testimony of my respect and esteem, that I now lay before you, the most that I know (and all that was ever published in the world) concerning a matter, which I have been an occasion of its being pretty much talked about. If upon mature deliberation, you should think it advisable to be proceeded in, it may save many lives that we set a great value on. But, if it be not approved of, still you have the pleasure of knowing exactly what is done in other places.

He then described the process of inoculation and concluded: "But see, think, judge; do as the Lord our healer shall direct you, and pardon the freedom of, Sir, Your hearty friend and Servant. . . ." [17]

Boylston was not lacking in courage, an attribute attested to by William Douglass. He was intelligent, experienced, and skillful, and was being encouraged to act by Cotton Mather, an influential citizen of the town. He recognized that, because of his calling, his household was more than ordinarily exposed to contagion. "Mature deliberation" did not take long. On June 26 he inoculated his six-year-old son Thomas and two of his Negro slaves—Jack, aged thirty-six, and Jacky, two and a half. He would doubtless have selected himself as a subject but he was presumably already immune, having survived an attack in 1702.

His action was not without risk. Thomas Hutchinson wrote:

> Inoculation was introduced on this occasion contrary to the minds of the inhabitants in general, and not without hazard, to the lives of those who promoted it, from the rage of the people. . . . [T]he vulgar were raised to that degree that his family was hardly safe in his house and he often met with affronts and insults in the streets. . . . Many sober, pious people were struck with horror, and were of opinion that if any of his patients should die, he ought to be treated as a murderer.[18]

This attitude on the part of the people is confirmed by entries in Cotton Mather's diary for July 16 and 18:

. . . I have instructed one physician in the New Method used by the *Africans* and *Asiatics,* to prevent and abate the Dangers of *Small-Pox,* and infallibly to save the Lives of those that have it wisely managed upon them. The Destroyer, being enraged at the proposal of any Thing, that may rescue the Lives of our poor People from him, has taken a strange Possession of the People on this Occasion. They rave, rail, they blaspheme; they talk not only like *Ideots* but also like *Frantics.* And not only the Physician who began the Experiment but I also am an Object of their Fury; their furious Obloquies and Invectives.

. . . The cursed Clamour of the People strangely and fiercely possessed by the Devil, will probably prevent my saving the lives of my Two Children, from the Smallpox in the way of Transplantation.[19]

Boylston's original inoculations having proved successful, on July 12 he inoculated Joshua Cheever; on the 14th he treated John Heyler and another Negro; on the 17th his thirteen-year-old son John; and on the 19th three more people.

Boylston essentially followed the method outlined by Timoni in the *Philosophical Transactions.* He obtained his viruses from the pustules of a person with a mild case of smallpox (inoculated or natural) who was otherwise healthy. Taken on the ninth to fourteenth day after eruption, the infected matter was stored in a closely sealed vial. Unlike the Turks, who made scratches on the skin, Boylston made two incisions with a lancet, either on the outside of the arm above the elbow or on the inside of the leg. Pus was inserted into the incisions, which were then covered with a simple dressing. Subsequent treatment was largely symptomatic.

On July 21 Boylston invited his fellow physicians to examine the seven inoculated patients under his care. Only one, a Dr. White, accepted.

A few days later the selectmen and several justices of the peace met with members of the medical profession. The doctors accepted Dal 'Honde's statement that inoculation had produced horrible consequences in Italy and Spain. They reached the conclusion that inoculation "has proved the Death of many Persons [and] Tends to spread and continue the Infection." Thus fortified, the selectmen and justices "severely reprimanded [Boylston] for spreading the Small-Pox; . . . and with high Menaces warned him against proceeding with his practice any farther." [20]

A letter, written in the style of William Douglass but signed W. Philanthropos, appeared in the *Boston News-Letter* for July 17–24, 1721. It attributed to Cotton Mather "a Pious and Charitable design of doing good" but held only contempt for Dr. Boylston. Douglass, in fact, was contemptuous of everyone who did not have a medical degree. He never let his hearers forget that he had studied at Leyden and Utrecht.[21]

A Leyden degree did not intimidate everyone. Increase Mather, Cotton Mather, and four other so-called "inoculation-ministers"—Benjamin Colman, Thomas Prince, John Webb, and William Cooper—were quick to reply with a lengthy letter in the *Gazette*. Its third and fourth paragraphs were clearly aimed at Douglass:

> The Town knows and so does the Country how long and with what *Success* Dr. *Boylston* has practis'd both in *Physick* and *Surgery;* and tho' he has not had the honour and advantage of an *Academical* Education, and conse-

quently not the *Letters* of some *Physicians* in the Town, yet he ought by no means to be called *Illiterate,* ignorant, &c. Would the Town bear that Dr. *Cutler* or Dr. *Davis* should be so treated? No more can it endure to see *Boylston* so spit at. . . .

The meanwhile we heartily wish that Men would treat one another with decency and charity, meekness and humility as become fallible creatures, and good Friends to one another and their Country.[22]

Backed by these six ministers, Boylston disregarded the selectmen's orders and on August 5 resumed inoculating.

The debate continued through a variety of media until the epidemic abated in the early summer of 1722. By then 286 persons had been inoculated (247 by Boylston), of which 281 "had a perfect Smallpox by Inoculation." [23] Six of these inoculatees (or about 2 per cent) died. By contrast, of 7590 Bostonians who contracted smallpox, 844, almost 12 per cent, died. Here for the first time was evidence based on a sufficiently large sampling that inoculation was effective. By January 1722 Dr. Douglass was willing to admit that inoculated smallpox was frequently more favorable than natural smallpox and might, with improvement, become a specific preventive. "For my own Part," he said, "till after a few years, I shall pass no positive Judgement of this bold Practice." [24]

Boylston's success, reported back to England, encouraged first English and then continental physicians to re-evaluate the practice of inoculation, a rare instance at so early a date of scientific knowledge flowing in reverse. Full acceptance by the people at large came painfully slowly, but some progress was evident when Boylston visited England in 1725.

ADAM THOMSON'S METHOD

Under the circumstances in which Boylston worked he had no opportunity to prepare his patients for the inoculation; and in his opinion, healthy people of good habits did not really require any preparation. In Adam Thomson's opinion, they did.

Beyond the fact that Adam Thomson was born and educated in Scotland, nothing is known of him prior to his settling in Prince George's County, Maryland, early in the eighteenth century. He moved to Philadelphia in 1748. Thomson was influenced by the work of Hermann Boerhaave (1668–1738) of Leyden, who was described by his most famous pupil, Albrecht von Haller, as "the general teacher of all Europe."

In 1709 Boerhaave published his *Aphorisms on the diagnosis and treatment of diseases*. Aphorism No. 1392 stated: "Some success from antimony and mercury prompts us to seek for a specific for the small-pox in a combination of those two minerals, reduced by art, to an active, but not to an acrimonious or corrosive state." [25] This hint was enough to encourage Dr. Thomson to initiate in 1738 his method of preparing the body for smallpox inoculation. His two-week "cooling regimen" involved a light, non-stimulating diet, a combination of mercury and antimony as medication, and moderate bleeding and purgation.

Following this preparatory treatment, Dr. Thomson inoculated the leg, being of the opinion that the site of local reaction should be as far removed as possible from the brain and vital organs. To prevent or remedy a troublesome sore, he prescribed "about 3 or 4 drams of Jesuit's bark [quinine] given at so many doses during the day." Dr. Thomson favored inoculation over exposure to smallpox. In his experience, inoculatees escaped severe sore throat and experienced a milder form of the disease than those allowed to contract it by direct contact.[26]

In a *Discourse on the Preparation of the Body for the Small-pox,* delivered by Thomson to the Academy of Philadelphia on November 21, 1750 (and printed by Benjamin Franklin the same year, reprinted in London in 1752 and in New York in 1757), the doctor reported: "On every occasion, for the space of twelve years that I have been called upon to prepare people for the small-pox, either for receiving it in the natural way, or by inoculation (for I have prepared many for both), I have constantly us'd such a medicine as mention'd [mercury and antimony], and I can honestly declare that I never saw one so prepar'd in any considerable danger by the disease." [27]

It was Thomson's belief that the blood of every human being carried a greater or lesser amount of "variolous fuel," dormant in the body until it was activated by the "variolous contagion." Subsequent immunity resulted from the total elimination of the variolous fuel in the course of the disease. He further believed that mercury and antimony reduced the potency of the variolous fuel.[28]

While there was some opposition to the Thomson method, the *Discourse* was well received both in America and Europe. In fact its acceptance was so great that the year 1762 found Dr. Thomson complaining in a "long and scholarly letter," which appeared in the *Maryland Gazette* for November 25, that his method was being employed by quacks as "a matter of merchandize." In the same letter he thanked "Dr. Alex. Garden of Charleston, S.C. for his honesty in stating in public that the uncommon success following the inoculation of a great number of individuals during a very fatal epidemic of small-pox in 1759, was entirely due to the employment of the method recommended in the Discourse." [29]

Had Dr. Thomson's method "not been superceded by vaccination, the American method of preparing the body for small-pox would have remained, with but slight modification, the most rational means of reducing the mortality during disastrous epidemics. . . ." [30]

THE SUTTON METHOD

There is considerable evidence that the Thomson method was the basis for a "new" method announced in England in 1757 by "an unqualified practitioner" named Robert Sutton. Within eleven years Sutton inoculated more than twenty-five hundred individuals, assisted by his sons Robert and Daniel. In 1796 Daniel Sutton wrote a book that claimed to "fully set forth in a plain and familiar manner" the "Suttonian System of Inoculation." His preface opened with the statement that the "practical part of the following Work is the result of a very extensive practice and an unremitting attention to the small-pox for near forty years, founded neither on ancient nor modern authorities, but deduced from observations of my own: not that I had neglected to consult, or held in contempt, such valuable relics. . . ." [31]

Despite Sutton's denial of "modern authorities," his "purging powders" contained "Calx of antimony washed, ten drachms, Calomel [mercurous chloride], eight drachms." Moreover, he stated that little need be said about inoculation itself "as the manner of performing the operation is now familiar to almost everyone. . . ." He differed from Thomson, however, in making "the puncture not more than two or three inches above the joint of the elbow, on the upper part of the arm of an adult; if on infants, not more than an inch above it," in contrast to Thomson's preference for the leg.[32]

If Sutton, in preparing his 1796 publication, did not read Thomson's *Discourse,* he must at least have examined an essay written in 1767 by Dr. Thomas Rushton, which began:

> The method of preparing in inoculating for the small-pox, of which I propose to speak in the following treatise, was first practised in America, about the year 1745, which was long before it was made use of in any part of Europe. It is somewhat uncertain, who first gave the hint of it, though it would be well worth our while to know, to whom we are so much indebted for this discovery; for gratitude to the author of one, so useful to mankind, ought to be engraven on our, and his name should be most respectfully held in perpetual rememberance. To Dr. Murison, however, of Long Island, and Dr. Thomas of Virginia, we lie principally under obligations, for first making the public experience the benefit of it.[33]

(Dr. Rushton's error in describing Dr. Thomson of Maryland as Dr. Thomas of Virginia was attributable to his source of information. Dr. Benjamin Gale [1715–1790] of Connecticut, in the 1765 *Transactions* of the Philosophical Society, referred to " 'Dr. Thomas of Virginia,' who . . . began the 'new method' with Dr. Murison of Long Island and several others in 1745." Even the date 1745 is wrong because "Dr. Thomson started his preliminary treatment seven years previously, in the Province of Maryland and carried on this pioneer work unaided by others." [34])

In addition to the essay proper, in which Dr. Rushton described the American method, including the preparatory use of antimony and mercury, which "are known to be the most useful and powerful evacuants of any we are acquainted with," there was "An Appendix, Containing A Chymical Examination of Mr. Sutton's Medicines." Rushton wrote: "Since the foregoing sheets were committed to the press, a very ingenious gentleman, who is well acquainted with Mr. Sutton, and has been much conversant among his patients, brought me a quantity of the medicines which he uses in inoculating for the small pox, and which were prepared by himself." Six experiments brought Rushton to the conclusion that the basis of Sutton's powder was calomel.[35]

If the method was Thomson's, Sutton nonetheless made a major contribution of a different kind. His book, with its 8-by-5-inch page, contains a folded insert opposite the final page. This insert, on 10½-by-7¾-inch sheets, consists of four pages of detailed "Instructions for The Conduct of Patients under Inoculation." The first page deals with Preparatory Diet, detailed to the point of "For Breakfast," "For Dinner," "For Supper," and "Not allowed during Preparation." The second covers "Alterative White Powders and Purging," and the third, air, exercise, and cleanliness, the rash, and convulsions. The final page, quite remarkable for its day, is a detailed Record of Proceedings form, "to be returned to the Operator at the close of the cure, and by him to be filed as a record, should it be required." [36]

VACCINATION

Vaccination has been described as "simply inoculation with a safer virus." [37] The safer virus was that of cowpox, a disease that has existed among cows from earliest times.

Edward Jenner (1749–1823), an English physician, is usually credited with being the discoverer of vaccination, announcing his discovery in 1796 or 1797, but his claim has been disputed on behalf of Benjamin Jesty (1737–1816), a farmer and cattle dealer of Yetminster in Dorset, England. Jesty is hailed on his tombstone at Maltravers, near Swanage, "for having been the first Person (known) that introduced the Cow Pox by inoculation, and who, from his great strength of mind, made the experiment from the Cow on his wife and two sons in the year 1774." [38] Also, a medical practitioner named Nash, who died in 1785, left the following notes, written about 1781:

> I never heard of one having the smallpox who ever had the cowpox. . . . I have now inoculated about sixty persons, who have been reported to have had the cowpox, and I believe at least forty of them I could not infect with the variolous virus. The other twenty, or nearly that number, I think it is very reasonable to presume (as they were no judges), had not the real cowpox. . . . My principal intention in publishing being to recommend to the world a method of inoculation that is far superior . . . to any yet made known. [39]

Naming any particular person as the discoverer of vaccination seems pointless, since there is "abundant proof of the disorder being known, and of its preventive power, long before Dr. Jenner's name was heard." [40] Jenner's merit "rests upon the fact that . . . he started out with the hope of making his thesis a permanent working principle in science, based upon experimental demonstration, and he succeeded to the extent of

231

carrying his inoculations successfully through several generations in the body and, above all, in overcoming the popular aversion to vaccination." [41] Jenner considered cowpox and its relationship to smallpox for upward of thirty years before he performed his first vaccination on May 14, 1796. He published his first book on vaccination, based on twenty-three cases, in 1798. Word quickly reached America. In December 1798 the New York *Medical Repository* reprinted from the *Analytical Review* an account of the Jenner book.

ᐱ

As with other deadly plagues, including bubonic plague itself, people tend to think of smallpox epidemics and pandemics as a thing of the past. The decision of the Public Health Service in 1971 to recommend that general vaccination be discontinued may be overconfident. Infectious diseases have a way of reappearing. The case against these recommendations was discussed in a letter from Dr. Lamson Blaney of Greensboro, which appeared in the *North Carolina Medical Journal* of December 1971. His reasons were:

1. Reporting of smallpox cases on a world-wide basis is of questionable accuracy.

2. Immunization of all travelers from endemic areas is not reliable.

3. Smallpox recently imported into Europe entered a population rendered relatively immune by previous vaccination.

4. Smallpox is extremely infectious and carries a high mortality rate.

5. Importation of smallpox into the U.S. at a later time when the general population is unprotected would be

akin to the introduction of a highly contagious disease among the aborigines of North America in colonial times—disastrous.

6. The potential threat of a widespread epidemic would be more likely than now, making necessary the maintenance of an imposing emergency control system to meet such an eventuality.[42]

A month later *Time,* in reporting the action of the Public Health Service, noted a marked drop in smallpox cases worldwide and stated that the "improvement results almost entirely from vaccination. In the U.S., where immunization of infants has long been routine, there has not been a recorded case of smallpox since 1949. . . . In virtually all of the U.S. state or local regulations still demand that school-age children be vaccinated. However, at least 15 state legislatures are now considering bills to relax that requirement. The U.S. Center for Disease Control in Atlanta believes that by the end of [1972] most states will have given up mandatory vaccination." [43]

With smallpox essentially eliminated, it seems preferable to the authorities to rely on very rapid immunization on a mass scale in times of epidemics rather than perpetuate the risk of adverse reactions to routine vaccination, which may include death.

{(14)}

The Scourge of
Yellow Fever

Yellow fever, often confused with dengue and infectious jaundice (hepatitis), was carried from Africa to Spain and Portugal in the sixteenth century. Contemporary physicians in England, France, and Germany seem to have been largely unaware of the disease, which would come to be regarded as a scourge of the New World. Consequently yellow fever was first studied in America.

Outbreaks of what may have been yellow fever were reported in the West Indies as early as 1635, and by the second half of the seventeenth century the disease was well known there and had spread to Central and South America. Alleged outbreaks among New England Indians in 1618 and Martha's Vineyard Indians in 1643 have been discounted on the ground that "isolation . . . from the known centers of the infection

234

makes this assumption untenable." Nor was the attack of "bilious fever" that hit New York in 1668 yellow fever because the characteristic "black vomit" was absent. The same could not be said of a Boston outbreak in 1693. When a British fleet out of Barbados anchored in the harbor, Cotton Mather described the resultant "Distemper, which in less than a Week's time usually carried off my Neighbors, with very direful Symptoms, of turning Yellow, vomiting and bleeding." [1]

The disease hit Philadelphia and Charleston in 1699 and probably New York three years later. Then for thirty-five years, while present off and on in the West Indies, it apparently reached no farther north than Charleston, with epidemics in 1706, 1728, and 1732. The next northern appearances were in Philadelphia in 1741, 1747, and 1793, and in New York in 1743, 1745, and 1748. New Orleans suffered its first outbreak in 1796. Throughout the nineteenth century the disease arrived almost every summer, intermittently reaching epidemic proportions.

It has been suggested that yellow fever in the West Indies was not endemic but subject to periodic reinfection from Africa and the Spanish continental colonies, and therefore the area was not a persistent source of infection for the American seaboard. A factor in the incidence of epidemics may have been the wars between European powers during the period, which brought numerous unexposed soldiers and sailors from Europe to the Caribbean.[2]

Quarantine regulations were established in Boston as early as 1647 and in Pennsylvania around 1700. By 1790 rudimentary regulations existed in almost all American ports. In light of modern knowledge, it seems clear that stricter quarantine measures would have gone a long way toward keeping yellow fever out of northern seaports; but evaluation of such measures was part and parcel of the controversy over whether the fever was contagious or spontaneous, imported or local.

The effectiveness of the measures varied with need. In New Orleans the measures were rigorously enforced. The same was true of New York when it was badly hit in 1819–22. By then the great majority of physicians elsewhere were anticontagionist and antiquarantine. Baltimore virtually abolished its quarantine system in 1808. In Philadelphia in 1820 an anticontagionist president of the Board of Health applied "localist principles" and virtually ignored the quarantine laws still on the books. In Boston around the same time the Board of Health, under attack for its quarantine procedures, was abolished by a new city government, which promptly relaxed quarantine regulations.

The first American writer to draw attention to the disease was John Mitchell (c.1680–1768) of Urbana, Virginia, whose unpublished manuscript, "An Account of the Yellow Fever Which Prevailed in Virginia in 1737, 1741 and 1742," did not come to light until after his death. Then it "fell into the hands of Dr. [Benjamin] Franklin, who communicated it to Dr. [Benjamin] Rush. Dr. Rush not only read the essay with interest, but acknowledges that he derived from it hints which assisted him in detecting the true nature of the method of treating the yellow fever as it appeared in Philadelphia in 1793." [3] In the meantime, John Lining (1708–1760) had in 1753 "published a history of the yellow fever, which was the first account of that disease that was given to the world from the American continent. He seems to have been satisfied that this disorder affected the system but once in life. . . ." [4] The name yellow fever was first applied to the disease by the English naturalist Griffith Hughes in the account of a Barbados epidemic that occurred in 1715 which was included in his book *Natural History of Barbadoes,* published in 1750.[5]

PHILADELPHIA, 1793

Mathew Carey, a Philadelphia publisher, and Benjamin Rush wrote graphic accounts of the Philadelphia epidemic of 1793. Carey's picture of the largely deserted city might have described Florence, Italy, in 1348 at the height of the plague:

> The consternation of the people . . . was carried beyond all bounds. Dismay and affright were visible on the countenance of almost every person. Most people who could . . . fled the city. Of those who remained, many shut themselves in their houses and were afraid to walk the

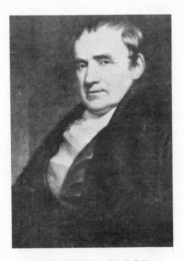

MATHEW CAREY

streets. . . . Many were almost incessantly purifying, scowering, and whitewashing their rooms. Those who ventured abroad, had hankerchiefs or sponges impregnated with vinegar or camphor at their noses. . . . The corpses of the most respectable citizens, even if they did not die of the epidemic, were carried to the grave, on the shafts of a chair, the horse driven by a negro, unattended by a friend or relation, and without any sort of ceremony. People shifted their course at the sight of a hearse. . . . Many . . . went into the middle of the streets, to avoid being infected in passing by houses wherein people had died. . . . The old custom of shaking hands fell into such general disuse, that many were affronted at even the offer of a hand.[6]

Rush, not quite so vivid, might have been describing London during the plague of 1665:

The streets every where discovered marks of the distress that pervaded the city. More than one half the houses were shut up, although not more than one third of the inhabitants had fled into the country. In walking for many hundred yards, few persons were met, except such as were in quest of a physician, a nurse, a bleeder, or the men who buried the dead. The hearse alone kept up the remembrance of the noise of carriages or carts in the streets. . . . A black man, leading or driving a horse, with a corpse on a pair of chair wheels, . . . met the eye in most of the streets of the city . . . while the noise of the same wheels . . . kept alive anguish and fear in the sick and well, every hour of the night.[7]

Carey was the eyewitness and critic. Rush, no less of a commentator, was also the man of action. His letters to his wife, Julia, who, with the younger children, was away from Philadelphia between August 21 and November 12, 1793, "vividly reflect the mental state of the sensitive, high-strung physician, overworked to the verge of collapse, desperately fighting the disease that was killing half his friends." [8]

There was a great diversity of opinion as to the cause of the epidemic. Dr. James Hutchinson maintained that it was not imported while most Philadelphians felt the disease came from outside the city.[9] Rush adopted Hutchinson's view. "It is supposed to have been produced by some damaged coffee that putrefied on one of the wharves," Rush wrote his wife on August 21.[10] "Supporters of the local origin of the fever rallied to the banner of Benjamin Rush, while the foreign origin found its chief proponents in the College of Physicians. Possibly no great harm would have resulted from this professional difference had the public press not published from day to day and indeed frequently in the same issue the divergent views of the leaders in medicine. Rush with characteristic vigor maintained the local origin of the epidemic through the public press." [11]

On September 4 Rush wrote to his wife: "The disease spreads, but its mortality is in proportion to the number who are affected. The jalap and mercury cures 9 out of 10, of all who take it on the day of the attack." On the 13th he reported: "Yesterday was a day of triumph to mercury, jalap and bleeding. I am satisfied that they saved in my hands only nearly one hundred lives." [12]

Rush's cure for yellow fever, based on intense bleeding and purging with calomel (mercurous chloride), has not been recognized by modern evaluators, and there was considerable disagreement over it at the time. It had the support of a number of influential practitioners and of Rush's former pupils, but his "radical measures" were not generally accepted by the profession. "Dr. Kuhn called it a murderous dose. Dr. Hodge called it a dose for a horse. Dr. Hutchinson who is nearly as large as Goliath of Gath, and quite as vauntful and malignant, even threatened" to flog him.[13]

Hutchinson, who had been the first to point to damaged coffee as the cause, disagreed with Rush's treatment. The attack by Adam Kuhn particularly incensed Rush, who asserted that Kuhn's experience with yellow fever was limited to seven cases.

"So tired and irritable from overwork was Rush that he viewed the opinions and theories of his opponents as personal affronts. . . . [He] had been working fifteen to eighteen hours daily for weeks; and, having seen a high percentage of his patients recover, he became convinced of the curative value of his treatment. Even if there was another side to the question he was too exhausted mentally to follow its argument. . . . The attacks on his opinions of origin and treatment so embittered him that, on November 5, he resigned from the College of Physicians, the organization which he had helped to found."[14]

As a corollary to the question of cause, eighteenth-century physicians disputed whether yellow fever was contagious or spontaneous. Rush was a leader in the anticontagion school. Though he noted that those who lived and worked in smoky houses escaped the disease—it was already known that smoke discouraged mosquitoes—he ignored the mosquitoes, preferring to believe that smoke kept away the putrid exhalations of decayed animal and vegetable matter (miasma) that were, in the opinion of his school, the cause of the disease.

Rush was a man who not only stuck religiously to his views but applied them with zeal. "When faced with the horrors of yellow fever, Rush drew heavily on his most valuable tool—observation, reason, and a stubborn belief in himself." The fact that his ideas proved to be wrong in this case does not reduce the eminence of his place in American medicine. "His contribution to the Art of Medicine is measurable in the obvious sacredness in which he held human life and his really heroic efforts to preserve it." [15]

CAUSE AND CURE

It was a contemporary of Rush, John Crawford (1746–1813) of Baltimore, who pinpointed mosquitoes as the source of malaria, yellow fever, and other diseases. In a long series of articles Crawford considered a variety of related matters (including the history of quarantine), rejected Rush's miasma theory, and advocated the avoidance of the breeding grounds of mosquitoes. "Crawford attributed to insects too large a role in the genesis of human suffering and misinterpreted the mechanism by which they transmit yellow fever, but he was the first to turn from the hazy concepts of miasma and contagium to a tangible intermediate carrier, the insect." [16]

In 1848 Josiah Clark Nott (1804–1873) of South Carolina came closer to suggesting the mosquito's role in the transmission of yellow fever, but it remained for the Cuban Carlos Juan Finlay (1833–1915) to put the theory of transmission of yellow fever by the *Aëdes aegypti* mosquito to the test. Finlay began his experiments in 1881; they proved to be inconclusive because, for inoculation purposes, he used mosquitoes contaminated only two to six days previously, not being aware,

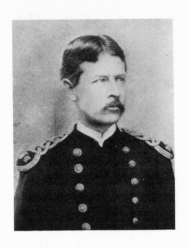

as the army commission led by Walter Reed (1851–1902) would show, that the mosquito was not able to transmit the disease by stinging for eleven days. But Finlay's "was a cogent and brilliant deduction from the spare data then available." [17]

Reed's experimental work was started under more propitious auspices. He was in the position to make use of experiments and epidemiological observations of other researchers during the last two decades of the nineteenth century. He knew, for example, that the culex, anopheles, tick, and tsetse fly were instrumental in transmitting filariasis, Texas fever, nagana, and malaria; that the malaria parasite taken in with the blood entered the stomach wall of the mosquito and then needed twelve days before it was ready for transmission into man's blood vessels; that the time interval between the first case of yellow fever in an isolated farmhouse and the first secondary case in the same house was two to three weeks, despite the fact that incubation was known to require only one to seven days, the time difference pointing to a maturation period in the intermediary host; that ticks too needed a maturation period before spreading cattle fever.

Experiments with contaminated mosquitoes, carried out by the U.S. Army Yellow Fever Commission between December 5, 1900, and February 7, 1901, established the role of the *Aëdes aegypti* mosquito and confirmed Finlay's theory.

The commission found that "vomit, stool, and soiled bedding were innocuous and epidemiologically irrelevant." As early as December 1900 Reed wrote his wife: "How General [George M.] Sternberg and hosts of others could have believed in the contagiousness of clothing and of the stools of yellow fever patients I cannot possibly see. . . . A little careful testing of this theory has served to knock it completely into smithereens." [18]

The commission concluded that: "The mosquito serves as the intermediate host for the parasite of yellow fever, and it is highly probable that the disease is only propagated through the bite of this insect." [19]

The discoveries of the Yellow Fever Commission were followed shortly by a dramatic demonstration of yellow-fever control, engineered by William Crawford Gorgas (1854–1920) of the American Medical Corps. By September 1901 he had completely eradicated yellow fever from Havana through a program of antimosquito measures directed against *Aëdes aegypti*. He repeated this demonstration in Panama. Oswaldo G. Cruz (1872–1917) had a like success in Rio de Janeiro, and control measures were established in most tropical ports of the New World.

In 1916 the Rockefeller Foundation Yellow Fever Commission was formed, with General Gorgas one of its members, and was instrumental in eradicating yellow fever in many

Latin American countries. In the mid-1920s commissions supported by the foundation went to West Africa, the cradle of yellow fever. A permanent West African commission was established at Yaba, near Lagos, Nigeria.

In 1927 three Nigerian physicians, Adrian Stokes (1887–1927), Johannes H. Bauer, and N. Paul Hudson confirmed that the yellow-fever agent was a filterable virus. They showed too that, once infected, mosquitoes remain infective for their life span.

In the mid-1930s the internationally known epidemiologist Fred L. Soper defined a new concept, jungle yellow fever, as "yellow fever occurring in rural, jungle and fluvial zones in the absence of *A. aegypti.*" [20] Although verification of this concept has put an end to dreams of totally eradicating yellow fever, the vaccine developed in 1937 by Max Theiler, a South African microbiologist working at the Rockefeller Foundation laboratories, has proved to be effective.

NEW ORLEANS, 1905

In May 1905 an infected passenger or an infected mosquito slipped past the quarantine station on the river below New Orleans and brought yellow fever into the city. The population at that time was about 375,000, with less than one-fourth immunized by prior attack. By the time the epidemic had run its course there had been 452 deaths out of 3402 cases in Orleans Parish.

One would have expected that by this time, four years after the report of the Yellow Fever Commission, the city would have undertaken an antimosquito campaign. It had not. The people refused to believe that this small, familiar pest, annoying though it might be, was the agent. Even the medical profession was divided. In its report for 1900–1901 the Louisiana State Board of Health declared: ". . . we Southern Health officers, charged with the grave duty of protecting our people against the most dreaded of all diseases, are unwilling to accept the dictum of the experimenters that yellow fever can be conveyed by no other agency." [21] There were exceptions, such as Dr. Quitman Kohnke, chairman of the New Orleans Board of Health, who, impressed by the results of Gorgas' work in Havana, tried to promote a similar movement in New Orleans.

It took the epidemic of 1905 to change people's minds. By installing municipal drainage, sewerage, and water systems in the next few years, the favorite breeding grounds of the mosquitoes were eliminated. Since 1906 Louisiana has been free of the disease.

This was the last yellow-fever epidemic in the United States.

Federal direction of maritime quarantine was achieved early in the twentieth century over the protests of states' righters, and yellow fever has been kept out of the country by vigilant quarantine authorities and the careful supervision of travel to and from the yellow-fever zones of Latin America and Africa. Beyond these protective barriers danger still lurks.

⑮

The Battle against Widespread Diseases

Smallpox and yellow fever were not the only communicable diseases to hit a burgeoning America. In fact, epidemic disorders visited the colonists with relentless regularity. In the Civil War the 224,000 deaths from disease were more than double the deaths in action and from wounds received in action.

TYPHOID, TYPHUS, AND DYSENTERY

These diseases were not readily identifiable in the seventeenth and eighteenth centuries. Typhoid fever "was undoubtedly present among the American colonists, but just how extensive it was and how early it appeared is still debatable. The symptoms . . . resemble those of both dysentery and typhus, a fact which adds to the difficulties confronting the student of these three diseases. The fever, cramps, diarrhea, and bloody discharge of dysentery often characterize typhoid, and the mild skin eruption of typhoid was occasionally confused with typhus rash." [1]

Typhus was relatively unknown in the American colonies. It was a disease resulting from overcrowding, poverty, and filth—transmitted by lice—and largely agricultural America did not present these conditions. Typhus could prove fatal on the voyage from Europe in dirty, overloaded vessels, but its appearance on shore, certainly in epidemic proportions, was rare.

In 1836 an outbreak of typhus at the Pennsylvania Hospital enabled the resident physician, William Wood Gerhard (1809–1872), who had seen both diseases while studying in Paris, to distinguish between typhus and typhoid. Gerhard found "that in the typhus fever the intestines were more free from lesions than in any other disease accompanied by a febrile movement." Such lesions as were present "were as different . . . as the pustules of smallpox are unlike the eruption of measles." [2] Clinical differences involved the appearance of the eyes, the degree of stupor, abdominal symptoms, and skin eruptions.

A few years later Elisha Bartlett (1804–1855) of Rhode Island, in the first complete account in English of typhoid and typhus, concluded that typhoid "differs essentially from all others in its causes, in its symptoms, in its lesions." [3]

During the Civil War there were 75,368 cases of typhoid and 27,056 deaths (in contrast to 2501 cases of typhus with 850 deaths.) Nearly a hundred years would elapse before Dr. Theodore E. Woodward of the University of Maryland, and his associates, found in the antibiotic chloromycetin, developed in the 1940s, a remedy for typhoid.

The symptoms of dysentery are similar to those of typhoid and typhus—"fever, diarrhea, cramps, and . . . bloody flux. . . . More than likely some of the virulent outbreaks of bloody flux" diagnosed as dysentery were "typhoid or some form of cholera." [4]

The first outbreak of dysentery may have occurred during the original colonists' initial summer in Virginia. George Percy, one of the first settlers at Jamestown, reported that the men were destroyed by such cruel diseases as burning fever, swellings, and fluxes. The most that can be said with any certainty is that dysentery was present, sometimes in epidemic proportions, throughout the seventeenth and eighteenth centuries.

If the Civil War figures are any criterion, the mortality rate in dysentery cases did not begin to approach that of typhoid and typhus fever. Only 4084 deaths were reported out of 233,812 cases of acute dysentery; 3299 out of 25,670 cases of chronic dysentery. Joseph Janvier Woodward (1833–1884), writing in 1863 on the "chief camp diseases of the . . . present war," remarked that "the malignant dysentery of European armies had not yet made its appearance among our troops." By the end of the war the total number of dysentery cases was 1,739,135 (with 44,558 deaths), in which Woodward apparently included diarrheas as dysenteries.[5]

In 1901 Simon Flexner (1863–1946), the distinguished American pathologist and bacteriologist, reported on a comparative study he had made of dysenteric bacilli. He found "that the acute dysenteries . . . whether in the Far East, Germany, or the West Indies are due to the same organism. . . .

There is little doubt that the acute epidemic dysenteries in this country are caused by the same micro-organism." [6]

CHILDREN'S DISEASES

Diphtheria and scarlet fever also were confused in the eighteenth century. Several factors contributed to this. "Neither of these diseases . . . ranked with smallpox and other major contagions of the colonial period. They were restricted largely to children and were neither so universal nor so virulent as some other sicknesses. It was not until the mid-nineteenth century, when it assumed its present-day form, that diphtheria became a serious threat. Scarlet fever was of even less significance" in colonial times.[7] The decline of scarlet fever in the twentieth century is attributable to the discovery of penicillin, which has revolutionized the treatment of the disease.

The specific treatment for diphtheria was developed by Emil von Behring (1854–1917), a Prussian army surgeon who resigned from the service in 1890 and went to work at the Koch Institute for Infectious Diseases in Berlin. Here, working with Shibasaburo Kitasato (1852–1931), he demonstrated that the serum of animals immunized against attenuated diphtheria toxins could be used as a preventive or therapeutic inoculation against diphtheria in other animals, through a specific neutralization of the toxin of the disease. After trying out the remedy in man, von Behring in 1894 began to produce his antitoxin on a grand scale. He continued to study diphtheria and, before his death, recommended immunization of children with a mixture of toxin and antitoxin.

One of the first American physicians to use this antitoxin was pediatrician Abraham Jacobi. Since little was known about how the material should be administered, or its possible side effects, most physicians, jealous of their reputation, were wary. "The hazards Jacobi risked (and physical violence in the tenements of New York was not the least of these) have never been placed in print, nor was he a man to recount them himself. It will be sufficient to say that it was owing to his efforts and the careful calculations of the diplomatic [William Hallock] Park [of the New York City Health Department], and the support of the latter's associates, . . . that antitoxin therapy was rapidly placed at the disposal of American physicians." [8]

Measles received little attention in the eighteenth century. Its relatively low mortality rate in a day when smallpox and other disorders reduced the population by the hundreds relegated it to a minor role. Yet measles ranks with smallpox, with which it was confused well into the seventeenth century, as one of the most infectious diseases. Adding to the confusion is the fact that there are three kinds of measles: measles proper, which run for about ten days; rubella, or German measles, with ordinarily a three-day duration; and roseola, a mild form that attacks infants.

Francis Home (1719–1813), a native of Scotland, in 1759 vaccinated children with material from measles and apparently produced some degree of immunity.

In 1896 Henry Koplik (1858–1927) of Mount Sinai Hospital (New York) found that before the rash breaks out, small red spots with bluish-white centers appear on the mucous membrane of the mouth. The presence of these "Koplik spots" makes possible a positive early diagnosis.

From 1905 to 1919 Ludvig Hektoen (1863–1951), the eminent American pathologist and bacteriologist, experimented with measles by blood-injection. From 1917 to 1927 Ruth Tunnicliff (1876–1946) of the John McCormick Institute for Infectious Diseases in Chicago worked on serum therapy.

The effective use of gamma globulin prophylactically or in the treatment of measles was reported in 1944 by Joseph Stokes, Jr. (1896–1972), professor of pediatrics in community medicine at the University of Pennsylvania and physician-in-chief at Children's Hospital, Philadelphia, and his associates. They found that exposed children who received the serum were almost always protected; those to whom the serum was given after Koplik's spots or the characteristic rash had appeared seemed to suffer less severely.

In the 1960s a measles vaccine was produced by Joseph Stokes and John F. Enders, who had together previously developed immunization procedures against mumps. Without Enders' work in growing viruses in tissue culture, little progress would have been made in the fight against this and other viral diseases, including polio.

RESPIRATORY INFECTIONS

Reports of respiratory diseases came from the colonies within fifteen years after the first settlers arrived in Virginia. Colonial records were "replete with notations of epidemic sicknesses called 'pleuretical disorders,' 'pleurisies,' or 'peripneumonies,' and fatal illnesses were frequently described as 'a kind of Pleurisy,' or 'a sort of Pestilential Pluriticle feaver.' Certainly various forms of pneumonia must have reached epidemic proportions on many occasions among a population undernourished from a restricted winter diet. . . . Using contemporary colonial descriptions, it is almost impossible . . . to distinguish between attacks of pneumonia, pleurisy, or influenza." [9]

Nor is differentiation by the layman much easier today. Put as simply as possible, pneumonia involves inflammation or acute infection of the lung itself. There are over fifty causes. Pleurisy involves an inflammation of the membrane lining of the lungs. Influenza involves inflammation of the respiratory mucous membranes.

Most eighteenth-century writers believed that pneumonias began with a certain amount of pleurisy. (Leopold Auenbrugger [1722–1809], who developed percussion as a means of distinguishing the healthy from the diseased side of the chest, was an exception.) There was considerable disagreement, however, as to whether pleurisy inevitably led to pneumonia. Between 1830 and 1840 it was finally accepted that this was not so.

Pneumonia. The usual eighteenth-century therapeutic procedure in pneumonia was bleeding, of which William Cullen (1712–1790) of the University of Glasgow said: ". . . upon the recurrence of the urgent symptoms, the bleeding should be repeated at any period of the disease, especially within the first fortnight; and even afterwards, if a tendency to suppuration be not evident, or if, after a seeming solution, the disease shall have again returned." [10] Cullen advised against the withdrawal of more than four or five pounds of blood in the course of two or three days.

While diagnostic methods improved, thanks largely to René Théophile Hyacinthe Laënnec (1781–1826) and his invention of the stethoscope, treatment measures lagged, and it was not until the 1890s that the golden age of serum therapy had its beginnings.

The Klemperers, Georg (1865–1931) and Felix (1866–1932), of Berlin were among the first to attempt systematically to immunize animals against pneumococcal infection; in their preliminary observations in man, they found that a dose of pneumococci fatal for a rabbit could with impunity be injected subcutaneously into a man (1891). In 1913 Rufus Cole of the Hospital of the Rockefeller Institute presented two principles in the serotherapy of pneumonia: treatment should be begun as early as possible (otherwise it would likely prove ineffective); large doses of potent serum should be used. Additional studies of pneumonia were made around 1917 by Oswald T. Avery and his associates at the Rockefeller Institute. Ultimately serum therapy was replaced by antibiotics.

Influenza was so named in 1767 by John Huxham (1694–1768) of Plymouth, England, in an account of the "vernal catarrh" of 1743.

Between 1597 and 1693 there were epidemics of influenza in Spain and England; it was pandemic in Europe between 1707 and 1743, and epidemic in 1762, 1767, and 1775. The disease usually appeared in America a year after it had attacked Europe.

Periodically influenza sweeps through the civilized world attacking up to 40 per cent of the inhabitants of affected areas. The pandemic of 1918 was truly global. Boston, New York, San Francisco, London, Paris, Berlin, Bombay, and Calcutta were hit severely; such widely separated countries as Russia, Argentina, Australia, and the Philippines were attacked. In the American army 24,000 died of influenza in contrast with 34,-000 killed in battle. In all, more than ten million people died of the disease.

With so many cases to study it is reasonable to suppose that the army would have learned something about cause, prevention, transmittal, and control of the disease, but the epidemic came and went with these mysteries unsolved. The army found that the agent identified as the influenza bacillus by the German Richard Pfeiffer in 1892 was present so irregularly that it could only be regarded as a secondary invader. Opinion began to develop that influenza was caused by a filterable virus. In 1933, three English physicians, Wilson Smith, Christopher H. Andrewes, and P. P. Laidlaw confirmed this.

During the first few years of study of the influenza virus, it was thought that there was only one type. Strains isolated in England, in the United States, in Puerto Rico, and elsewhere were shown by immunological tests to be identical. In 1940 the virologist Thomas Francis, Jr. (1900–1969) isolated from an outbreak in New York State an agent that produced the typical reactions of influenza in ferrets but that, by all existing immunological criteria, could not be the previously identified virus. It turned out to be another type of influenza virus. At about the same time T. P. Magill, who had done earlier work with Francis in the study of influenza, arrived at a similar conclusion. Yet the diseases produced by the two types (A and B, as they were designated—Type C would be uncovered later) were clinically indistinguishable.

To complicate matters there were strains within the types, and it was found that immunity as a result of a bout of the disease was effective only if the individual had had the particular type *and* strain. When a vaccine was developed, it also immunized only against one type and strain. The pandemic of 1957–58 was caused by the Asian Type A strain, which was novel, and vaccines based on previous Type A strains were ineffective.

The vaccine to be used for checking a specific epidemic

has to be on hand long enough in advance for a sizable portion of any population to be inoculated at least two or three weeks ahead of an outbreak; but when a new strain emerges there just is not enough time to develop and administer a vaccine before the epidemic strikes. To make matters worse, there is no specific treatment for influenza—vaccines are useless once the disease has taken hold. Treatment, therefore, must be symptomatic.

Relief may be on the way. In August 1972 scientists of the National Institute of Allergy and Infectious Diseases announced the preliminary success of a new vaccine that uses a combination of live viruses (in contrast with the customary killed virus) and can be produced quickly enough to meet an influenza threat. Live viruses can be used because the vaccine is extremely sensitive to heat and cannot survive in the temperature of the lungs, where flu viruses ordinarily settle to bring on illness. Field trials had to be conducted before the new vaccine could be employed extensively, but there was cautious confidence that the vaccine would be licensed before the next flu epidemic. It was not. The London flu of 1972 swept through America late that year and early in 1973.

Tuberculosis is an infectious disease caused by one of several closely related moldlike bacteria. Although it usually involves the lungs, it can produce gross lesions in other organs and tissues. There is evidence that the disease has plagued man since earliest time, but it was not subjected to concentrated investigation until the beginning of the nineteenth century, when important work was done in France and Germany.

In 1882 the German bacteriologist Robert Koch (1843–1910) discovered the tubercle bacillus. The curative material (later named "tuberculin") he subsequently developed proved to be a failure in therapy but is none the less in use today in testing for tuberculous infection.

Shortly after Koch's announcement of his cure in 1890, Edwin Livingston Trudeau (1848–1915), reported that his work on essentially the same material was also fruitless. But Trudeau was by then making a greater contribution to American medicine than his scientific investigations. He was the founder of the sanitarium movement in this country.

In 1873, while practicing in New York, he was told by his physician that he had pulmonary tuberculosis. Advised to seek mountain air, he wintered in the Adirondacks, then decided to remain there. In November 1876 he began his life work at Saranac Lake, New York. The Adirondack Cottage Sanitarium was opened in 1885. The sixteen-acre site on which it stood had been presented to him by a number of local guides and their families grateful for the free professional services with which he had provided them. He personally begged for construction funds. The result was "probably the most complete institution of its kind in the world," in which the best means of combating tuberculosis were developed.[11]

In the 1940s, H. C. Hinshaw and W. H. Feldman of the Mayo Clinic began to investigate antibiotic therapy in tuberculosis. In 1945 they cautiously announced that small doses of streptomycin produced a limited suppressive effect in man.

By 1953 standardized schemes of antibiotic therapy in tuberculosis had been worked out. Isoniazid, para-aminosalicylic acid, and ethambutol (in addition to streptomycin) are the antibiotics most often used today in the treatment of tuberculosis.

Brucellosis. In 1911, during routine tests for tubercle bacilli in milk, Ernest Charles Schroeder (1865–1928) and W. E. Cotton of the U.S. Bureau of Animal Industry encountered curious lesions resembling tuberculosis of the bones and joints in the animals used for testing. Milk from perfectly healthy cows, tuberculin-negative, sometimes produced these lesions. In 1918, Alice Evans of the Research Laboratories of the Dairy Division of the Bureau of Animal Industry showed that the bacillus that infected cow's milk was closely related to the organism that commonly infected goat's milk on the island of Malta. Malta fever was not unknown in this country. Thomas L. Ferenbaugh, an army surgeon, had in 1911 encountered it among young men working in goat camps in southwest Texas and among persons who had drunk unboiled goat's milk.

This disease has been named brucellosis (from the generic name of three species of bacteria involved). It is transmitted from animal to man, through direct contact with secretions or excretions, or ingestion of milk or milk products, but rarely from person to person. Whenever a fever of unknown origin occurs, brucellosis is considered. The most important prophylactic measure is pasteurization of milk. Persons handling animals or carcasses should wear rubber gloves. Treatment involves such broad spectrum antibiotics as chlortetracycline and oxytetracycline for moderately ill patients; steroids such as cortisone and hydrocortisone (used in conjunction with antibiotics) for severely ill patients.

PELLAGRA

Any account of the attempts to determine the cause and prevention of pellagra, a disease first thought to be infectious, must read like a medical detective story. Pellagra was first de-

257

scribed in 1735 by a Spanish physician, Gaspar Casal y Julian (1691–1759), although his book was not published until 1762, three years after his death. While widely known in Europe, pellagra did not strike the United States until 1907, when it was reported in several southern states. Between 1909 and 1913 two surveys were conducted, one in Illinois and the other in southern textile-mill towns. Both groups concluded that pellagra was an infectious disease. The rapid and widespread advance of the disease prompted the Public Health Service to enter the picture. Its approach to finding a cause of the disease was based on the conclusion of the survey teams—that pellagra was infectious.

Rarely has a governmental agency chosen so wisely as the Public Health Service did in 1914 when it selected Joseph Goldberger (1874–1929) to undertake the investigation. Born in Hungary, one of the many children of a poor tenant farmer, Joseph was seven when, with the aid of money from relatives already in America, the Goldbergers moved to New York. At the age of sixteen Joseph went to the City College of New York to study civil engineering. Two years later, in 1892, his choice of a career changed after hearing the well-known clinician Austin Flint, Jr. (1836–1913), deliver the Harvey Lecture at the Bellevue Hospital Medical College. Joseph turned his thoughts and energies toward medicine.

In 1895 Joseph graduated from the medical college second in his class. He took first place in the highly competitive examinations for internships at Bellevue Hospital. During his internship his intellectual curiosity and attention to detail made him a master at writing up case histories.

After two somewhat boring years in private practice in Wilkes-Barre, Pennsylvania, Goldberger entered the Public

Health Service in 1899 and was assigned to the quarantine station on Reedy Island in the Delaware River. From 1900 to 1905 he worked on yellow fever in Mexico, Puerto Rico, and the southern states, becoming an authority in this field. The next five years he spent studying parasitic worms, doing outstanding and imaginative work.

In 1909, while at Woods Hole, Massachusetts, Goldberger became acquainted with Howard Taylor Ricketts (1870–1910), and went with him to Mexico City to work on a typhus epidemic. It was Goldberger, in fact, who first showed that Mexican typhus and Rocky Mountain spotted fever were separate diseases. Both Goldberger and Ricketts came down with typhus and were deathly ill. Ricketts, unfortunately, did not survive the attack, dying at the age of forty, but his outstanding work on Rocky Mountain spotted fever and typhus has kept his name alive.

In 1910 Goldberger became the first to inoculate monkeys with measles, opening the way to effective studies of that disease. Three years later he investigated an epidemic of diphtheria and developed new methods for studying and controlling that elusive affliction.

With this background Goldberger was a natural choice for solving the pellagra problem.

While Goldberger's pellagra investigations were spread over many of the southern states, in the early stages he devoted most of his time to the State Asylum at Milledgeville, Georgia, and the Methodist Orphan Asylum in Jackson, Mississippi.

Characteristic gastrointestinal disturbances and butterfly-like skin eruptions made pellagra relatively easy to identify. At Jackson, Goldberger soon began wondering why the children under six and over twelve did not have pellagra, while a high proportion of those between six and twelve did. In addition, he noticed that none of the personnel at the two institutions suffered from the disease. Careful study of the diets of these categories identified deficiencies in the six-to-twelve age group. By appropriately supplementing the diet of this group, Goldberger was able to wipe out the disease. This was certainly a novel way of curing an infectious disease!

The next step was to reproduce the disease. With the support of Dr. E. H. Galloway, secretary of the Mississippi State Board of Health, and Governor Earl Brewer, Goldberger was permitted to ask for volunteers among the long-term convicts at the Rankin State Prison Farm. Twelve prisoners agreed to undergo dietary experiments that would run for no more than six months, at which time they would be granted unconditional pardons.

The spring of 1915 dragged into summer. None of the convicts developed symptoms of pellagra. Goldberger, sure he was on the right track, became despondent. Then, shortly after the start of the fifth month, the symptoms began to appear. By the end of the sixth month five of the convicts definitely had pellagra.

The infectious-disease theory did not die easily. Goldberger was accused of conducting half-baked experiments, even of having faked the entire program at Rankin. In an attempt to win over the "infection" group, both Goldberger and some of his co-workers subjected themselves to a variety of attempts to transmit the disease. These included the transfer of nasal secretions, the swallowing of capsules containing feces and urine from sufferers from pellagra, and even injections of blood from the diseased. Pellagra did not develop.

Goldberger extended his experimental work to dogs and

rats and by 1922 the "P-P" (pellagra prevention) factor was felt to be an amino acid. In 1923 brewer's yeast was identified as a carrier of this substance and preventive measures became much simpler.

Goldberger did not live to see the final steps in the mystery. The "P-P" factor was first named Vitamin G, as a tribute to Goldberger, and subsequently became Vitamin B_2, or riboflavin. In 1937 Conrad Elvehjem of the University of Wisconsin demonstrated that the factor was actually a fraction of the original Vitamin G, namely nicotinic acid.

Pellagra was the first metabolic disease to be untangled. It had killed tens of thousands in Europe and the United States and had made the lives of millions unpleasant and even unbearable. It had been a catastrophe in both human and economic terms. Thanks to the imagination, scientific ability, and perseverance of Joseph Goldberger, pellagra has disappeared from the list of dangerous diseases.

${(16)}$

Toward a Public Health Service

Attempts to protect the public health by government action date back to the seventeenth century.

In 1647 the Massachusetts General Court, hearing reports of a devastating epidemic in the West Indies (almost certainly yellow fever) and "having cause to feare least our sinnes may provoke the Lord to lay more heavy corrections upon us," first appointed a day of fasting and then ordered a quarantine of all ships coming from the West Indies. In May 1649, "seeing it hath pleased God to stay the sickness," the quarantine order was repealed—to be revived, again for a two-year period, in 1665 when plague was raging in London.[1] As we have seen, this haphazard pattern of quarantine continued into the nineteenth century not only in Boston but in other port cities.

Another area of public concern was care of the sick poor,

including the mentally ill. In New England and New York this was considered a responsibility of town or county government; the physician was paid on an individual case basis. Gradually one physician tended to take over most local cases, and the practice arose of engaging a "town physician" who was paid an annual salary. For those of "poor account" in the Province of Georgia money was voted for "food, apothecaries, drugs, attendance midwife, nurses, burying dead. . . ." [2] In Pennsylvania public funds supplemented public subscription to maintain the Pennsylvania Hospital.

What was probably the first board of health was set up in Petersburg, Virginia, in 1780, and by the turn of the century New York, Baltimore, and Boston had followed suit.

On a federal level, public health services had their beginning in 1798 when President John Adams signed an act establishing the Marine Hospital Service for "the relief of sick and disabled seamen." Hospitals were acquired or erected in various port cities. Originally the service was financed by a deduction of twenty cents a month from the wages of each seaman on all ships docking in American ports. (It has been pointed out that this "was the first prepaid medical care program established in the United States." [3])

THE NATIONAL QUARANTINE AND SANITARY CONVENTIONS

By the 1850s there was general dissatisfaction with such maritime quarantine laws as existed. Merchants and tradesmen were unhappy because of delays in the movement of goods; at the same time the regulations failed adequately to protect port city dwellers; furthermore, practices considered safe in Baltimore were condemned in New Orleans, and so on.

In 1856 Dr. Wilson Jewell (1800–1867), who had several years' experience as a health officer in Philadelphia and who knew the defects of the quarantine laws, proposed to the Philadelphia Board of Health that a national convention be called for the purpose of establishing a uniform set of quarantine laws. On October 29 the board appointed a committee to sound out the attitude of the boards of health of New York, Boston, Baltimore, and New Orleans.

The first convention met in Philadelphia in May 1857. There were seventy-three delegates representing twenty-six authorities in nine states. A second convention was called for the next year in Baltimore; the third, the following year in New York. The fourth was held in Boston in 1860. Cincinnati was to be the next in May 1861, but Fort Sumter intervened in April, and the convention never reassembled.

"Like Peter Pan, the organization never grew up, but twelve years after its last meeting four men who had attended one, two, or all four conventions met in New York with six other men and organized a new public health association. Three of its first five presidents were alumni of the old conventions. To use a favorite allusion of Osler's, perhaps the convention did the Phoenix trick, and, consumed by the fire of war, there rose out of its ashes the great American Public Health Association." [4]

PROGRESS IN SANITATION

In 1850 Lemuel Shattuck (1793–1859), a prime mover in the field of public hygiene in America, brought to the attention of the Massachusetts Sanitary Commission a report by Edwin Chadwick, a member of the British Poor Law Commission, in which the relationship between poverty and disease was discussed. Chadwick blamed the high mortality rate among the city poor directly on "atmospheric impurities produced by decomposing animal and vegetable substances, by damp and filth, and close and overcrowded dwellings." [5] The majority of doctors came to subscribe to the Chadwick theory. Homes, they said, must be well ventilated; refuse must be removed from streets and alleys, streets must be paved, a plentiful supply of pure water must be provided, sewerage must be constructed, damp areas must be drained, and so on. It was an ambitious program that could only be attacked piecemeal. In a first rush of enthusiasm cities began extensively to develop water supplies. From a total of thirty-two waterworks in 1825, the number increased to 162 in 1865, 598 in 1880, and 1878 in 1890. Greater emphasis was put on the number of systems in operation than on the quality of the product, and so great was the belief in the self-purification of running water that it was not until 1871–72 that the first filtration plant was constructed in the United States, at Poughkeepsie, New York. "Whether or not the early waterworks offered protection against infections, they at least promoted cleanliness." [6]

THE AMERICAN PUBLIC HEALTH ASSOCIATION

The American Public Health Association was founded in 1872 and, according to its first president, Stephen Smith (1823–1922), "had its origin in the natural desire which thinkers and workers in the same fields, whether of business or philanthropy, or the administration of civil trusts, have for mutual council, advice and cooperation." [7] An introductory note to the second volume (1874–75) of *Public Health,* the association's publication, put the body's purposes quite succinctly:

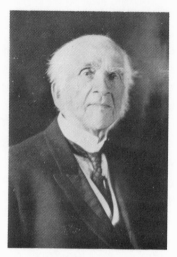

STEPHEN SMITH

The widely expressed interest in public health questions, the tendency to sanitary organization, and to various works for the improvement of public health of cities and large towns, the recognition of inevitable but hitherto neglected relations of hygiene to social progress and human welfare, and the necessity which is now felt for sound legislation and organization of competent sources of advice and authority relating to the protection of the public health in several States, called this Association into existence and now govern its policy.[8]

Prior to 1872 only Massachusetts (1869), California (1871), Virginia (1871), and the District of Columbia (1870) had established state boards of health. In 1873 there was some form of health board in 124 cities in the United States.

On a national level very little had as yet been done. In 1879, in face of an impending yellow-fever epidemic, Congress created a National Board of Health, but it was allowed to pass out of existence four years later. The Marine Hospital Service, which had been established by Congress in 1798, was in no sense a federal health department. It was in existence eighty years before it was finally granted authority to impose quarantines to prevent disease entry from abroad, and another dozen years elapsed before it was given like authority to prevent interstate spreading of disease. (In 1902 its name was changed to the Public Health and Marine Hospital Service, and in 1951 the U.S. Marine Hospitals became U.S. Public Health Service Hospitals.)

Seven years after the Association was founded, Smith said:

Beneficial as has been the work of the Association, and important as are the reforms which it has achieved, it can but be in the infancy of its usefulness. However perfectly our system of public health service may become organized there will always be need of consultation and cooperation among those devoted to official duties, as also the discussion of theoretical and practical subjects by sanitary students.[9]

These words are as appropriate today as they were then.

THE HYGIENIC LABORATORY

In the 1880s a young medical officer of the Marine Hospital Service, Joseph J. Kinyoun (1860–1919), visited European medical centers and watched the great bacteriologists of the day demonstrate their new methods of controlling infectious disease. Back in the United States in 1887, he opened a one-room laboratory (probably the first bacteriological laboratory in the country) at the Marine Hospital on Staten Island,

New York. In the course of his initial year he isolated and observed the cholera organism brought in by immigrants.

In 1891 his laboratory was moved to Washington, D.C., so that his abilities could be made available to others in the service. Things went well at the Hygienic Laboratory, as it came to be known, until Kinyoun correctly identified a 1900 San Francisco epidemic as bubonic plague. An irate community accused the health officer of dishonesty and corruption and brought pressure on Washington through the governor of California. Kinyoun was fired. He was replaced by Milton J. Rosenau (1869–1946), who would make an important contribution to the study of allergic shock reaction to serum (anaphylaxis).

In 1902 Congress created a division of zoology in the Hygienic Laboratory. This allowed the service to undertake research in parasitology. The new division was headed by Charles Wardell Stiles (1867–1941), who held the position for thirty years. In 1947 the division of zoology became the Laboratory of Tropical Disease, a department of the National Institutes of Health, as the Hygienic Laboratory had been reconstituted in 1930.

THE PURE FOOD AND DRUG LAW

The passage of this law in 1906 was the culmination of a long struggle with private commercial interests that claimed the right to sell whatever they wished. Even then, its sphere was restricted to proper labeling, and its inadequacy became apparent with the blossoming of mass advertising. Still the law was not amended to include regulation of advertising until 1938. At the same time cosmetics were brought within its scope.

While all new drugs must receive the stamp of safety from the federal government before being admitted to interstate commerce, the law offers many loopholes and weak points. As Milton I. Riemer of the Public Health Service wrote in 1945, "the greatest abuses of America's drug consumption are due to factors that cannot be legislated away. They depend rather on an inadequate provision of medical care that forces people to resort to the corner drug store as a cheap substitute for medical attention." [10]

The battles for better public health and freedom from infectious diseases are still being fought on many fronts. While improved legislation, education, and enforcement will help, the foundation of success is enlightened public opinion. Without public understanding of the problem, informed action is impossible.

Part V

ADVANCES ON
SEVERAL FRONTS

❧(17)❧

Research on a
Sound Foundation

Writing in 1958, medical historian Morris C. Leikind stated that "the history of research in general and of medical research in particular has still to find its historian." The urgent need for a historian had been voiced before. Speaking at the opening of the William Pepper Laboratory of Clinical Medicine in Philadelphia on December 4, 1894, William H. Welch had pointed out that "the evolution of the modern laboratory still awaits its historian." In 1946 psychiatrist and historian Iago Galdston wrote an article titled: "Wanted—a History of Research." Though Richard H. Shryock's *American Medical Research Past and Present,* which appeared in 1947, was "a most useful introduction to the history of the subject," it did not answer "the plea of Dr. Welch and Dr. Galdston . . . in a satisfactory fashion." [1]

There has been understandable confusion and disagreement as to what constitutes medical research and when it began. Shryock says, "Without any attempt at exact definition, it can be said that the word [research] means a more or less systematic investigation of phenomena intended to add to the sum total of verifiable knowledge." [2] Leikind accepts this definition.

Writing in 1876 of American medicine during the hundred years that had elapsed since the birth of the United States, Professor Edward H. Clarke (1820–1877) of Harvard cautioned: ". . . let us remember that a large amount of scientific work cannot justly be expected of the medical profession in a new country. When the nation had acquired its independence, its population extended along a narrow coast-line from what was then known as Massachusetts, now Maine, to Georgia. The inhabitants had the Atlantic Ocean in front of them, and in their rear the unexplored forests, filled with aborigines that stretched far away towards the Pacific. As a matter of necessity they were obliged to occupy themselves almost exclusively with the task of obtaining a secure existence in a new country. For the first fifty years of the nation's life, the necessities of the present left little leisure for the cultivation of the arts and sciences. The medical profession were compelled by their position to devote themselves exclusively to the practice of their profession and to leave scientific investigation and discovery to a later period. There was no superabundance of educated physicians." [3]

The well-known Philadelphia physician Samuel Jackson (1790–1872), addressing the 1840 graduating class of medical students at the University of Pennsylvania, spoke favorably of contemporary German research and then declared: "Not one man is now considering similar studies in the United States." He ascribed this inertia to a "commercial spirit" that offered the true scientist neither income nor prestige, reward being chiefly measured in financial terms.[4]

In the opinion of Dr. Henry E. Sigerist, "Whoever gave up money-making to live for science was considered a crank. . . . An American of that day missed beyond everything else intellectual resonance, a mutual reverberation of ideas." [5] Leikind says it was the "tradition of learning" that was lacking. "The isolated investigators [such as Beaumont and Drake] who did make major contributions were so few as to be almost the exception to prove the rule." [6]

THE SMITHSONIAN INSTITUTION

In 1835 the United States Legation in London had been informed that James Smithson (1765–1829), an accomplished British chemist and mineralogist, had willed his entire fortune, slightly in excess of $500,000, "to the United States of America to found at Washington, under the name of the Smithsonian Institution, an establishment for the increase and diffusion of knowledge among men." [7]

Nobody knows why Smithson made this extravagant gesture, but speculation has run in at least two directions. It has been conjectured that Smithson was acquainted with the American poet and diplomat Joel Barlow (1754–1812) and had learned of his plan to carry out at the nation's capital the project outlined by George Washington in his Farewell Address: "Promote, then, as an object of primary importance, institutions for the general diffusion of knowledge: in proportion as the structure of a government gives force to public opinion, it is essential that public opinion should be enlightened." [8] Or it may be that Smithson felt that the needs of England were well met and acted to express his faith in a poor but growing nation. However motivated, the bequest was a generous one.

Acceptance of the bequest was rigorously opposed in Congress by Senator John Caldwell Calhoun (1782–1850), who insisted that it was beneath the dignity of the United States to accept presents. Three years elapsed before the thoughtful and persuasive arguments of Representative John Quincy Adams (1767–1848) prevailed. On September 1, 1838, the proceeds of the legacy were delivered to the Philadelphia mint. Then it took another eight years for the nation's leaders to decide what to do with the money. Finally, the Smithsonian Institution was formally established by act of Congress on August 10, 1846.

Now scientific research had substantial financial backing, and under the leadership of Dr. Joseph Henry (1797–1878), the Smithsonian's first secretary, and his successors, the institution began to foster research and disseminate the results. The fledgling institution, animated by three major ideas —record, research, and education—had a profound influence on the growth and effectiveness of science throughout America. Medicine was not a direct beneficiary under Smithson's will, but the institution's work in general science encouraged the advancement of medical research.

THE ROCKEFELLER INSTITUTE FOR MEDICAL RESEARCH

The American scene changed radically with the founding by John D. Rockefeller in 1901 of the Rockefeller Institute for Medical Research. According to Simon Flexner, who gave up the chair of pathology at the University of Pennsylvania to become the first director of the institute:

> The Rockefeller Institute for Medical Research was conceived not by physicians or scientists, but rather by laymen who studied the state of medical knowledge at the end of the nineteenth century and concluded that the time was favorable for the establishment in the United States of an institute devoted exclusively to medical research, just as institutions devoted to physical or chemical research might be founded.[9]

John D. Rockefeller (1839–1937) was born on a farm in Tioga County, New York, and grew up in Cleveland. By the age of twenty-five he was a respected businessman. When he retired in 1911, an oil magnate, he was considered the richest man in the world.

Rockefeller regarded charity as a dictate of conscience, a serious responsibility. By 1891 his philanthropic activities were absorbing so much of his time that he was forced to place their conduct in the hands of Frederick T. Gates, who had been secretary of the American Baptist Education Society. Rockefeller described Gates as "the guiding genius in all our giving. He combines business skill and philanthropic aptitude to a higher degree than any other man I have ever known." [10]

Among the first acts of this new partnership was the founding of the University of Chicago, which would assume a position of leadership in higher education and research. (By 1910 Rockefeller had contributed $35,000,000.)

The Institute for Medical Research was conceived in 1901. At about the same time Rockefeller and Gates extended their interest to education at large. The General Education Board was incorporated in 1903 and within six years had received $53,000,000, of which more than $13,000,000 went to Chicago, $10,000,000 to the Rockefeller Institute for Medical Research, and $16,000,000 to medical schools, college endowments, Negro education, and like projects. In 1909 Rockefeller and Gates conceived the idea of a Rockefeller Foundation designed to contribute to the well-being of mankind throughout the world, but, because of extreme opposition (largely unrelated to philanthropy), incorporation was not accomplished until 1913.

Rockefeller was not the only wealthy man to engage in multimillion-dollar philanthropy. His institute was followed in 1902 by the Andrew Carnegie Institution of Washington, which, while primarily concerned with the physical sciences, gave some funds to such fields as embryology and nutrition; and by the John McCormick Institute of Infectious Diseases in Chicago. The activities of Rockefeller, Carnegie, and McCormick attracted the interest of other wealthy men. Such names as Morgan, Stanford, Sage, Guggenheim, Havemeyer, Bamberger, Huntington, Rosenwald, and Duke have become associated in the public mind with giving. "This was a period when medicine, offering new hope, captivated the imagination of wealthy benefactors somewhat as religion had once done in a less secular age. Instead of building churches and monasteries, philanthropists now endowed hospitals and laboratories or set up foundations to do this for them." [11]

The Rockefeller Institute, while conceived by laymen, was created by a group of scientists—William H. Welch of Hopkins; pathologist T. Mitchell Prudden (1849–1924); pediatrician and infant nutritionist L. Emmett Holt (1855–

1924); bacteriologist and epidemiologist Theobald Smith (1859–1934); biologist Christian A. Herter (1865–1910); public health pioneer Herman M. Biggs (1859–1923); and Simon Flexner.

The purposes of the institute, which have continued unchanged, were "to conduct, assist and encourage investigations in the sciences and arts of hygiene, medicine and surgery, and allied subjects, in the nature and causes of disease and the methods of its prevention and treatment, and to make knowledge relating to these various subjects available for the protection of the health of the public and the improved treatment of disease and injury." [12] The first step was the opening of a laboratory.

In the progressive view of the day, medicine's great hope lay in an experimental approach to clinical problems. Areas immediately under study included pathology and bacteriology, physiology and pharmacology, biological chemistry, and experimental surgery. To extend fundamental studies clinically "under conditions as near as possible to standards of laboratory exactness and efficiency," a hospital unit was added in 1910.[13] In 1916 a department of animal pathology under Theobald Smith was established three miles from Princeton University. This department, and the department of plant pathology created in 1931, were brought into the parent laboratory in New York in 1950.

The achievements of the scientists working at the Rockefeller Institute during the first half of the twentieth century covered a wide range. Among these were the effective study of epidemic cerebro-spinal meningitis, with the experimental production of the disease in monkeys, and the development by Simon Flexner and James W. Jobling (1876–1961) of an antimeningococcic horse serum (1905), which was regarded as most helpful until the introduction of the sulfonamides thirty years later; the program of bacterial and pathologic research into poliomyelitis begun in 1907 and continued for thirty years; the work of Alexis Carrel (1873–1944), the father of organ transplantation, on culturing living cells, tissues, and organs; the investigations (until his death from yellow fever in Africa) of Hideyo Noguchi (1876–1928) in the areas of syphilis, yellow fever, Oroya fever, and trachoma; the work of Peyton Rous (1879–1970) on malignant tumors produced by a filterable virus; the study of the influenza virus, begun at the time of the 1917–18 pandemic; the work of Rufus Cole and Oswald T. Avery on pneumococci; the work of Homer Swift (1881–1953) and Alfred Cohn (1879–1957) on rheumatic fever and heart disease; the studies of living processes undertaken by Jacques Loeb (1859–1924).

Simon Flexner, the first director of the Institute, retired in 1935 and was succeeded by Dr. Herbert S. Gasser (1888–1963), who served until 1953. Under his stewardship the research continued to grow in breadth and volume until its influence on research in general, the training of investigators, and the medical progress of the nation was inestimable.

THE NATIONAL FOUNDATION FOR INFANTILE PARALYSIS (NFIP)

The Rockefeller Institute and Foundation and similar institutions have essentially, and providentially, made research possible in many areas of medicine. Still other foundations and associations, philanthropically supported, direct their efforts toward a single disease or organ—the National Tuberculosis Association, the American Cancer Society, the American Heart

Association, and the National Foundation for Infantile Paralysis (since 1969 the National Foundation).

Of these, the last is probably the best known because of the publicity that attended its activities from its inception in 1938 to the Salk-Sabin polio-vaccine dispute in the 1960s. The other associations have been more conservative in making claims and less spectacular and flamboyant in their pronouncements. Each has made substantial progress toward the control and eradication of its specific disease.

The National Foundation for Infantile Paralysis was an outgrowth of the Warm Springs Foundation, which maintained a treatment center for polio victims in Warm Springs, Georgia. A frequent visitor was Governor Franklin D. Roosevelt of New York, a victim of the disease, who had helped organize the foundation.

By 1934 the Warm Springs Foundation was in financial trouble, and it was decided to raise funds by soliciting contributions from the public—a method that had proved successful for the National Tuberculosis Association. The accession of Roosevelt to the presidency that year provided a focus for the fund-raising campaign. A series of balls were planned in various cities to celebrate his birthday and raise funds at the same time. The first balls were held on January 30, 1934, and were successful. The Birthday Ball Commission allocated some of the funds for research. Its first grants to medical investigators were made in 1935—sixteen of them, totaling close to a quarter of a million dollars.

When the balls in 1935 and 1936 proved disappointing, other means of financing research had to be found. The solution was the National Foundation for Infantile Paralysis, which would be supported by appealing directly to the people for small contributions. At the head of it was Basil O'Connor, Roosevelt's former law partner, who had been active in the Warm Springs Foundation and the Birthday Commission.

For the years 1938 through 1962 the foundation raised roughly $630,000,000. The largest portion of this income (59 per cent) was spent on medical care for polio victims; 8 per cent went for educational programs, 13 per cent ($80,-000,000) for fund-raising, and 9 per cent for administration. The remaining 11 per cent ($69,000,000) was set aside for research.

Thomas M. Rivers (1888–1962) came from the hospital of the Rockefeller Institute to head the National Foundation's Committee on Scientific Research. At the first meeting of his committee, in July 1938, unsolved problems were enumerated and priorities established. "And yet in the early 1940s an uneasy feeling prevailed among clinical investigators that the home and the fountainhead of this disease had somehow been removed to chromium-plated headquarters at 120 Broadway in downtown New York City, quite remote from the hospital wards with all their worries and activities, not to speak of the background grinding noises of respirators known then as iron lungs, which were a constant source of sweat and tears." [14]

Whatever the reaction of workers in the field, the public viewed the foundation as an organization equipped and ready to lead the fight against poliomyelitis, providing financial funds where needed.

After World War II medical research increased remarkably, with the government contributing much of the funding, especially through its National Institutes of Health. This has had far-reaching effects both on medical education and practice, to the extent that, during the late 1960s, physicians and administrators began to fear that the balance between education, practice, and research was being destroyed. This has led in part to the dramatic cutbacks in the support of medical research that occurred in 1971 and 1972. Only time will show if the pendulum has swung too far.

$\{(18)\}$

The Fight against Polio

Poliomyelitis (infantile paralysis) is a contagious, epidemic viral infection, often resulting in sudden paralysis, that affects infants, children, even adolescents, and occasionally young adults. The first epidemic in the United States hit Vermont in 1894. Of 132 cases, the largest number in any one year anywhere in the world, ninety were in the under-three age group, twenty were between nine and twelve.

The Bible and Homeric literature speak frequently of lameness or a withered limb in a child, but the references are too brief to permit the pinpointing of poliomyelitis as the cause. An Egyptian stele dating from B.C. 1580–1350 depicts a deformity characteristic of poliomyelitis, but a case can hardly be made from an isolated depiction.

If poliomyelitis existed in Greek times, it was not epidemic. Hippocrates did not describe it in his *Of the Epidemics,* though he spoke elsewhere of crooked legs crippled by disease occurring in an advanced period of youth. Paralytic poliomyelitis was not described with any degree of accuracy until the end of the eighteenth century.

It was a London physician who specialized in obstetrics and pediatrics, Michael Underwood (1738–c.1810), who recognized a relationship between fever and the onset of lameness. In the first American edition (1793) of his *Treatise on Diseases of Children* he wrote of a disorder that "seems to arise from debility, and usually attacks children previously reduced by fever; seldom those under one, or more than four or five years old." [1] The *Treatise* ran through twenty-five editions, including several American and German ones, and Underwood progressively clarified the picture as his clinical experience increased. His findings must have come to the attention of many physicians in Europe and America, but few took advantage of them. The same was true of the *Istituzioni Chirurgiche* of Giovanni Battista Monteggia (1762–1815) of Milan, the second edition (1813) of which contained a detailed and accurate description of poliomyelitis.

The beginning of the breakthrough came in 1840 when the German orthopedist Jacob von Heine (1800–1879) published a monograph that offered the fruits of a meticulous, systematic, discerning, personal investigation. Von Heine concluded that the total symptomatic picture pointed to an infection of the central nervous system involving the spinal cord. The word "poliomyelitis" comes from the Greek and means "inflammation of the gray matter of the spinal cord."

In 1886 Mary Putnam Jacobi (1842–1906), then professor of therapeutics at the Woman's Medical College of New York, wrote an article covering all medical knowledge of poliomyelitis to date. The evidence "led, not unnaturally, to the theory that all cases of acute infantile paralysis are due to a specific infecting agent, some as yet unknown member of the great class of pathogenic bacteria." [2] Toward the end of 1908 Karl Landsteiner (1868–1943) of Vienna (who would join the Rockefeller Institute in 1922) showed on microscopic slides of the spinal cords of a human and two monkeys typical poliomyelitis lesions. The two monkeys had been injected with bacteriologically sterile material obtained from the spinal cord of the fatal human case. Within a year he had confirmed the assumption that poliomyelitis was caused by a virus.

Almost from the time that acute poliomyelitis was accepted as a distinct disease, the possibility that polio could be prevented through immunization attracted the attention of experimenters. Simon Flexner was quick to grasp the implications of Landsteiner's work. It was thought that polio would yield to research methods similar to those used in the successful attack on meningococcal meningitis. Although Flexner made pioneer contributions in the field of experimental poliomyelitis, among them his discovery of polio-virus antibodies, his early hopes were not realized.

Flexner and Paul A. Lewis (1879–1929) were the first to produce active immunity in monkeys (1910), but their results were irregular and the technique was hazardous. A dozen years later, with Harold L. Amoss (1886–1956), a nonfatal form of the experimental disease in monkeys was achieved. It provided immunity to subsequent inoculations of a more virulent strain, but injections of live polio virus proved risky. (If in the 1920s a different species of monkey had been used and the virus administered orally the outcome might have been different.) [3]

In 1935 there were two ill-fated vaccine trials. Dr. Maurice Brodie, originally from Montreal, working with William H.

Park of the New York City Health Laboratory, inoculated three thousand children. The vaccine they used had been tried on only twenty monkeys, none of which showed any harmful effects; Brodie had also tried it on himself. Several children, however, came down with polio and one died.

John A. Kolmer (1886–1962) of Philadelphia was more conservative. He tested his immunizing procedure on forty-two monkeys, then on two adults, himself included, his two children (aged eleven and fifteen), and on twenty-two other children. Some thousands of children were then given the vaccine. At a meeting in St. Louis in November 1935 James P. Leake of the Public Health Service criticized Kolmer's activities. After mentioning twelve cases, six of them fatal, Dr. Leake concluded: "Paralytic poliomyelitis was not epidemic in any of the localities at the time of the occurrence of these cases. . . . The likelihood of whole series of cases having occurred through natural causes is extremely small. Although any one of these cases may have been entirely unconnected with the vaccine the implication of the series as a whole is clear." [4]

The effect on the scientific world of the Brodie and Kolmer experiences was a wave of revulsion against human vaccination that persisted for many years.

When the National Foundation for Infantile Paralysis was founded in 1938, there was still not much basic scientific knowledge on the disease, and to overcome this the foundation allocated funds to interested investigators. In 1948 the foundation financed a program to type the various strains of polio virus. This was later described as "the greatest single piece of developmental research that the NFIP was to accomplish during the years of its existence" [5] since it automatically opened the way to all subsequent developmental projects. Hitherto, in preparing vaccines, the mixture of virus strains was largely ignored. The Committee on Typing and Strains (which included Jonas E. Salk and Albert B. Sabin) started with 250 strains of polio virus of unknown type from different geographic areas and different parts of the bodies of the subjects. These strains were reduced to 100 (86 per cent from the United States and the rest from around the world) and later increased to 196. In 1953 the committee announced that the strains could be classified into three types (I, II, and III), in the ratio of 82.1 per cent to 10.2 per cent to 7.7 per cent. The success of this undertaking gave the foundation the confidence to go on.

The Committee on Immunization, formed in 1951, was found to be too cumbersome, and in 1953 a smaller Vaccine Advisory Committee was set up. Two types of vaccine were possible: an inactivated vaccine, such as Jonas Salk was working on, which uses a virus that has been killed, usually by chemical means (formalin in the case of Salk); and an attenuated vaccine, which uses living infectious virus considerably weakened in strength.

Jonas Salk, born in New York City in 1914, began his work in virology in the field of influenza. Here he revealed himself as a resourceful, independent research worker, and he became expert on the technicalities of vaccine production and evaluation. It was not therefore surprising to find him assuming a position of leadership in the typing program or for the foundation to recognize in him a keen young man who knew his business and with whom it could work.

On July 2, 1952, Salk inoculated thirty children at the D. T. Watson Home for Crippled Children in Leetsdale, Pennsylvania. He was taking a minimal risk because the subjects were all afflicted with polio-related paralysis and were therefore immune. Salk's objective was to find out if his inactivated vaccine would raise the antibody level. If this occurred it would be a sign that his vaccine could cause poliomyelitis. There were no bad reactions. By the following January, Salk had inoculated ninety-eight subjects at the home and sixty-three at Polk State School—there were no convalescent poliomyelitis patients among them. In subsequent months he advanced the total of inoculated children to around five thousand.

Meanwhile two investigators, Herald Cox and Hilary Koprowski, were working on an attenuated vaccine for Lederle, a division of American Cyanamid Company, and the foundation was anxious to be first. The Vaccine Advisory Committee committed itself to the Salk vaccine and began preparations with pharmaceutical houses for the manufacture of the Salk vaccine for use in field trials.

Although the foundation continued to support research on the attenuated vaccine, "it would have been inadvisable to postpone the inactivated vaccine until the other approach had produced more solid evidence of its safety and effectiveness." [6]

Dr. Thomas Francis, Jr., chairman of the Department of Epidemiology at the University of Michigan's School of Public Health, was invited to take charge of nationwide field trials. He accepted, subject to the provisions that the children involved should be divided into two groups, one to be injected with an inert solution (placebo) as a control group; that the two groups be followed identically; and that there be absolutely no interference by the foundation. The children participating in the field trial, which began on April 26, 1954, were first, second, and third graders. Dr. Francis spent nearly a year evaluating the results. On April 12, 1955, he stated positively that the vaccine developed by Dr. Salk was a success: ". . . extensive examination of available data [essentially complete] has yielded no evidence that cases of poliomyelitis attributable to the inoculation of vaccine occurred during the 1954 Field Trials." [7]

The controversy over live- versus killed-virus vaccine continued nevertheless. Sabin, supported by the foundation, had begun to work seriously on an attenuated vaccine in 1953, and in a few years developed an oral vaccine. From 1957 to 1959 his vaccine received extensive field testing in the Soviet Union, Czechoslovakia, Mexico, and Singapore. In July 1959 the Vaccine Advisory Committee "praised the new Sabin vaccine, . . ." but believed "it would be unwise to embark at this time upon mass vaccination . . . in the United States." [8]

In 1961 the U.S. Public Health Service licensed the Sabin vaccine. This cleared the way for the manufacture of the oral vaccine and was viewed as an official replacement of the Salk vaccine. An editorial in the *Journal of the American Medical Association* summed up the situation:

> This has become a highly controversial and emotionally charged field, and it is difficult to get agreement, even in small groups, as to the indications for use of the oral vaccine under this or that circumstance. On the one hand, it would seem that in those countries where the killed Salk-type vaccine has not been widely and successfully used, there is little question as to the desirability of the immediate introduction of the oral polio-virus vaccine. On the other hand, in those countries where a well-established program entailing the use of the Salk-type inactivated polio-virus vaccine has been successful, there may be a real

question as to whether an immediate switch to the oral vaccine is indicated. Undue haste is always undesirable." [9]

Once the effectiveness of the oral vaccine was proved it seemingly had some advantages over the Salk vaccine, which had to be injected. It was easier to administer. It produced immunity more promptly. The immunity produced was believed to last longer. It was effective in halting incipient epidemics. In any event, by 1963 the Sabin-vaccine had become the vaccine of choice in the United States.

Though it is generally believed that "to all intents and purposes the disease has been conquered, . . . in the developing countries of the world this is not the case, and it is clear that a new array of techniques and approaches, administrative and otherwise, will have to be found." [10]

⟨ 19 ⟩

Investigation of
the Brain

THE DEVELOPMENT OF NEUROSURGERY

Three discoveries of the nineteenth century made neuro-surgery possible: "anesthesia (1846), asepsis (1865), and cerebral localization. Without asepsis (or antisepsis) surgery of the brain would never be possible. With asepsis and without cerebral localization, it could be of little value. With both asepsis and cerebral localization and without anesthesia, it would be possible but greatly limited." [1]

Other factors have been the discovery of the roentgen ray by Wilhelm Conrad Roentgen (1895); the numerous technical devices introduced and the clinicopathological entities elaborated upon by Harvey Cushing during a long and fruitful career (1901 to 1939); the revolutionary method of identifying and localizing brain lesions by means of cerebral aerography instituted by Walter Dandy (1918), and the histological classification of the cerebral gliomas by Percival Bailey and their clinical correlation by Cushing (1925).[2]

Although phrenologists Franz Josef Gall and Johann Caspar Spurzheim had in a four-volume work (1810–19) adumbrated the concept of cerebral localization, it was Paul Broca (1824–1880), the French founder of modern surgery of the brain, who in 1861 first dealt with the idea scientifically. In his concept the center of articulate speech was localized in the third left frontal convolution. On this basis, Broca concluded that a patient suffering from what he termed *aphemia* or *motor aphasia* (loss of speech due to impairment of the word-memory center) had a cerebral abscess, which he located and removed. Broca's work led to a systematic mapping of the various areas of the brain on the basis of their function, an approach fundamental to successful brain surgery.

In 1870 Gustav Fritsch (1836–1897) and Eduard Hitzig (1838–1907), by applying an electric current to isolated points on the exposed brain of a dog, showed that local bodily movements and convulsions can be produced by stimulation of definite areas of the brain (always identical in animals of the same species) and that removal of these areas produced paralysis or loss of function in corresponding parts of the body. Sir David Ferrier (1843–1928) extended their investigation to mammals, birds, frogs, fishes, and other creatures; he inferred that the human brain had similar properties.

Robert Bartholow (1831–1904) of Cincinnati was the first actually to extend the investigation to the human brain. Bartholow had an opportunity for clinical investigation similar to that of Beaumont a half-century earlier. In 1874 he had under his care a patient with a large cranial defect that exposed parts of each cerebral hemisphere. Bartholow was able to stimulate the brain and observe reactions, experiments that, unfortunately, were cut short by the patient's death from meningitis. Seventy-four cases of cortical stimulation of the exposed human brain were reported during the next thirty years.

Lister's introduction of the antiseptic principle reduced the hazards of surgery. By the 1880s removal of brain tumors had become frequent if not commonplace. In 1886 England's Sir Victor Horsley (1857–1916) reported ten operations; two years later Sir William Macewen (1848–1924) of Scotland announced that he had undertaken twenty-one brain operations with eighteen recoveries. The same year William Williams Keen (1837–1932) of Philadelphia, pioneer American neurosurgeon, successfully removed a tumor at the junction of the spinal cord and the brain—the patient survived for thirty years. In 1891 Keen reported five additional cerebral operations.

The results reported by Horsley, Macewen, Keen, and others were promising. In the next half-century through the work of Harvey Cushing (1869–1939), knowledge of the nervous system and surgical techniques were vastly increased.

Harvey Cushing's "early interest in brain surgery cannot be attributed to any given circumstance or to a particular personality, but it is possible to trace the growth of the interest during the years of training." [3]

Cushing had done his undergraduate work at Yale, where, in 1890, he had removed a dog's brain and dissected the cranial nerves of a frog for George T. Ladd, professor of mental and moral philosophy.

In his senior year Cushing took a course in physiological

chemistry with Russell H. Chittenden (1856–1944); this "really stirred him and centered his energies on the study of medicine." On March 22, 1891, Cushing wrote to his father: "Prof. Ladd wants me to come back next year and go on with the work [with Chittenden]. We have just been working on the Chemistry of the tissues and are now working on brain tissue which we will about finish by Easter." In April, Chittenden offered him a position as assistant in the laboratory if he would come back for a graduate year, but Cushing turned this down and went on to the Harvard Medical School.[4]

Here Cushing was fascinated by the physiology of the nervous sytem, for which his lecture notes were "particularly full, and one finds him redrawing diagrams of the brain in which indication is given of the motor area as it was understood in those days." [5] In his second year a large part of his time was spent administering ether for John Wheelock ("Jack") Elliot (1852–1925), who was interested in cerebral localization as a result of having met Horsley in England in 1889. Elliot asked his colleagues to turn over to him any cases of brain tumor that might come their way, but not until 1895 did he have the opportunity successfully to operate on an intracranial tumor.

During the summer after graduation Cushing assisted Elliot at two such operations, noting on the back of one case history: "Elliot never had less bleeding in opening [a] skull." Later he spoke of Elliot as "one of the most brilliant and daring surgeons of his day, [who] ventured twice to trephine the skull for tumors involving the brain." [6]

After graduation in 1895 Cushing served as a house pupil at Massachusetts General Hospital from 1895 to 1896. During this year he helped launch the clinical use of X-rays. On February 15, 1896, he wrote to his mother: "Everyone is much excited over the new photographic discovery. Professor Röntgen may have discovered something with his cathode rays which may revolutionize medical diagnosis. Imagine taking photographs of gall stones in situ—stone in the bladder—foreign bodies anywhere—fractures &c &c." On May 10 he informed her: "We have at last succeeded in having an X-ray machine put in." [7]

Cushing had his mind set on a residency in general surgery at Johns Hopkins Hospital, and after some uncertainties he received a place on Halsted's service, effective October 1896. Later that year he set up an X-ray unit there. In May 1897 he made a first formal report to the Johns Hopkins Medical Society on the successful use of X-rays, based on two neurological cases of gunshot wounds of spine.

In his four years under Halsted, Cushing was introduced to a new type of surgery: absolute control of bleeding, painstaking care in the handling of tissue, slow deliberate technique. Cushing himself became an advocate of careful, diligent surgery, clearly an essential approach in brain operations.

The turn of the century found Cushing drawn more and more into the neurological field. He began concentrating on disorders of the central nervous system; he himself wrote careful histories of cases instead of leaving them to junior house officers. In April 1900, at the invitation of Dr. Keen, he presented to a joint meeting of the Philadelphia Neurological Society and the College of Physicians a paper on the surgical relief of severe facial pain. While the procedure was originally suggested by the Philadelphia neurologist William G. Spiller (1863–1940) and developed by a number of his contemporaries, Cushing's paper was an important landmark in the history of neurosurgery because of its unusual detail and because of the admirable illustrations he prepared.[8]

Following his residency, Cushing went abroad for fourteen months. He planned to study with such men as Theodor Kocher (1841–1917) of the University of Berne, acknowledged at the time to be the foremost surgeon in Europe, whose treatise on lesions of the spinal cord had served Cushing as a handbook in such cases; Victor Horsley of University College Hospital, London, considered to be at the height of his career; and Charles Scott Sherrington (1857–1952), then occupying the chair of physiology at Liverpool, whose fundamental investigations of the nervous system would earn him a Nobel prize in 1932.

Cushing arrived in London on July 3, 1900, and was invited to breakfast with the Horsley family the following morning. "He found Horsley living in seemingly great confusion; dictating letters during breakfast to a male secretary; patting dogs between letters; and operating like a wild man. [Cushing] gave him a reprint of his paper on the Gasserian ganglion, whereupon Horsley said he would show him how to do a case. They drove off the next morning in Horsley's cab, after sterilizing the instruments in [the] house and, packing them in a towel, went to a well-appointed West End mansion. Horsley dashed upstairs, had his patient under ether in five minutes, and was operating fifteen minutes after he entered the house; made a great hole in the woman's skull, pushed up the temporal lobe—blood everywhere, gauze packed into the middle fossa, the ganglion cut, the wound closed, and he was out of the house less than an hour after he had entered it. This experience settled [Cushing's] decision to leave London; for he felt that the refinements of neurological surgery could not be learned from Horsley." [9]

After a slow, instructive progress through France, Cushing reached Switzerland at the end of October. In Berne he divided his time between experimental work in the laboratory of Hugo Kronecker (1839–1914), professor of physiology at the University of Berne, and Theodor Kocher's clinic. Cushing asked Kocher for a problem to work on. Kocher agreed but took three weeks to produce one, by which time Cushing had about decided to go on to Heidelberg. The problem involved intracranial pressures—valuable information for a would-be neurosurgeon. Within an incredibly brief space of time Cushing assembled a body of highly significant data.

Cushing went next to Italy, primarily to visit Angelo Mosso (1846–1910) of Turin, a gifted physiologist whose major investigations involved fatigue, circulation, and respiration. Mosso was also interested in cerebral circulation and the temperature of the brain and had studied a group of individuals with bony defects of the skull. At Mosso's "asylum" Cushing "made the acquaintance of a few hundred crazy people, among whom was a man with a hole in his skull." [10] His observations led him to conclude that there must be a reciprocal relation between the vasomotor nerves of the body as a whole and those of the head.

On July 7, 1901, Cushing reached Liverpool, where he was to work with Sherrington. On the 14th he wrote to his father:

> I have been having the most curious experiences during the past three days. I never expected to be called upon

298

to trephine a gorilla but yesterday had that extraordinary experience. Sherrington has been going over the old cortical localization observations with some new methods and on the higher apes and seems to be finding some new things of considerable importance. I happen to have come just in time to see the work and to be of some assistance. In fact it takes many hands. Yesterday seven of us worked from two in the afternoon until ten in the evening in a hothouse room over the hardest kind of application—concentrated observation. I'm glad however that I do not have to take the responsibility of sacrificing these poor hairy *ape-like-men,* for such they seem.

Thursday a chimpanzee—Friday an orang-utang—yesterday a gorilla. Pretty expensive research is it not? The gorilla cost over $1000. . . .[11]

"Cushing had turned up at a psychological moment in Sherrington's epic research, for there was probably no one anywhere in the world better qualified to make a surgical exposure of an anthropoid brain than he. . . . Sherrington was grateful not only for the surgical assistance which Cushing gave, but also for the remarkably clear drawings of the anthropoid brain which Sherrington later used when he [and his assistant] came to report their results." [12]

Cushing returned to Johns Hopkins in 1901. He was to have the neurological side of the clinic. "I must work in the neurological dispensary mornings with Dr. Thomas," he wrote, "and try to learn something in general about nerve cases—then I will have entry into the wards to see the house cases and one clinic a week with the 4th year surgical group on this material and a chance to operate on them once a week." [13]

Throughout his teaching career he advised medical students and house officers that their first objective should be to become good physicians. If they had a bent for neurological surgery, they must first become proficient in general surgery. They must be as much "at home" in the abdomen as in the head. "And so in his own career he started as a general surgeon, and continued to operate in the wider field long after he had begun to concentrate on the brain and the spinal cord." [14]

In 1903 Cushing reported his first successful case of regeneration of the motor nerves of the face. In 1904, in an address before the Academy of Medicine in Cleveland, he attempted "to formulate some personal views concerning a branch of surgery [neurological] which, in this country at least, largely owing to the allurement of other and more promising fields of operative endeavor, has hardly received the attention it deserves." [15] In 1905 he produced several chapters and diagrams for that year's edition of Osler's *Principles and Practice of Medicine.* In 1906–1907 he contributed a 276-page monograph with 154 illustrations to William Williams Keen's *System of Surgery.*

Between 1900 and 1908 Cushing succeeded in making brain surgery a recognized specialty. He began with decompressive procedures for the relief of increased intracranial tension and operations on the Gasserian ganglion (the mass of nervous tissue that supplies the ophthalmic, maxillary, and mandibular nerves). On February 21, 1902, he undertook his first brain operation. During 1902 and 1903 he did seven operations for intracranial tumor; 1904 saw four more such cases, 1905 eight, 1906 and 1907 ten in each year. At first his mortality rates were so high that he was often discouraged and sometimes questioned whether he was justified in proceeding, but in time his successes outweighed his failures. In 1908 surgery of the pituitary gland at the base of the brain began actively to engage his attention.

Cushing remained at Johns Hopkins until 1911, when he was called to Harvard as professor of surgery. He was the "first to devote himself entirely to the surgical problems of the nervous system. . . . He trained surgeons from all parts of the world and carried out research on the pituitary, intracranial tumors, and many other problems, as well as introducing revolutionary surgical procedures." [16]

Working under Cushing, Walter Edward Dandy (1886–1946), who received his M.D. degree at Johns Hopkins in 1910, and Kenneth Daniel Blackfan (1883–1941), established the site of formation of cerebrospinal fluid and its circulation. This information was vital to neurosurgery.

In 1918 Dandy introduced ventriculography or cerebral aerography, a method of X-raying the brain by injection of air into the spinal cord.

Percival Bailey worked with Cushing at Harvard on the classification of cerebral tumors from 1919 to 1928. Their *A Classification of Tumors of the Glioma Group* was published in 1926.

NEUROPSYCHIATRY

The first successful removal of a spinal tumor, in 1887, brought "a cry of outrage from the medical establishment. Horsley had gone too far, it was said, in encroaching on the canal that carried the spinal cord. When operations of the head were performed in increasing numbers they dealt at first only with clots of blood, abscesses, tumour, or cranial nerves. The ethics of such ventures were hardly in doubt, though the early results were so poor that they were greeted with considerable and not always surreptitious cynicism. It was after the introduction of prefrontal leucotomy [lobotomy] that the ethical controversy really got under way. Here was a deliberate intervention directed at changing the individual's mentality by a physical operation on the brain." [17]

The brain is, of course, the physical organ of the mind. With neurosurgeons successfully excising brain tumors, why should attention not be turned to that part of the brain responsible for mental illness? Certainly little else was being done for the mentally ill. By the 1870s the humanitarian efforts of Dorothea Dix (1802–1887) to get the insane out of the poorhouse, the county home, and the private home and into the newly constructed asylums were counteracted by the conditions in these hospitals. Patient populations of a thousand or more, "personnel problems, budgetary difficulties, . . . overcrowding, the large proportion of chronic cases, and a dogmatic depersonalized theoretical orientation to insanity led to . . . therapeutic nihilism. Hospitals became more isolated from the general medical community, and often hospital management could clearly be characterized as inhumanity and neglect." [18] The decline in recoveries that began in the final quarter of the nineteenth century continued into the twentieth. "Out-of-mind, out-of-sight, typified the obscured public visibility of the mentally ill." [19]

In 1935, working at Yale, John Farquhar Fulton (1899–1960), Sterling professor of physiology, and Carlyle F. Jacobsen, assistant professor, observed that primates who had undergone a bilateral prefrontal lobotomy were not easily made neurotic by the presentation of difficult problems. About the same time Egas Moniz (1874–1955) of Portugal was undertaking his first prefrontal lobotomy. A paper he published in Paris in 1936 reported twenty cases on which he had operated with good results. Walter Jackson Freeman of California and James Winston Watts of Washington, D.C., popularized the procedure in the United States. The prefrontal lobotomy was widely practiced till the advent of tranquilizers in 1952. Since then it has been the general opinion of psychiatrists that the risks of such surgery far outweigh the anticipated benefits, especially since the damage is not reversible.

The early 1930s saw the adoption of another approach —convulsive or shock therapies, also known as assault therapies. Actually, as far back as 1785 a certain W. Oliver reported that convulsions produced by camphor had a therapeutic effect on psychiatric patients. A century and a half later, psychiatrists observed that patients who developed spontaneous convulsions, as in high fevers, seemed to become less depressed.

Shock therapy throws the body into a brief convulsion. No one knows why the treatment helps, but it often does. It may be that "shock turns off the mind and stops the patient from thinking about whatever it is that he is preoccupied with"; or perhaps it shakes up the brain so that things fall back into their normal places.[20]

In 1933 Ladislaus von Meduna of Budapest revived the Oliver approach, inducing convulsion by intramuscular injections of a 25 per cent solution of camphor in oil. This method of treatment proved so unpredictable that he turned in 1935 to Metrazol, a synthetic camphor preparation. Though this substance was "superior to camphor," many patients were terrified; they "experienced feelings of impending death and sudden annihilation during the interval between the injection and the convulsions." [21]

Manfred Sakel (1900–1957) of Berlin and H. Steck of
Lausanne began experimenting with insulin therapy around
1927, independently reporting their initial findings in 1933
and 1932 respectively. Before this, insulin had been used in
small doses for various symptoms, but pains had been taken to
avoid coma. Sakel accidentally found that insulin coma led to
marked improvement in some cases, so much so that in 1950
the International Conference of Psychiatry declared insulin-
coma therapy the best available treatment for early schizophre-
nia. This form of chemical shock therapy remained popular
until it became apparent that the relapse rate was high. By
1971 it was "almost completely abandoned." [22]

In 1938 two Italians, Cerletti and Bini, conceived the
idea of inducing convulsion by passing a small electric current
through the patient's brain. "At its best the treatment is very
distasteful, even terrifying, because, though it seems to be pain-
less, patients awaken afterward with temporary loss of memory
and frightening feelings of disorientation in time and space. At
its worst, it can have dangerous side effects in damaged muscles, bones, or brain tissue." In the 1950s new sophisticated
drugs largely replaced chemical and electric-shock treatments.
Electroconvulsive therapy "has given way, for the most part,
to anti-depressant drugs, while insulin and Metrazol therapies
have largely been abandoned in favor of strong tranquilizers." [23]

By 1972 "prevailing medical sentiment seems to have
shifted to the idea that shock therapy ought to be only an
emergency measure or one of last resort, on the theory that psy-
chotherapy alone can get at the underlying causes of the
depression. . . ." [24]

PSYCHOPHARMACOLOGY

Prefrontal lobotomies and the several forms of convulsive therapy were for mental patients ill to the point of a lesser or greater degree of incapacity. What about the vast majority of Americans who, far from being severely ill, have nonetheless been disturbed from time to time—anxious or apprehensive—and need help, but help short of hospitalization or protracted psychiatric or psychoanalytic treatment? The answer has been tranquilizers. One practitioner of internal medicine who was seeing forty patients a day was asked how he could possibly do this. He replied: "I give them all Miltown." The inference, of course, was that most of his patients were suffering from psychosomatic disturbances. In a practical sense, if not an entirely acceptable medical one, he was right.

The modern era of psychopharmacology dates from 1951 when the Frenchman Henri Laborit synthesized chlorpromazine, intending to use it in the management of general anesthesia. Chlorpromazine of the phenothiazine group of major tranquilizers was quickly joined by reserpine of the rauwolfia group, and by 1956 researchers V. Kinross-Wright, J. A. Barza, and the American Nathan S. Kline were reporting remarkable results from their use.

By 1958, in the United States, "the consumption of psychotherapeutic drugs for tranquilization, or ataraxia of the human mental state, or for 'peace of mind,' [had] soared at an alarming rate since the hesitant introductions of such medicaments in 1954. According to some reports, in total sales, tranquilizers [were] exceeded only by antibiotics and vitamins. Consequently, the production and marketing of ataractic drugs has become typical American 'Big Business.' " [25]

305

There are a number of minor tranquilizers, used to control anxiety, apprehension, agitation, and general nervous disorders, of which the best known to the public is meprobamate—Miltown and Equanil. Despite their wide use and great popularity, much less is known about the minor tranquilizers than the major ones. Changes brought about by their use are less marked and therefore more difficult to measure and evaluate. In fact, "there is really no substantial evidence for their effectiveness. . . . The widespread use of weak tranquilizers must be seriously challenged," but, in spite of a "lack of objective and scientific evidence, the great popularity of the minor tranquilizing group does support the contention that they are of value in relief of many nervous symptoms." [26]

Part VI

INTO THE MODERN AGE

┇(20)┇

In Defiance of Obsolescence

In the past, the decline of living things once they reached maturity was partly attributable to "external attack." By the 1970s, as a result of spectacular advances "in therapeutics, particularly in chemotherapy, over the last half century," the picture has changed. "The plagues and diseases that once claimed large numbers of people are now either defeated or, at worst, manageable. Many other afflictions of mind and body have yielded to drugs, diets, and careful regimes. . . . Paradoxically, our increasing success with therapeutics has thrown an even greater burden on surgery. People who might once have died of a communicable disease before their thirties are now living on into middle and old age and becoming candidates for degenerative diseases and disorders, which can be thought of as the premature aging of one organ or part of the body." [1]

To restore a degree of function to a bodily part that has been severely damaged or is failing will usually involve surgery and may take one of two forms: an artificial part applied externally or internally; or an organ from the body of another person, living or dead.

SPARE PARTS OUTSIDE THE BODY

Artificial limbs were known to the Greek historian Herodotus in the fifth century B.C. and to the Roman Pliny six centuries later. They seem to have been largely neglected from then until the fourteenth century, when crutches and wooden legs were mentioned by chroniclers and contemporary frescoes depicted them. The first picture of an iron hand dates from 1400. A century later Götz von Berlichingen, a German feudal knight, lost his right hand to a musket-shot and had several replacements made. They had movable joints and flexible fingers and were capable of closure. Ambroise Paré's collected works, first published in 1575, included illustrations of artificial hands, arms, and legs.

The peg-leg and the iron hook in the adventure stories read in childhood were forerunners of the artificial limbs of today. The peg-leg gave place to the wooden leg, a prosthesis revealed by some awkwardness in the wearer's gait. The more recent flexible legs made of lightweight metal have brought walking close to normal and allow all sorts of previously barred activities. The iron hook of the pirate chief is reflected in the metal hand of today. The modern artificial hand, while it may be dressed up cosmetically, acts on the same general principle as the "hands" used in atomic laboratories to handle hot material from behind a shield. Prostheses have been designed "to use two kinds of 'hand.' The hook, giving a firm three-point grip of up to ten pounds, which is generally preferred for work, can be unplugged and exchanged for a 'cosmetic prosthesis' in the shape of a Dorrance hand, where thumb and the first two fingers are 'active' and move . . . in a caliper motion, to provide a maximum fingertip force of six pounds. Power is drawn from a twenty-ounce battery strapped to the back of the wearer, along with the fifteen-ounce control unit." [2]

One approach to the powering of artificial limbs was cineplasty—modifying the muscles of the stump by surgery so that, when flexed, they would pull upon a control cable. When tested, difficulties arose that were both medical (keeping the area free from infection) and psychological.

Pneumatic powering (by a gas such as carbon dioxide stored under pressure) and electric-battery powering have been tried but their advantages were offset by significant limitations. Powering by small electrical signals (up to twenty-five millivolts) generated by the contraction of muscle fibers has also been tried. It was Norbert Wiener (1894–1964), the American cyberneticist, who first suggested the use of myo-electric currents, as these are called, in the early 1950s.

The status of prosthetic development is not yet satisfactory. The present hand, "for all its complexity, satisfies no one except amputees who until now have had to use even poorer hands." In the 1970s and 1980s it is expected that "a prosthetic hand with many paired movements" will be developed, "including rotation, for the moderately disabled. For the severely disabled chairbound amputee . . . the 'hand' will be part of the 'chair' (which may, in fact, be a walking bed) and it will be capable of many programmed movements, stored in computer-type stores and activated and controlled by master signals from the amputee." [3]

It is better, of course, to restore a severed limb than to replace it with a prosthesis. The first time a severed limb was "put back" was in Boston in 1962. One day on his way home from school Everett Knowles, a twelve-year-old Little Leaguer, leaped on the ladder of a slow-moving freight train. Moments later he was crushed against a tunnel entrance. His right arm was cut off at the shoulder. He was rushed to Massachusetts General Hospital with the arm still in the sleeve of his coat. In a three-and-a-half hour operation, bones, arteries, and veins were rejoined and nerve ends tied. (Some of the nerve work was not completed until a year later.)

When all was over, Everett still had his arm. It was no longer a pitching arm and it was not as strong as his left arm, but it was usable and his own.

There have been other successful cases—not many, because the severed part must be available for replacement, and too often in accidents it is crushed beyond recognition. There is also a time factor: the part to be restored must be "fresh."

THE BEGINNINGS OF HEART SURGERY

Of all man's essential organs—heart, brain, liver, and at least one of his lungs and one of his kidneys—the heart was the first to attract surgeons.

In 1824 Dominique Jean Larrey (1766–1842), the greatest French military surgeon of his day, drained off an excess of liquid that had, as a result of war wounds, collected between the two layers of the fibrous sac surrounding the heart and was exerting pressure on the heart. As we have seen, in 1893 the American Negro Daniel Hale Williams sewed up a wound in the pericardium. Early operations on the heart itself involved repair of the damage of stab wounds. Attempts in 1895 and 1896 by a Norwegian, Axel Cappelen (d. 1919), and an Italian, Guido Farina, failed; in 1896 the German Ludwig Rehn (1849–1930) successfully repaired a wound in the right ventricle of a man who had been stabbed in the chest and left for dead.

In the early 1890s Sir William Arbuthnot Lane (1856–1943) worked out a method for the surgical treatment of mitral stenosis, a condition involving the scarring of the valve between left atrium and ventricle, but no one would allow him to try it on a living patient; in 1902 Sir Thomas Lauder Brunton (1844–1916) was shouted down when he sponsored the same idea; and it was not until 1925 that their proposal was carried through by Sir Henry Sessions Souttar (1875–1964), whose nineteen-year-old patient enjoyed good health for another five years. Still, most doctors would not accept the method, and it was not again employed until 1948, when it was successfully followed by Sir Russell Claude Brock of London, Charles B. Bailey of Philadelphia, and Dwight E. Harken of Boston. Thereafter the Lane-Brunton-Souttar method became the accepted procedure for mitral stenosis.

In the late 1930s and early 1940s some attempts were made to correct a variety of heart defects. Heart surgeons worked under a great handicap: they had to perform "blind." This working by touch alone defeated the first principle a surgeon learned—to see what he was doing. Furthermore, as he worked, the heart continued to pump gallons of blood through the body. To remedy this situation required lengthening the period (ordinarily two or three minutes) for which the brain, the liver, and the kidneys could get along without the food and oxygen supplied by the blood; this meant finding a means of substituting an extrinsic pump for the action of the heart to provide a temporary bypass.

In 1950 Wilfred G. Bigelow of Toronto and William O. McQuiston of Chicago conceived the idea of hypothermia, the reduction of body temperature so that the period for which the brain can get along without oxygen is prolonged. In 1952 and 1953, respectively, F. John Lewis of the University of Minnesota and Henry Swan of the University of Chicago employed this technique in closing a hole between the atria of a heart.

There are two levels of hypothermia—mild and profound. In mild hypothermia the body temperature is reduced from the normal 98.6° F to around 86° F, extending the brain's tolerance of interrupted blood supply to ten minutes; profound hypothermia, in which the patient is cooled to between 45° F and 60° F, raises the period to about one hour. "Ten minutes is long enough to allow a nimble surgeon to close a hole between two chambers of the heart, or to cut back muscle tissue that may be interfering with a valve or close a complex hole in the heart." [4]

THE WORK OF ALEXIS CARREL

Attempts to replace parts inside the body and to keep defective organs functioning really began with the work of Alexis Carrel.

Born at Sainte-Foy-les-Lyon, France, Carrel received his M.D. degree from the University of Lyon in 1900. In 1902 he published a paper on the uniting of blood vessels and the transplanting of organs. His method of anastomosis (uniting of blood vessels) involved three sutures that created a triangular opening instead of the usual round one. This laid the groundwork for future developments and earned him a Nobel Prize in 1912.

Carrel left Lyon because none of his professors were interested in his proposed research in these areas. In 1904 he arrived at the University of Chicago where he worked in the Hull Physiology Laboratory. He was joined by Charles Claude Guthrie (1880–1963), a physiologist. In 1906 they summarized their work in a paper on the uniting of blood vessels by the "patching method" and on kidney transplantation, in which they set forth their definitions, aims, techniques, results, and conclusions.[5]

In 1906 Carrel left Chicago for the Rockefeller Institute, where he remained until he retired in 1939. Guthrie moved on to the chair of physiology and pharmacology, first at Washington University (St. Louis) and subsequently at the University of Pittsburgh. Guthrie continued his work on vascular anastomoses and on structural changes and survival of cells in transplanted blood vessels.[6] Beginning in 1912, Carrel attempted to maintain living organs in glass containers, without success. He felt it was "futile to try to cultivate whole organs, until incomparably more efficient means for the artificial circulation under sterile conditions of a nutrient fluid through their blood vessels should be developed." [7]

The problem was solved by Charles A. Lindbergh (of aviation fame) in 1931. Lindbergh designed a coil apparatus that could be kept sterile; pressure was maintained by the head of liquid, and the liquid was raised and kept in circulation by placing the apparatus on a tilted base. In 1934 he designed a pump by which a pulsating circulation of nutrient fluid, properly oxygenated, could be maintained through an organ. Early in 1935 he designed a new type of organ chamber, and on

April 5 a whole organ (that of a cat) was successfully culti-
vated in a glass container for the first time. Writing in 1938,
Carrel and Lindbergh offered these conclusions:

> While the method, in its present state, is capable of
> being applied profitably to the whole field of organ nutri-
> tion, it is not as yet fully developed. Machines are always
> in the process of becoming. . . . The construction of
> larger pumps may lead to other applications of the
> method. We can perhaps dream of removing diseased or-
> gans from the body and placing them in the Lindbergh
> pump as patients are placed in a hospital. Then they
> could be treated far more energetically than within the or-
> ganism, and if cured replanted in the patient. . . .[8]

MEDICAL TECHNOLOGY

Carrel's experiments largely involved animals. John H.
Gibbon, Jr., of the Jefferson Medical College in Philadelphia
produced a machine that would put oxygen into a human's
blood and bloodstream while bypassing his heart and lungs.
Gibbon and his wife began work in 1937. One of their major
problems was avoiding damage to red blood cells and the element in the blood responsible for clotting. It was not until May
6, 1953, that Gibbon successfully used the machine to bypass
the heart of an eighteen-year-old girl while he closed a large
hole between her atria. In the next ten years the heart-lung machine was considerably improved, particularly by C. Walton
Lillehei and his team at the University of Minnesota.

Machines so far can replace only three bodily processes
—pumping blood, exchanging its gases, and removing its

wastes. The artificial kidney, like the heart-lung machine, functions outside the body, but it cannot be considered a temporary replacement because, in chronic cases, once used, it must be used regularly.

The vital function of the kidneys is to filter the blood and the body fluids contained in it, removing poisonous waste and passing it out as urine. They also maintain the water content of the body and the level of chemicals, essential to life but harmful in excess. In a sense the kidneys dictate health and illness, life and death. If one kidney becomes incapacitated, the other can assume the full load. If both are destroyed, the patient is condemned to a slow, pitiful death—unless a substitute kidney is available.

In 1913 three Americans, John Jacob Abel (1857–1938), Leonard George Rowntree, and B. B. Turner of Johns Hopkins, attempted to construct an artificial kidney but they could find no material capable of performing the filtering function.

In 1938 a young Dutchman, William J. Kolff, after losing a twenty-two-year-old patient to kidney failure, determined to find a solution. A former professor introduced him to a remarkable new material called cellophane. This proved to be the material that Abel, Rowntree, Turner, and others had sought in vain.

Kolff built several machines but none was constructed well enough to be clinically reliable. In May 1940 when the Germans invaded Holland, Kolff continued his work underground and evolved a seemingly satisfactory machine. However, of fifteen patients treated between March 17, 1943, and July 27, 1944, only one survived. After World War II Kolff brought his artificial kidney to the United States, where he joined the Cleveland (Ohio) Clinic. Later he moved to the University of Utah.

Because the early Kolff machines were large and costly to produce, they were scarce. Only 1400 individuals a year could get dialytic (flushing of the kidneys) treatment until Kolff, Dr. William G. Esmond of the University of Maryland, and Dr. Morrell M. Avram of Long Island Hospital (New York) found a way to produce less costly machines. Still, the requirement of two or three treatments a week keeps a patient largely tied to his unit, whether it is at his home or in a hospital. The day may come when there will be dialysis hotels (human laundromats) where patients will check in for the night, have their kidneys flushed while they sleep, and leave in the morning. "The perfect dialyzer" has not yet been invented. There are possibilities in an implantable dialyzing membrane that will eliminate the need for skillful medical supervision and in a "small plastic unit worn like a sleeve" that the patient can empty into any drain and fill at any tap.[9] A step in the direction of the second proposal was taken in 1966 when a team headed by Ted Blaney of the Chemical Engineering Science Group at Case Institute projected to the American Society for Artificial Internal Organs the idea of a dialyzing unit encircling one arm and attached to a fluid reservoir containing activated charcoal, which has been found to be an alternative filtering agent, worn around the waist.

KIDNEY TRANSPLANTATION

On June 19, 1950, the *Chicago Sun-Times* reported: "A healthy kidney was removed from the body of a dead woman and used to replace the diseased kidney of a dying woman in a historic 90-minute operation by two teams of doctors in the Little Company of Mary Hospital."

The patient had consulted urologist Patrick H. McNulty who, finding that both her kidneys were diseased, the left one hopelessly, discussed the case with surgeons Richard H. Lawler and James W. West of the hospital staff. Lawler had often thought of attempting to transfer the healthy kidney of a deceased person to a fatally ill patient, foreshadowed by Carrel's experiments with animals. He was now ready, providing a woman-donor of matching blood group was found.

Thirteen months after the transfer, on May 23, 1951, the *Chicago Tribune* reported: "The first attempt in history to transplant a kidney from one human to another has ended in failure. . . . Inability of tissues of one person to be compatible when transplanted to another was given as the reason for failure. . . . Seven weeks ago an exploratory operation was performed and found that the organ had shrunk from the size of a grapefruit to a small hazel nut." Nevertheless the patient lived almost four years longer; she finally succumbed to pneumonia related to her chronic kidney ailment. Transfers by French doctors, from an executed criminal to a twenty-two-year-old girl in January 1951, and from a mother to her sixteen-year-old son in December 1952, also ended in failure.

In 1954 a team of doctors at Boston's Peter Bent Brigham Hospital, headed by Joseph E. Murray and John P. Merrill, "were confronted with a unique opportunity. . . . David Miller, an alert physician in a nearby U.S. Public Health Service hospital, was caring for a young veteran who was dying of severe kidney failure and high blood pressure. A daily visitor to his bedside was his apparently identical twin. Miller knew of the work on kidney transplantation. He also knew that biological incompatibility was the reason transplantation of tissues generally failed. He reasoned that if the two young men were identical twins, their tissues might not be biologically incompatible. As is well known, identical twins develop from a single fertilized egg; they not only resemble each other in appearance but also have a high degree of biological identity." [10] On December 24 the first successful kidney transplant operation was performed.

On January 24, 1959, a similar transplant was done with non-identical twins by the Peter Bent Brigham team. Massive doses of X-rays were used all over the patient's body to suppress rejection response.

In January 1967 a thirty-two-year-old woman, who had been diabetic since she was a child, was dying from kidney failure. Dr. Richard C. Lillehei and Dr. William D. Kelly decided in favor of a double transplantation—kidney and pancreas, the seat of diabetes. The patient lived for four months, during which time she required no insulin, the specific for diabetes, and had adequate kidney function. The doctors found, however, that it was harder to get a pancreas out of a donor than into a recipient, and this limited the number of cases undertaken. By the end of 1969 Dr. Lillehei had underway a program of pancreatic transplants for young diabetics. Six out of eight recipients died, but none from rejection of the pancreas. The other two were released from the hospital and have needed no insulin since their transplants.

THE PROBLEM OF TISSUE REJECTION

From 1954 through 1968 several thousand kidney transplants were performed, many unsuccessful. Since 1969, through the use of antilymphocyte serum, or globulin (ALG), to curb rejection, results have improved. The survival rate for cases undertaken by Dr. Richard C. Lillehei of the University of Minnesota has been over 90 per cent in blood-related transplants, 50 per cent in other cases.

As early as 1935 Carrel had recognized and described immune rejection reaction in kidney transplantation:

> As a rule the tissues of one individual refuse to accept those of another individual. When, by the suture of the vessels, blood circulates again in a transplanted kidney, the organ immediately secretes urine. At first, it behaves normally. After a few weeks, however, albumin, then blood, appear in the urine. And a disease similar to nephritis rapidly brings an atrophy of the kidney. . . . Obviously, the humors recognize, in foreign tissues, certain differences of constitution, which are not revealed by any other test. Cells are specific of the individual to whom they belong.[11]

Immune reaction "is the instant and overpowering rejection of anything that our lymphocytes recognize as not-self." The lymphocytes or white cells are scavengers that circulate in the bloodstream, engulfing and digesting invading organisms, whatever their size. "The body's inner defense mechanisms are not concerned with any philosophical contrast like 'living or dead,' 'friendly or antagonistic.' Their activity is triggered by one single event: the appearance in the body of a chemical entity that the body can recognize as *not-self.*" [12]

When a surgeon plans to replace a defective organ with a good one, he must find a graft material as close as possible in type to the host material, the perfect match being between identical twins. Since the science of tissue typing is relatively primitive, he cannot be sure that he has a compatible graft. Although immuno-suppressive drugs help in minimizing rejection, they inhibit the division of lymphocytes; while the transplanted organ thrives, the patient is vulnerable to everyday diseases. The use of ALG also has drawbacks; it has been found that some transplant patients permanently on ALG become allergic to it.

"The rejection of tissue grafts involves a mechanism of daunting complexity, the full subtleties of which lie way beyond our present grasp. To cover its full ramifications will call for a great deal more work. But to discover its secret machinery and to put it to work on our behalf will surely be a matchless prize." [13]

HEART TRANSPLANTATION

South Africa's Christiaan N. Barnard and his team, on December 3, 1967, performed the first successful human-to-human heart transplantation. The recipient, Louis Washkansky, survived for eighteen days and died from lung complications, seemingly brought on by early overuse of immuno-suppressive drugs as a prophylactic measure, rather than by failure of his acquired heart.

But for differing concepts of medical ethics and philosophy, the credit might have gone to Dr. James D. Hardy, chief of the surgical department, University of Mississippi Medical Center, and his team. On the evening of January 22, 1964, the would-be recipient of a heart, a man in his late sixties, was at the point of death. In the intensive care unit a young man with fatal brain injuries was being kept alive by artificial respiration.

All brain function had ceased, but the heartbeat could not be expected to fail in time for the heart to be of value unless mechanical respiration was withdrawn. Hardy would not even consider such a step. As an alternative he used the heart of a large chimpanzee. Unfortunately the ape's heart did not have enough strength to maintain human circulation.

Barnard, when he was ready to transfer the heart of his donor, had artificial respiration suspended, bringing about the cessation of the heartbeat. For the rest, his surgical technique showed no important advance on techniques worked out by Hardy and other Americans.

By the end of 1967 twenty or more surgical teams at centers around the world were waiting—and may have been waiting for weeks, months, even years—for the coincidence of the need for and availability of a human heart. Three days after the Washkansky transplant, on December 6, Dr. Adrian Kantrowitz of the Maimonides Medical Center (Brooklyn, New York) transplanted the heart of a child who had died of brain damage to a seventeen-day-old boy. Dr. Norman E. Shumway of Stanford University (California) made his first attempt on January 6, and Kantrowitz his second on January 10. None of these was successful. Barnard's second transplantee, Philip Blaiberg lived for 594 days after his operation on January 2; during this time he drove his car, drank beer, ate heartily, and wrote his autobiography. On the first anniversary of Barnard's operation the score was ninety-five heart transplantations with a survival rate of 50 per cent. In 1969 transplants fell off to forty-six. Doctors were discouraged by the fact that not many recipients survived longer than six months. They were beginning to recognize that anyone sick enough to qualify for a transplant was already too sick to live; that anyone well

enough to live should not face the risks of what was still experimental surgery. There have been exceptions.

On August 24, 1968, Louis B. Russell, Jr., a black school-
teacher from Indianapolis was given the heart of a seventeen-
year-old boy (who had died from a gunshot wound in the head)
by Dr. Richard Lower at the Medical College of Virginia in
Richmond. In April 1970 Russell surpassed the survival record
set by Blaiberg. *Time* magazine reported:

> Beyond mere survival, Russell has set another note-
> worthy record for heart-transplant recipients. None of the
> others has worked so strenuously at his old job—and
> taken on other tasks besides. Russell, a skilled carpenter
> who teaches industrial arts at a boys' junior high, repaired
> the roof of his two-story house ten months after his opera-
> tion. He keeps busy on remodeling jobs or making
> furniture—except when he is touring the country to
> give speeches about his heart transplant. Last month Rus-
> sell, who has two children living at home, found room in
> his new heart for still another burden. He and his wife
> became foster parents of a 13-year-old boy who had been
> in trouble with the authorities.[14]

Russell had several advantages over Blaiberg. When he
received his new heart he was fifteen years younger than Blaiberg had been. Blaiberg's long-standing heart disease had damaged other organs prior to the transplant. Russell's heart attacks in 1962, 1965, and 1968 had caused no such damage.

The lack of success so far in lung transplantation has
deterred surgeons from undertaking more heart transplants. It
is generally felt that at least one lung (or a major part of it)

should be transplanted along with a heart; in most candidates for hearts the lungs, more than any other organ, also suffered damage.

LIVER TRANSPLANTATION

People can be kept going with a heart-lung machine or an artificial kidney, but there is no artificial substitute for a liver, and without a functioning liver an individual can exist only for about a day and a half. Dr. Thomas E. Starzl of the University of Colorado pioneered liver transplants, of which less than fifty had been undertaken by the end of 1968. At first the best Dr. Starzl could hope for was life-prolongation for a month; at the end of August 1968 he had eight patients living, one of whom, a two-and-a-half-year-old girl, had survived a full year. She died a month later from a resurgence of the cancer that had made the transplantation necessary; her acquired liver was still working well. The general picture continues to be disappointing.

PSYCHOLOGICAL REJECTION OF TRANSPLANTS

Apart from the danger of rejection of the foreign organ, there is the possibility of psychological rejection of the transplant procedure and its implications. New techniques have been developed so rapidly that society has not yet time to cope with their philosophical, psychological, social, ethical, and legal significances.

Perhaps no other recent development in surgery has made the surgeon more aware of the need for psychiatric assistance than organ homotransplantation. The complex phases of treatment include prolonged technical preparation, the sequence of operations, the recovery period when large doses of immuno-suppressive drugs are used, and continuous follow-up outpatient care. Each has its own stresses that tend to produce fear, pain, anxiety, depression, and dependency. . . .

A number of issues present themselves when the donor is a live relative: Does the person have the right to sacrifice an organ and risk his life for another person? On the other hand, does one have the right to deny to another person a vital organ that is not needed to maintain the donor's life?

Such organ transplants affect all members of the family, not just the donor and recipient. The patient's emotional response to this procedure depends on the maturity of the patient, the donor, and the entire family because they must withstand many stresses. . . .[15]

MAN-MADE REPLACEMENT PARTS FOR THE INNER MAN

Until it becomes possible to store human organs relatively indefinitely (still largely a dream of the future, notwithstanding the fact that it was Carrel's dream half a century ago), human organ transplantation must remain a hit-or-miss proposition since there will presumably never be enough suitable donors at the right place at the right time. Major reliance therefore has been placed on man-made replacement parts.

To make this feasible, there must be materials that the body will not reject. The search has proved less difficult than might have been expected. Certain plastics are not rejected. Sprayed-on plastic has been used in brain surgery, clear plastic to replace eye corneas. Stainless steel has been found acceptable, as has a kind of silicone rubber used by plastic surgeons to give shape to reconstructed ears, chins, breasts, and so on. In the late 1950s Dr. Michael E. DeBakey of Baylor University (Houston, Texas) found that failing arteries, a main cause of death, could be replaced by Dacron tubing without immune reaction. Dacron was subsequently joined by Teflon.

Much of the work on replacement parts has centered on acceptable materials for the heart. Dependent as life is on it, the heart is nothing more than a pump. Its muscles, the expansion and contraction of which provide its pumping action, act in response to tiny electrical signals from the brain, received by the heart's switchboard, the sinoatrial node. When disease or injury cuts off impulses directed to the muscles, the heartbeat drops to about one-half of the normal rate—insufficient to provide the necessary flow of oxygen to all parts of the body. To put the heart back into good working order, an artificial pacemaker is necessary.

At the beginning of 1957 Dr. C. Walton Lillehei and two electronic engineers produced an electronic pacemaker into which the patient could be plugged by means of silver-plated wires passing through the chest and stitched to the surface of the heart. The next step was to produce a pacemaker small enough to be implanted in the body. This was achieved by Dr. Ake Senning of Sweden, closely followed by a number of American surgeons, including Dr. William Chardack of the Veterans Administration, who, with his engineer-associate Wilson Greatbach, produced a five-ounce, battery-powered package. But it was "obviously unsatisfactory to have to cut open a patient every so often, take out a costly and still functioning pacemaker with spent batteries, and replace it by a new pacemaker with full batteries." [16] An early attempt to use nickel-cadmium cells that could be recharged by high frequency electromagnetic waves was abandoned when the accumulator was found to be unreliable. The next move was to a button-size mercury battery, like that used in an electric watch. It had the advantage of maintaining its voltage till almost the end of its life (the approach of which a user could anticipate from a change in his pacemaker frequency). While theoretically such a battery should last four or five years, its limit in practice was two to three years.

The answer may lie with radioisotopes. It has been calculated that a pacemaker powered by plutonium 238 will continue to work for ten years. Only time can prove this. In May 1970 the first such pacemaker was implanted in a sixty-eight-year-old Frenchwoman. In July 1972 Dr. Chardack, by now chief of thoracic surgery at the Veterans Administration Hospital in Buffalo, New York, and Dr. Andrew Gage, chief of surgical services, implanted the first two nuclear-powered pacemakers in the United States.

Someday there will be pacemakers powered by the body's electrical impulses. These, it is claimed, will never need to be recharged.

All heart problems do not originate in the heart's switchboard. Parts wear out and have to be replaced.

In 1953 Dr. Charles A. Hufnagel of the Georgetown University Medical Center replaced a heart valve with an artificial one for the first time, in a research project funded by the National Institutes of Health. By the end of the 1950s all four heart valves were being replaced regularly, but never more than one or two to a patient.

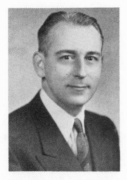

CHARLES A. HUFNAGEL

In the early 1960s DeBakey set his team to develop an auxiliary pump that could be implanted in a patient who had undergone heart surgery and left there for a matter of days, perhaps weeks. (Use of the heart-lung machine is limited to a few hours.) DeBakey tried out his pump on a man *in extremis* in July 1963. The patient died three days later. An autopsy revealed deficiencies in the materials that would have to be overcome; the pump had worked and temporarily achieved its objective. In February 1966 Adrian Kantrowitz announced the development of a bypass pump similar to DeBakey's. Despite the fact that the patient on whom it was used survived only twenty-four hours, the incident convinced DeBakey that he was on the right track. On April 21 DeBakey planted an improved pump in a patient to serve while he replaced one of the heart valves. When the patient died in the early hours of the 26th, the pump was still functioning well. DeBakey felt that considerable knowledge had been gained and planned, after further modifications of the pump, to try it again. In May he was again unsuccessful. In August his persistence was rewarded. The patient was a 37-year-old woman, victim of rheumatic heart disease, named Esperanza del Valle Vásquez. On September 6, less than a month after surgery, Mrs. Vásquez, the first patient to survive the use of the bypass and now the possessor of two artificial heart valves, left the hospital and flew home to Mexico City, where she resumed the running of her beauty parlor and was soon putting in an eight-hour day, largely on her feet.

On April 4, 1969, Dr. Denton A. Cooley of St. Luke's Episcopal Hospital (Houston, Texas) replaced a heart with an artificial device. The patient was waiting for a donor, but surgery could not be indefinitely postponed. The patient was given to understand that, if Cooley attempted conventional repair of the heart and failed, he would die unless a human heart was available or a mechanical device was used. The operation showed that the heart was beyond redemption. Cooley worked for an hour in an attempt to restore it to function; then and then only did he remove it and substitute an artificial heart, weighing eight ounces, to keep the patient going until a donor could be found. A forty-year-old woman was found; she was in a Boston suburb, being kept alive by artificial respiration. It was questionable whether she would survive the plane trip, but she did. Sixty-three hours after the artificial heart was implanted in the patient it was replaced by a human heart. Twenty-four hours later the patient was dead from pneumonia and kidney failure.

A wave of criticism swept over Cooley. It was variously stated that the use of an untested device on a human was criminal; that the surgeon's aim was to prolong life, not to prolong dying; that he was guilty of a murderous attack upon medical science.

The shock that greeted the failure of this great adventure subsided. The importance of prolonging life by means of a perfected artificial heart, which must someday supplant the transplanted heart, came to be recognized. Cooley, DeBakey, and teams in Salt Lake City, New York City, and many other cities across the United States have redoubled their efforts to fulfill this dream.

{(21)}

Aerospace Medicine

Aerospace medicine may be defined "as that specialty of general medicine which concerns itself with the problems of aviation." [1] It has two subdivisions—aviation medicine and space medicine.

Aviation medicine "deals with the devices, techniques, and other preventive measures needed to protect man within the region that is now regarded as being relatively close to the earth's surface." Aerospace medicine and space medicine are "logical extensions of aeromedical objectives. Reaching beyond the clinical and preventive medical requirements of man in atmospheric flight, aerospace medicine also encompasses the research, development, and test programs necessary to explore his capabilities and limitations in near-space and space-equivalent environments. Its ultimate aim is to promote the safety and effectiveness of man while he is exposed to stresses of acceleration, weightlessness, heat, noise, vibration, confinement, and radiation, all of which he is likely to encounter in aerospace flight." [2]

332

Aerospace medicine, "like other fields of human endeavor, has produced its own giants. While some of their contributions seemed relatively insignificant at first, when taken in context with subsequent breakthroughs and achievements, they were later recognized as the basic building blocks in the over-all picture of progress. Some other accomplishments were of such fundamental importance, however, that manned flight of significant duration and beyond what are today considered modest altitudes would not be feasible without them. . . . But far above the large group of experimenters and researchers looms the figure of Paul Bert, who, in retrospect, became the adopted godfather of aerospace medicine." [3]

Paul Bert (1833–1886), born in Auxerre, France, was the favorite pupil of the great French physiologist Claude Bernard and in 1868 succeeded his preceptor in the chair of physiology at the Sorbonne.

Bert was thirty when he obtained his M.D. degree, having previously studied engineering and law. He became interested in barometric pressure, especially with its effect on men engaged in mountain travel, caisson work, and ballooning. The results of his 670 laboratory experiments undertaken between 1870 and 1878 were published in *La Pression Barométrique* (1878).[4] It was "a masterly presentation of research recorded in an orderly, clear, concise and logical manner [1178 pages and 89 illustrations] which anyone would do well to utilize as a model for any similar task." [5]

In 1874 two experienced balloonists, H. Theodore Sivel and Joseph E. Crocé-Spinelli, invited Bert to expose them to very low barometric pressure in a chamber he had recently constructed. Their aim was to prepare themselves for high-altitude flights, a precaution prompted by the near-fatal experience of

James Glaiseer and Henry Tracy Coxwell twelve years earlier, when the balloon's ascent had gone out of control. When the aneroid barometer they had aboard indicated 29,000 feet, Glaiseer became unconscious from lack of oxygen. "Coxwell lost the use of his limbs but was able to seize the balloon's relief valve rope between his teeth. With his remaining strength he pulled the cord. Sufficient gas was vented to cause the balloon to descend, and both aeronauts soon recovered. There is some reason to suspect that the barometer gave an inaccurate reading—according to today's evidence, it is most unlikely that the altitude recorded is survivable for a significant length of time without oxygen for life-support." [6]

In Bert's chamber, Sivel and Crocé-Spinelli were subjected to a pressure-equivalent of 23,000 feet and learned how to use oxygen to prevent the effects of hypoxia. On March 22, 1874, they successfully undertook a flight aimed at reaching a like altitude. They were equipped with bags of oxygen-nitrogen supplied by Bert. On April 15, 1875, accompanied by Gaston Tissandier, they embarked on a more ambitious undertaking. Their aim: 26,240 feet. Bert was absent from Paris when they made their plans. A letter warning them that the three bags of 72 per cent oxygen they were taking along were manifestly insufficient arrived too late. Despite adverse effects, they pushed up to 28,820 feet. Only Tissandier lived to tell of the tragedy. "Other balloonists have been killed by falling to the ground; Sivel and Crocé-Spinelli were the first to die while rising." [7]

In 1957 Dr. David G. Simons of the United States Air Force used a balloon to get a man (himself) to a space-equivalent altitude and keep him there long enough to determine how the environment would affect his mind and body. On August 19, dressed in a pressure suit and other protective garments and sealed in a capsule (which could be released from the balloon in case of in-flight emergency), Simons was carried to 101,516 feet and "became the first man to see, describe, and photograph the incredible views of the earth from the stratosphere." [8]

Well in advance of the first moon landing in 1969 aerospace medicine was studying the problem of how to maintain the astronaut's health as he journeyed through outer space. To be able to do this, it had to determine the effect of forces (or the lack of them) not previously experienced by man. Another of its problems was how to prevent astronauts landing on the moon (or any planet) from bringing home unfamiliar bacteria or viruses that might be lurking there.

The long and so far generally fruitless struggle against influenza viruses illustrates what might happen if a strange virus from the moon should reach earth. Possibilities were raised, precautions discussed, and plans formulated by space-program doctors and scientists. The program decided upon involved quick transfer of the astronauts to the quarantine vehicle, careful decontamination of the re-entry vehicle and of everything with which the astronauts had had contact en route or in landing, and immediate isolation of moon rocks in cabinets containing germ free mice. If the mice succumbed, it would have to be due to an extraterrestrial cause. The outcome of the several moon landings has reasonably satisfied the scientists that the moon is germ- and virus-free, but no one could have guaranteed this in advance.

Man in his space vehicle faced many new situations, some merely disturbing, some restrictive of mental and physical action, some even frightening. There were problems related to acceleration, deceleration, and decompression. There were the effects on vision of changed night-day cycles and of the earth's appearing to roll across the sky overhead. There were the psychological factors of being confined in cramped quarters and being separated for long periods of time from female companionship. There was the dull, limited diet involving synthetics and concentrates. Waste products of the body had to be disposed of. There were sound and heat barriers to be crossed, cosmic radiation to be dealt with. There was disturbance in the established rhythms of daily life. There was danger of fatigue and boredom. There was even anxiety.

As one moves away from the earth, atmospheric pressure is reduced, reducing the pressure of oxygen. Too little oxygen can threaten performance, can even prove fatal. This problem was met by the rigid pressure cabin and the pressure suit (or flexible pressure cabin).

The force of gravity is comparable to a pit 4000 miles deep out of which man must climb to reach outer space. To escape from the pit, a vehicle must reach a velocity of 25,000 feet per second within a matter of miles. (A car traveling at 100 mph has a velocity of 146⅔ feet per second.) On re-entry into the earth's atmosphere at high velocity there is a deceleration problem. These challenges were met by having the astronaut lie in an essentially horizontal position with his heart on a level with his head and his legs higher. Out of the range of gravity, man is faced by a weightless condition in which his body continues to move in a straight line unless some force changes its speed and direction. Weightlessness has produced no major problem for men living and working in space.

An astronaut going aloft is wired like a pinball machine. Every breath, every pulse beat, and every muscle reaction is radioed back to earth for analysis. Prior to the Apollo 8 flight, while the astronauts remained aloft for days, they remained in the earth's orbit. If major trouble, mechanical or medical, developed, they could head for home. When flying to the moon (and beyond) there is a point of no return.

The star ships of science fiction boast crews of hundreds; the first three men to go to the moon did so in a cramped capsule. Care of their health had to be fully planned in advance. Anything that might upset normal body performance had to be fully anticipated.

The doctors of the Air Force Systems Command (at Andrews Air Force Base, Washington, D.C.), who, working with NASA, undertook the developmental work, recognized that many civilians were faced with problems similar to those that would face the astronauts, such as restricted activity. They expected to learn from civilian illnesses how to deal with side effects. To their surprise they found that little or nothing was being done, that the problems had never been the subject of controlled studies. In the final analysis, instead of aerospace medicine benefiting from the lessons of medicine, earth medicine has benefited from the lessons of space.

One finding is that an astronaut immobilized in his space capsule loses one pint of body fluid in the first twenty-four hours of flight (although the loss levels off after forty-eight hours). The heart patient who is ordered "bedrest" is in a similar situation. As a result of this space information, it has been recognized that the loss of color observed in recuperating bedridden patients (the "ten-day anemia") is not due to disease, but to the reduced volume of blood—about a pint—circulating through the body.

To avoid fluid loss, muscle tone must be maintained throughout the body. Isometric exercises, which can be performed in a relatively cramped position, were developed for the astronaut. Now certain patients are required to work for a set length of time each day with footboards and electric armpulls installed in regular hospital beds.

A gravity-free environment produces problems involving the heart, blood vessels, and muscles. In effect, body pressure becomes even and the muscles do not produce the driving force that ordinarily returns blood to the heart. The astronaut and the bedridden patient, who is also stretched out horizontally and therefore relatively gravity free, are in a similar situation. A pressure suit, built into the space suit, stimulates the legs and returns blood to the heart, and a similar device is being used on bedridden hospital patients.

Originally the astronaut was required to function in an atmosphere of 100 per cent oxygen, and his reaction to this was a matter for research. (After the disastrous Apollo spacecraft fire in January 1967, cabin atmosphere was reduced to 60 per cent oxygen, 40 per cent nitrogen, but the use of 100 per cent oxygen was continued in space suits.) As a byproduct of investigations in this area, techniques have been developed for the treatment of gangrenes caused by gas-producing bacteria and of carbon monoxide poisoning.

Hip surgery has also benefited from aerospace research. Because of the unusual amount of tissue exposed in hip surgery, the infection rate could be as high as 4 per cent. Early in 1970 at Hollywood Presbyterian Hospital in Los Angeles a method was devised for reducing the chances of infection. The entire area surrounding the operating table was tented with plastic, ultra-filtered air flowing in from above was completely changed every six seconds, and the doctors and operating-room staff were garbed in space suits.

In a confined space, as in a space capsule, noise and vibration seem greater than they actually are and the smallest recurrent noise will beat on the brain. Noise and vibration had to be minimized if an astronaut was to keep his reason. Sounds can prove as disturbing to patients in hospitals. The lessons learned in reducing sound and vibration in space vehicles have proved of great value in hospitals.

Noise and vibration could not be entirely eliminated from space crafts, and the remnant was found to interfere seriously with the monitoring of the astronaut's heartbeats. Existing types of stethoscopes proved useless, and a special instrument had to be created. The electronic stethoscope that was developed is in fact a miniature electronic computer. In hospitals, where some sound is inevitable, the electronic stethoscope has proved a major advance on the old-style acoustical stethoscope. In surgery, the miniature electronic computer (which has broader functions in and out of space than simply monitoring heartbeats) enables the surgeon to keep an eye on body functions and to know when danger points have been reached and passed.

The astronaut must be protected from impact with potentially dangerous objects inside the capsule. He must be protected from fire and radiation. Impact studies have pointed the way to improved automobile design and safety features; the lessons of fire protection are being applied in homes and hospitals; new methods are being developed to protect us from excessive radiation.

Doctors and scientists engaged in the solution of space problems had to face the question of the disposal of the waste products of the body. This involved more than getting rid of the liquids and solids discharged. The liquid lost had to be re-placed. A healthy individual needs an intake of about three quarts of water a day. Some of this comes through the food he eats. The astronaut is largely on a dehydrated diet, and most of his fluid has to come through fluid intake. In a small craft with limited storage facilities, carrying sufficient water is a major problem. It has been solved by processing and purifying waste liquid put out by the body and using it again for body intake. What has been learned in the space program about the re-use of body waste has a bearing on the treatment of garbage to avoid air and water pollution. Scientists are even looking for-ward to a day when, in isolated areas of the world where there are serious food shortages, solid matter put out by the body will, through a reconstituting process, be turned into food.

Among miniatures developed by the space program is an electrocardiograph machine the size of a matchbox. The usual instrument, which records electrical impulses from a series of heartbeats, is a cumbersome machine on wheels that has to be trundled to the patient lying on a doctor's examining table or to a hospital bedside. It can be used only when a patient is at rest. What the heart does during movement could not be stud-ied before the advent of the miniature machine developed for the space program. This can be worn during all activity, with the impulses it records transmitted to a central station. A doc-tor can follow what is happening to the heart of a patient who is jumping and jogging or engaging in any other activity.

Another practical spin-off has resulted from the method developed to improve the quality of television pictures from the moon. These pictures are "read" into a computer that has been programed to eliminate distortion. This process, called "computer enhancement," sharpens contrast and emphasizes fine lines. Similar fine lines occur in the X-rays of hairline fractures, especially of the hip and hand. In the past these fine lines were often unclear or did not even register on the X-ray film. Computer enhancement has greatly improved X-ray diagnosis of these troublesome fractures.

An electroencephalograph is a machine for recording waves in the brain. To establish electrical contact, it used to be necessary to shave the head and puncture the skin of the scalp. For astronauts, whose heads were in motion most of the time, the wires and electrodes attached to their scalps were a source of considerable irritation. This problem was overcome by the development of a simple adhesive solution that does not require shaving the head or breaking the skin. In civilian life it has proved particularly useful in handling younger children.

Another development is the brain helmet produced by the Brain Research Institute of the University of California at Los Angeles. It involves no skull attachments and can be used to monitor brain activities during sleep, fatigue, weightlessness, vibration, prolonged darkness, and so on. In an experiment a driver wearing a brain helmet drove a car on a busy freeway. He seemed unaffected by the traffic, but the brain recordings showed otherwise.

To determine the best-performing fuels for rockets, those under consideration had to be "taken apart." In the process, by-products that had no value as fuel were tested to find out for what they might be useful. Hydrazine, for example, has presented the possibility of slowing down certain types of tumor.

The astronauts and the space program have indeed made a major contribution to the welfare of mankind.

❧(22)❧

Nuclear Medicine

Nuclear medicine has been described as "a clinical specialty, meaning that it is concerned with patients and their problems. Its practitioners use radioactive tracers to try to find answers to the four basic questions: . . . What is wrong with the patient (diagnosis)? What is going to happen to him (prognosis)? What can be done about it (treatment)? Why did it happen (biomedical research)?" [1]

Nuclear medicine did not suddenly begin on August 2, 1946, when the first fission-produced radioisotope was shipped from the Institute of Nuclear Sciences at Oak Ridge, Tennessee, to Barnard Cancer Hospital in St. Louis. Nuclear medicine was made possible by the work of a number of scientists active in the late nineteenth and early twentieth centuries.

In 1896 the French physicist Henri Becquerel (1852–1908) found that some substances were radioactive (emit radiation). This was followed by the discovery by Marie Curie (1867–1934) and Pierre Curie (1859–1906) of radium and other radioactive substances.

The first significant North American work was undertaken during the early years of the century at McGill University (Montreal) by Ernest Rutherford (1871–1937), a New Zealand-born, English-trained physicist, and his English-born associate Frederick Soddy (1877–1956). Rutherford and Soddy developed the theory of atomic transformation. Previously physicists and chemists had held that atoms were indestructible and unchangeable—an atom of oxygen remained an atom of oxygen forever. Rutherford and Soddy showed that this was not true of radioactive atoms. Rutherford, in fact, arrived at the conclusion that the atom consisted of a central positively charged nucleus and outer negatively charged electrons—a concept still subscribed to by physicists.

By 1912 many scientists were on the track of isotopes, which are identical elements that differ only in their number of neutrons, the uncharged particles in the nucleus of an atom. Their discovery is generally credited to the Polish-American chemist Kasimir Fajans. As the story goes, while attending a performance of Wagner's *Tristan und Isolde* at the State Opera in Karlsruhe, Germany, Fajans' mind wandered to his work on various forms of radioactivity, and suddenly the whole pattern of isotopes and their behavior became clear to him.

By 1918 Rutherford was in England at the Cavendish Laboratory in Cambridge, conducting experiments that led to the fulfillment of that elusive goal of the medieval alchemists—the transmutation of elements. An atom of nitrogen bombarded by an alpha particle was converted into an atom of oxygen plus a left-over proton. "Not only was it possible to convert one familiar element like nitrogen into another like oxygen; bombardment also produced previously unknown species of matter—isotopes of the familiar elements, having the

343

same number of protons and electrons but different atomic weights. The oxygen produced by Rutherford's initial experiment, for example, was not ordinary oxygen-16, with an atomic weight of 16, but rather a heavier isotope, oxygen-17. A whole new world, it seemed, might be hidden in the interior of the atom." [2]

To learn more about the nucleus of the atom and to produce new isotopes more effective methods of bombardment were necessary. This called for the production of supervoltage —voltage in excess of anything so far produced. Scientists throughout the world engaged in the search for high-energy particle accelerators, or atom-smashers. Among them were four Americans: William David Coolidge, who in 1913 had developed the hot cathode tube for General Electric and between 1926 and 1930 the cascade tube, which emitted high-voltage electrons but not X-rays; Charles C. Lauritsen of the California Institute of Technology, who by 1933 had produced a tube made of porcelain rather than glass; Robert J. Van de Graaff (1901–1967), who, at Princeton in 1929–30, built an electrostatic generator that was simple, inexpensive, and portable in contrast with Coolidge's and Lauritsen's elaborate tube installations; Ernest Orlando Lawrence (1901–1958) of the University of California at Berkeley, who in 1932 produced the cyclotron, the first of the circular accelerators.

In 1911 Georg von Hevesy (1885–1966), a young Hungarian-born physical chemist from the faculty of the Technische Hochschule of Zurich, was asked by Rutherford to separate what was then called radium D from roughly a ton of lead chloride given Rutherford by the Austrian government. The lead chloride had been extracted from pitchblende, the Curies' original source of radium. The attempt failed, and radium D was considered inseparable from lead. Only later did it become apparent that radium D was the radioactive isotope of lead.

Hevesy continued to work on radioisotopes. By 1923 his experiments had led to the establishment of principles that have continued to underlie their use as tracers. One experiment had its amusing side: "While living in a boarding house in 1923, he had become suspicious of the cuisine. He therefore brought to the table with him a speck of one of the naturally occurring radioisotopes and deposited it in a scrap of meat which he left on his plate. Next day he brought a radiation detector—an electroscope—to the dinner table; sure enough, when the hash was served the electroscope revealed it was radioactive. Hevesy had used a naturally occurring radioisotope as a *tracer* to follow the course of the meat scrap from his plate to the kitchen, through the meat chopper, through the hash pot, and back to the table again." [3]

In 1926 three Harvard Medical School physicians, Hermann L. Blumgart, Soma Weiss, and Otto C. Yens, employed radioisotopes in human clinical research. In 1932 Professor Harold C. Urey of Columbia University discovered a stable isotope of hydrogen that, combined with oxygen, produced "heavy water." Two years later Hevesy and an associate performed the first tracer experiment with this fluid by drinking small quantities of it and monitoring its excretion in their urine.

To explore fully his tracer concept, Hevesy needed radioisotopes of phosphorus, sodium, and carbon. The breakthrough came as a result of discoveries made in 1933–34 by Irène Curie (1897–1956), and her husband Frédéric Joliot (1900–1958) at the Radium Institute at Paris. Still radioisotopes could only be produced in limited quantities, and many of those produced rapidly lost their radio-activity. Enrico Fermi (1901–1954), working in Rome, improved production methods and lasting quality, and by 1936 Lawrence was manufacturing in his cyclotron at least eighteen radioisotopes, notwithstanding the fact that a great number of them had a half-life too short for practical use.

RADIOISOTOPES IN THERAPY

The earliest medical use of radium and radioactivity was in the treatment of cancer. Then hyperthyroidism—a condition due to overworked thyroid glands—was treated radioactively from 1920 to 1930. Unfortunately it became apparent that X-rays, as then handled, were destroying healthy as well as defective tissue. Thereafter radioactive therapy was little used until the mid-1940s, when radioiodine, produced relatively cheaply at Oak Ridge, was substituted for X-rays.

Radioisotopes in therapy again ran into difficulty in the 1950s, when the public joined the government in a radiation (fallout) scare. Doctors hesitated to recommend radiation therapy except in hopeless cancer cases. Radioiodine treatment of hyperthyroidism was continued, as was the radiophosphorus treatment of leukemia introduced by hematologist John H. Lawrence of the University of California at Berkeley in 1936.

Radioisotope treatment involves the concentrating in malfunctioning tissue of an amount of radiation that will destroy the malfunctioning tissue without damage to healthy tissue.

RADIOISOTOPES IN DIAGNOSIS

The full diagnostic possibilities of radioisotopes were not recognized until around 1950, and it then took ten years to develop equipment.

Before radioisotopes, methods of determining whether an organ inside the body was performing properly were not fully reliable. X-rays were effective with bones but not as effective where tissue was involved. The doctor was forced to rely on palpation—what he could feel with his hands. Certain chemical tests might indicate that there was something wrong. No method was conclusive. Through the use of radioisotopes, more accurate diagnoses can be made.

When an isotope is introduced into an organ that is functioning normally, the organ will either retain it or dispose of it. If retention or disposal is greater or less than normal, the organ is not functioning properly.

To determine whether an organ is healthy, its size, shape, and method of functioning must be observed. Some organs cannot be X-rayed at all. Others do not show up well. Radiation passes through the patient and all that is left is a one-dimensional shadow on a film. When radioisotopes are introduced into the liver, thyroid, lung, spleen, kidney, heart, or pancreas, these organs can be seen clearly by using a specially designed scanner. What is more, these organs can be seen in function.

While bones show up well on X-rays, where there is cancer of the bone there are no definite clues until the damage is severe. Radioisotopes reveal change in the activity of the bone cells quite early.

Certain radioisotopes introduced into a patient's body find their way to certain organs. In diagnosis, the proper radioisotope is introduced and the organ scanned to see what happens when the radioisotope gets to it. Technologists explore thyroid glands with iodine-131, bone with fluorine-18, the liver with iodine-131 and gold-198. Isotopes of iodine, mercury, gold, copper, arsenic, and technetium are used to uncover brain tumors.

In 1949 Benjamin Cassen, a physicist at the University of California at Los Angeles, had the idea of moving a gamma-ray detector across a thyroid gland to detect iodine-131 activity. The principle was that of the Geiger counter used by uranium hunters.

Scanners have since been improved in a number of ways. There are compact machines which, with certain adaptors, do the work that until recently required three separate machines.

Faster results are now being obtained with radiation cameras that produce the image in fractions of a second instead of the scanner's fractions of an hour. The camera presents a picture in motion as opposed to the scanner's still pictures. However, such cameras are in their infancy.

Nuclear medicine began "as an exotic toy for endocrinologists . . . in thyroid work, then was taken up by hematologists . . . for the treatment of leukemia and . . . for the study of red cell production. When the rectilinear scanner and scintillation camera made radioactive imaging possible, radiologists entered the field. Clinical pathologists became involved with development of radioisotopes for in vitro studies. By now its uses span the entire field of medicine." [4]

{(23)}

The Future of
Medical Practice

A century ago medicine was a more personal profession. There was a one-to-one doctor-patient relationship. The family physician knew the family and its problems intimately, and all these factors left their imprint on health. He was of necessity and choice physician of the psyche as well as the body. The horse-and-buggy doctor may have been short on knowledge and techniques, but he was long on understanding and sympathy.

Almost fifty-years ago physiologist Howard W. Haggard (1891–1959), writing about faith healers, said:

> Diseases may be divided into three classes: first those which are entirely mental; second, those which are physical but tend to cure themselves; third, those that are phys-

ical but do not tend to cure themselves. Eighty to ninety per cent of all diseases belong to the first two classes. A man with a paralysis of his leg of mental origin, with a head cold, with lumbago, or with a stomach-ache from overeating gets well under the attention of a faith healer, a chiropractor, or even by taking patent medicine, and all but the paralytic will get well if nothing were done. On the other hand, such diseases as diphtheria, malaria, syphilis, cancer, diabetes, tuberculosis, and pernicious anemia do not get well with faith healing, chiropractic treatment, or psychoanalysis. If they are to be cured, the best medical attention is essential. The trained physician picks out from his patients the 10 or 20 per cent for whom his treatment may be life-saving. Under the ministrations of a faith healer these patients would die. But even if they did, the faith healer's result would be still 80 or 90 per cent effective.[1]

In the language of today, many of the problems patients present to their doctors are psychosomatic in origin. This does not mean, as many think, that the problem is imagined. The problem exists, as in the case of Dr. Haggard's man with a leg paralysis of mental origin. But the cause of the problem is not physical. The cause may, in fact, be imagination, a situation well defined by a male medical student working in the maternity ward who, asked why he was enthusiastic about obstetrics, said: "When I was on medical rotation I suffered from heart attacks, asthma, and itch. In surgery, I was sure I had ulcers. In the psychiatric wards, I thought I was losing my mind. Now, in obstetrics I can relax." [2]

With only 10 to 20 per cent of a doctor's practice calling

for knowledge beyond what the typical family doctor might possess, he did an amazingly effective job, even if some patients died that might have been kept alive by heroic measures. But the far-flung tentacles of medical research produced (for better or worse) more information than the busy general practitioner could sift, weigh, and utilize. He was faced by a choice. He could refer his problem patient to a specialist who might concentrate on one organ and ignore everything else; he could join with others to create what might be described as a conglomerate general practitioner.

THE MAYO CLINIC

English-born William Worrell Mayo (1819–1911), who arrived in America in 1845, settled in Rochester in southeast Minnesota in 1864. He had no dream of forming a clinic and was in fact a horse-and-buggy doctor in a very literal sense.

"In town he always made his calls on foot; for country trips he kept four or five horses of his own and sometimes had to rent others from a livery stable, for his daily rounds soon covered most of the roads radiating from Rochester. He would drive out on one road, come back, change horses, drive out on another and so on, until the necessary calls were made. And always he drove like mad. . . . Dr. Mayo's maxim was 'Don't spare the horses when a human life is at stake.' " [3]

The decisiveness of Dr. Mayo's brand of medicine was well illustrated in the case of young George Granger, future lawyer, judge, and legal advisor to the Mayos. On a professional visit to the Granger farm, Dr. Mayo asked young George a question. Hearing the answer he snapped, "Why that child is tongue-tied. Come here, George." The unsuspecting boy climbed on Dr. Mayo's knee and opened his mouth when told to. The doctor took a little pair of scissors from his pocket case and snipped the membrane under George's tongue. When the tongue healed the boy could speak like other children.[4]

Dr. Mayo was a typical frontier doctor, and an unusually resourceful one: when a young girl who had fallen off a horse three months earlier was brought to Dr. Mayo to see what could be done about the paralysis of one side of her face, he told her parents to use a galvanic battery and to come back if this didn't work. But this was not a brush-off. "Quere, where is the injury?" the doctor wrote in his ledger.

In another case, while Dr. Mayo was treating a badly infected leg with the patient partially under chloroform, the pulse stopped. The doctor dropped tincture of camphor between the man's lips and after fifteen minutes was able to resume the operation.

Not only did Dr. Mayo do his best under difficult circumstances (not the least of which was the fact that many of his patients were Norwegians who spoke and understood little or no English), but he was exceptionally thorough and inquisitive. He was very apt to note on the record card of a case presumably closed: "Left open for further thought and research." [5]

Dr. Mayo was a general practitioner, but surgery was what he wanted to do most. In the fall of 1869 he went to New York for a few months to study general surgery and gynecology. Before returning home he stopped off in Philadelphia to visit the Atlee brothers who had made the ovariotomy a matter of routine performance.

Twenty years later a new hospital, St. Mary's, opened in Rochester, created and administered by the Sisters of St. Francis of the Congregation of Our Lady of Lourdes. The professional staff consisted of three surgeons, Dr. William Worrell Mayo (now seventy), Dr. William James Mayo (1861–1939), and Dr. Charles Horace Mayo (1865–1939). The father, in view of his age, served largely as consulting physician and surgeon. William James had graduated from the University of Michigan Medical School six years earlier. "Dr. Will," as he came to be known, had joined his father in practice, and when asked by a family friend as to his plans for the future, he had replied: "I expect to remain in Rochester and become the greatest surgeon in the world." [6] Charles Mayo had received his degree from Chicago Medical College in 1888 and was still, therefore, a novice, the more so since his first year was marred by illness that led to a combination recuperative-investigatory trip abroad. Neither of the brothers had served as a hospital intern and they were acutely conscious of their limitations. Their beginning practice was general with emphasis on surgery. As time went by, they began to devote themselves exclusively to surgery, in which their skill and judgment were such as to raise them to the ranks of the great.

If one accepts the frequently made suggestion that the Mayo Clinic came into being with the opening of St. Mary's Hospital, then for its first dozen years the clinic was little more than what the Mayos claimed it to be—a well-organized surgical practice. In 1901 a new era began with the addition of laboratories of pathology and experimental medicine under the direction of Dr. Henry Plummer (1874–1936). By the middle of the decade the reputation of the Mayos had spread worldwide and the flow of patients was such that "every second house in Rochester had two or three of its rooms occupied by convalescent patients, their friends, and visiting surgeons." [7] Dr. Will proposed to hotelman John Kahler that he build a first-class convalescent hotel (that if need be could be turned into a hospital), and the Kahler House was opened in May 1907. At the same time, the professional staff was augmented by a variety of specialists until, by 1914, there was a permanent diagnostic staff of seventeen and eleven clinical assistants. The Mayo Clinic building opened in March 1914 provided space for medical research and medical education under the auspices of the Mayo Foundation. A still newer clinic building, completed in 1928, was fifteen stories tall and occupied almost an entire city block.

The Mayo Clinic has been described as "the most highly organized exemplar of group practice in existence." [8] But Dr. Will, commenting on the fact that he and his brother had been called the fathers of group medicine, said, "if we were we did not know it." They had "merely tried to solve the problems of their overwhelming practice in the way that seemed at the moment most likely to improve their surgery. . . . To be precise, the Mayos were not the fathers of group practice, but of *private* group practice. Cooperation of a sort among clinicians, surgeons, and laboratory men was taken for granted in municipal, state, and university hospitals; it was something quite new in private practice." [9]

Fathered or not by the Mayo brothers, private group practice has become the rule rather than the exception. Most groups operate on the fee-for-service basis customary among solo practitioners, but there have been other approaches based on other concepts. One is the Hunterdon Medical Center in New Jersey, conceived in the 1940s, which was designed to bring first-class medical care to an agricultural community under the sponsorship of the community. The most spectacular advances in the past forty years have been in the development of prepaid plans.

354

PREPAID HEALTH CARE

It has been said that patients at the Mayo Clinic pay "anything from nothing up to $10,000" and receive the same treatment.[10] This Robin Hood philosophy of "soaking the rich to take care of the poor" was fundamental to the economic development of private medical (and dental) practice, but it has become anachronistic in these days of high taxes and the welfare state. The man with money, earned or otherwise, is rightly resentful when he is taxed by his government and taxed again by his physician to take care of the poor. By and large the sliding-fee-scale in medicine is a thing of the past, retained only by a few star performers of surgery. However, the rising costs of medical care have made it essential that the average citizen be shielded from the financial disaster of prolonged illness. A partial answer is insurance—Blue Cross, Blue Shield, and commercial policies, which are in fact *sickness* insurance. Another is group medical practice involving prepayment.

In prepaid medical care plans a group of doctors receive a flat fee on a per capita basis to keep in good health a specified category of individuals (and usually their families also). While the originators of such plans may not have had in mind the old Chinese approach in which the doctor was paid as long as the client was well, physicians involved have had a financial interest in maintaining the health of their patients (more prevention meant less care for the same financial return). Thus the movement was toward true *health* insurance.

"The first successful prepaid group practice clinic (Ross-Loos, 1929) came into being and attracted some attention, but made only a minor impact on the medical profession's tradition of one-man, one-office, fee-for-service practice." [11] Other groups emerged in the depression years of the 1930s. Sidney R.

Garfield, of the University of Iowa Medical School and Los Angeles County Hospital, was convinced that good medicine meant group medicine centralized and streamlined under one clinic and hospital roof. In 1933 he "launched out as a sort of desert-rat doctor, to take care of men who had next to no money in a hot dusty region never meant by God for human activity or habitation. . . . Medically, the 5000 prospective patients were among the folks God forgot." [12]

These men were building a fresh-water aqueduct across the California desert to Los Angeles. Under the state's industrial compensation law, the injured were carted to Los Angeles (arriving alive if they were not too seriously hurt); if they took sick, it was just too bad—and, Garfield recognized, 90 per cent of their incapacities were just plain sickness. Garfield and a few doctors working for him set up an industrial accident and medical care plan. Management provided $1.50 per man per month, the workers a like sum—a nickel a day. "Workers, contractors, the doctors, and the insurance companies were happy with this plan, operated without charity or financial hardship on anyone. The key advantages of the scheme lay in predictability—in steady income for the medical group and in a ready source of care at low cost for the workers." [13]

Garfield found that his doctors were saving lives because, with no factor of medical cost to keep them away, people "came in before the chest colds progressed to pneumonia and their belly pains ended in ruptured appendixes." Kaiser-Permanente would publicize this concept in its slogan "Paying the doctor to keep you well." [14]

In 1938 Henry J. Kaiser and his son Edgar were completing the Grand Coulee Dam in the State of Washington. The unions were unhappy about the fee-for-service medical care that was being provided to the 10,000 workers and their families. Edgar Kaiser invited Garfield to take over. A group was formed under which care was provided for seven cents a day per worker, prepaid by the employer. Then the group was expanded to take care of wives for an equal sum and children for twenty-five cents a week.

In 1942 Henry Kaiser established the Garfield program in his World War II shipyards in California, Oregon, and Washington and in his steel mills in Fontana, California. "The shipyard workers included men and women from 16 to 80 years old, some of them physically handicapped and many 4-Fs. From a health insurance standpoint, they presented a complete set of bad risks. Nonetheless, the plan was not only a medical but a financial success and paid off bank loans, backed by Kaiser, to build and equip hospitals in Oakland, Vancouver [Washington], and Fontana." [15]

With the closing of the shipyards in 1945 the number of workers covered dropped from 200,000 to a few thousand, but ex-workers in the San Francisco-Oakland area (and their unions) wanted the plan to continue. Kaiser reached a decision unique in industrial health care—to throw the plan open to the public and see how it worked. The answer came in the next dozen years, during which the Kaiser Foundation Health Plan, Kaiser Foundation Hospitals, and Permanente Medical Groups fought their way to the enviable position in which they stand today.

"American public and private expenditures for health care reached an estimated $70 billion in 1970. Upwards of $45 billion of this amount were personal consumption expenses. From this financial base, it would be reasonable to suppose that the private health care industry would be capable of generating its own capital or reinvestment in research and development, including plant renewal, training, and the expansion and improvement of services. This, however, seldom occurs. . . . The operation of the medical profession and of free and private enterprise traditionally has depended on private philanthropic or public financing of capital requirements.

"The Kaiser-Permanente program, as a cooperative undertaking of doctors, hospitals, and health plan management, turns the traditional capital problem around. Through capitalization financing, all cash flows into the same pool. Performing as a corporate industry, although not for profit, the Health Plan resolves the need for capital by building this requirement into its rate/cost structure. The customer's own dollars assure the continued availability of the services he pays for, while at the same time assuring the financial security of the total system." [16]

A different approach was that of the Seattle-based Group Health Cooperative of Puget Sound, organized in 1944 by members of The Grange, the Aero-Mechanics Union, and residents of the area disenchanted by fee-for-service medicine. Its founding principles involved control of the organization by its members rather than its doctors; election of trustees and major policy decisions to be made on a one-member, one-vote basis; emphasis to be placed on health care and preventive medicine; a single monthly payment to cover all health costs for member families.

Each member invested $100 in the purchase of an existing clinic, and the cooperative formally opened for business in

1947 with an initial budget of $700,000. Twenty-five years later the budget was $28 million, the staff of doctors had grown from fifteen to 145, and hospital beds had risen to 302 from an original fifty.

The Group Health Cooperative provides full, unlimited medical, surgical, and hospital care, house calls by doctors and visiting nurses, all prescribed drugs (except tranquilizers), birth-control pills, dietary supplements, X-rays and laboratory services, physical therapy, worldwide emergency insurance, ten free psychiatric consultations ($5 a visit thereafter), and eye examinations.

While the bulk of the membership comprises individual family members and industrial and employee groups covered by contracts with employers, poverty families are cared for under contract with federal and state agencies. State officials find that Group Health is providing care to the public at 25 per cent less than what the state is paying elsewhere.

Other early plans include the Group Health Association of Washington, D.C., the Labor Health Institute in St. Louis, and the Health Insurance Plan of Greater New York (HIP).

A HEALTH MAINTENANCE ORGANIZATION (HMO)

The very term HMO is confusing, for the initials stand not for one thing but three: an idea in the heads of health planners; one of a number of already existing but substantially different health plan organizations; an entity in a number of legislative proposals that differ among themselves.[17]

The U.S. Department of Health, Education, and Welfare in a recent leaflet put out by its Health Services and Mental

Health Administration division states that a Health Maintenance Organization is based on four principles:

> It is an *organized system* of health care which accepts the responsibility to provide or otherwise assure the delivery of
>
> an agreed upon set of *comprehensive health maintenance and treatment services* for
>
> a voluntarily *enrolled group* of persons in a geographic area and
>
> is reimbursed through a pre-negotiated and fixed periodic payment made by or on behalf of each person or family unit enrolled in the plan.[18]

By contracting with subscribers to provide medical services, the HMO guarantees the delivery of such services. This is different from the other plans, such as Medicare and private health insurance, which provide patients with money to pay for care and leave them to seek care on their own.[19]

Consumers selecting the HMO option received their services in return for a fixed contract price, paid in advance through tax-supported health programs, various for-profit and nonprofit plans, payroll deductions, or out-of-pocket payment. There is little if anything new in the fundamental organization, management, and approach. What is new is the fact that this is the first time such theories have been embodied in a plan proposed by the administration for engineering major changes in the nation's medical care system.[20]

The proposed federal plan does not intend to set up HMOs exclusively for the old and/or the poor; such "subscribers" would be held below 50 per cent of an HMO's enrollment, in the belief that if not more than half the financing comes from government programs, the other half or more from private subscribers, dual standards in treatment will be avoided. It seems questionable, however, whether Congress will legislate a health-care delivery service that favors an elite population by limiting enrollment of high-risk groups, such as the very old, the very young, and the poor. Nevertheless the Nixon administration seems convinced that HMO offers a substantial hope for delivering a superior range and quality of services to large, diversified populations without excessive cost to the federal treasury. The administration makes the assumption that it can lure private capital to HMO development, thereby lessening the need for federal spending. The incentive: profit.

Organized medicine, however, "harbors a long-standing bias against commercialized medical care systems which are controlled by laymen. The American Medical Association warned many years ago that lay control and dollar compensation can sometimes lead to unethical business tactics, physician exploitation, and dangerously inferior health services." [21]

Government and organized medicine are both "seeking solutions to the same problem." The administration is "willing to gamble that HMOs—in whatever form they emerge—represent at least a partial solution to some of the most critical problems; organized medicine is wary of betting too many chips on one deal of cards." [22] The administration feels that "doctors all over the country, hospitals, medical schools, . . . will recognize the writing on the wall . . . and flock into these prepaid ameboid structures called HMO's. . . . Practicing doctors will examine the issue . . . and come up with a decision that will favorably affect their income. In some parts of the country, where group practices already dominate the scene (Midwest and Far West, for example) this will be easy. They will opt for HMO. In other parts of the country . . . the temptation to organize into groups or associated clusters of whatever kind will be resisted." [23]

Medicine in America is currently at a crossroads, with the path to the left leading to socialized medicine, the path ahead to the semi-federalized HMO, the path to the right following the *status quo*. The road the American physicians will choose is still uncertain.

Reference Notes
Selected Bibliography
Illustration Credits
Index

REFERENCE NOTES

1. THE VIRGINIA COLONY

1. Richard Harrison Shryock, *Medicine and Society in America, 1660–1860* (New York: New York University Press, 1960), p. 3.
2. Wyndham B. Blanton, *Medicine in Virginia in the Seventeenth Century* (Richmond: William Byrd Press, 1930), p. 6.
3. Captain John Smith, *General Historie of Virginia,* included in *Travels and Works of Captain John Smith* (Edinburgh: J. Grant, 1910), p. 392.
4. Alexander Brown, *The Genesis of the United States* (New York: Houghton, Mifflin Company, 1897), Vol. I, p. 329.
5. Edward D. Neill, *Virginia Carolorum* (Albany, N.Y.: J. Munsell's Sons, 1886), p. 130.
6. Thomas Jefferson Wertenbaker, *Virginia under the Stuarts* (Princeton, N.J.: Princeton University Press, 1913), p. 12; Blanton, *op. cit.,* p. 41.
7. Edward D. Neill, *History of the Virginia Company of London* (Albany, N.Y.: J. Munsell, 1869), p. 12.
8. *Supra,* note 3, p. 114.
9. *Ibid.,* pp. 427, 449.
10. Blanton, *op. cit.,* p. 11.
11. *Supra,* note 7, p. 48.
12. Shryock, *op. cit.,* p. 9.
13. *Records of the Virginia Company of London, The Court Book,* ed. by S. M. Kingsbury (Washington, D.C.: Government Printing Office, 1906), Vol. I, p. 517.
14. Alexander Brown, *The First Republic in America* (New York: Houghton, Mifflin Company, 1898), p. 454.
15. *Minutes of Council and General Court,* p. 58, quoted in Blanton, *op. cit.,* p. 19.

16. *Ibid.,* p. 117, quoted *ibid.,* p. 19.
17. *Supra,* note 3, p. 586.
18. Blanton, *op. cit.,* p. 31.
19. *Ibid.,* pp. 80, 148, 184.
20. Joseph M. Toner, *Contributions to the Annals of Medical Progress and Medical Education before and during the War of Independence* (Washington, D.C.: Government Printing Office, 1874), p. 106.

2. THE NEW ENGLAND COLONIES

1. Maurice Bear Gordon, *Aesculapius Comes to the Colonies* (Ventnor, N.J.: Ventnor Publishers, 1949), p. 58.
2. Quoted *ibid.,* p. 59.
3. Francis R. Packard, *History of Medicine in the United States* (New York: Paul B. Hoeber, 1931), Vol. I, p. 9.
4. *Ibid.,* p. 10.
5. James Thacher, *American Medical Biography* (Boston: Richardson & Lord and Cottons & Barnard, 1828), Vol. I, p. 267.
6. "Winslow's Relation" in *Chronicles of the Pilgrim Fathers* (London: Dent, 1910), pp. 309–10.
7. Quoted in Gordon, *op. cit.,* p. 61.
8. *Ibid.,* pp. 73–74.
9. Oliver Wendell Holmes, "Scholastic and Bedside Teaching," in *Medical Essays, 1842–1882* (Boston: Houghton, Mifflin Company, 1883), pp. 281–83.
10. Quoted in Packard, *op. cit.,* p. 25.
11. T [homas] Hutchinson, *The History of the Province of Massachusetts Bay from 1749 to 1774* (London: J. Murray, 1828), p. 174 *n.*
12. Thacher, *op. cit.,* Vol. II, p. 122.
13. Cotton Mather, *Magnalia Christi Americana* (Hartford, Conn.: S. Andrus & Son, 1855), Vol. III, p. 149.
14. Thacher, *op. cit.*
15. Mather, *op. cit.,* p. 152.
16. Quoted in Packard, *op. cit.,* p. 26.
17. *Ibid.*

3. INDIGENOUS REMEDIES AND PRACTICES

1. Claude E. Heaton, "Medicine in New Amsterdam," *Bulletin of the History of Medicine,* IX:2 (Feb. 1941), pp. 130–31.
2. John Josselyn, *An Account of two Voyages to New-England* (London: G. Widdowes, 1675), reprinted in *Collections of the Massachusetts Historical Society,* Ser. 3, Vol. 3 (Cambridge, Mass.: E. W. Metcalf, 1833), pp. 131–32 (298–99).
3. *Ibid.,* pp. 183–85 (333–34).
4. *Ibid.,* p. 60 (251–52).
5. *Ibid.,* p. 76 (262).
6. Bernard G. Hoffman, "John Clayton's 1687 Account of the Medicinal Practices of the Virginia Indians," *Ethnohistory,* XI:1 (Winter 1964), pp. 4, 5.
7. Quoted *ibid.,* pp. 5, 9, 11.
8. *Ibid.,* pp. 5–6, 25.
9. *Ibid.,* pp. 9, 10, 11–17, 18–19, 20, 28.
10. *Ibid.,* pp. 7–8, 26.
11. Quoted in Packard, *History of Medicine in the United States,* Vol. I, pp. 20–22.
12. *Ibid.,* p. 22.

4. COTTON MATHER, MEDICAL POLEMICIST

1. L. Sprague de Camp and Catherine C. de Camp, *The Story of Science in America* (New York: Charles Scribner's Sons, 1967), p. 6.
2. Otho T. Beall, Jr., and Richard H. Shryock, *Cotton Mather, First Significant Figure in American Medicine* (Baltimore: Johns Hopkins University Press, 1954), p. vii.
3. "Cotton Mather" (by Kenneth A. Murdock), *Dictionary of American Biography* (New York: Charles Scribner's Sons, 1933), Vol. XII, p. 386.
4. *Ibid.,* pp. 386–87.
5. *Ibid.,* p. 386.
6. Quoted in Beall and Shryock, *op. cit.,* p. 8.
7. Quoted *ibid.,* p. 15.
8. Quoted *ibid.,* p. 16.
9. Quoted *ibid.,* p. 35.

10. *Supra,* note 3, p. 389.
11. Mather, *Magnalia Christi Americana,* Vol. I, pp. 149–50.
12. *Ibid.,* Vol. II, p. 175.
13. *Ibid.,* p. 356.
14. Letter of July 13, 1716, in Beall and Shryock, *op. cit.,* pp. 46–47.
15. Mather, *op. cit.,* Vol. II, p. 606.
16. Quoted in Beall and Shryock, *op. cit.,* p. 50.
17. *Ibid.,* pp. 127, 131.
18. Quoted in Gordon, *Aesculapius Comes to the Colonies,* p. 190.
19. Quoted in Beall and Shryock, *op. cit.,* pp. 132, 144.
20. Quoted *ibid.,* pp. 145–46.
21. Quoted *ibid.,* pp. 149–50.
22. *Ibid.,* p. 152.
23. Quoted *ibid.,* p. 212.
24. Quoted *ibid.,* p. 217.

5. *HOSPITALS*

1. Heaton, "Medicine in New Amsterdam," pp. 140–41; Claude E. Heaton, "Medicine in New York during the English Colonial Period." *Bulletin of the History of Medicine,* XVII (Jan.–May 1947), pp. 10, 14–15.
2. John E. Ransom, "Beginnings of Hospitals in the United States," *Hospitals,* XV (Dec. 1941), p. 75.
3. D. G. Thomas, "History of the Founding and Development of the First Hospitals of the United States," *American Journal of Insanity,* XXIV (1867–68), pp. 131–32.
4. Ransom, *op. cit.*
5. [Benjamin Franklin], *Some Account of the Pennsylvania Hospital from its First Rise to the Beginning of the Fifth Month, Called May, 1754* (Philadelphia: Printed at the Office of the *United States Gazette,* 1817), pp. 3–4.
6. Quoted in Thomas G. Morton, assisted by Frank Woodbury, *The History of the Pennsylvania Hospital, 1751–1895* (Philadelphia: Times Printing House, 1895), p. 6.
7. Franklin, *op. cit.,* p. 6.
8. Morton, *op. cit.,* pp. 10–11.
9. Franklin, *op. cit.,* pp. 49–51.

10. Morton, *op. cit.*, p. 241.
11. Quoted *ibid.*, pp. 448–49.
12. Quoted *ibid.*, pp. 143–44.
13. Norman Dain, *Concepts of Insanity in The United States, 1789–1865* (New Brunswick, N.J.: Rutgers University Press, 1964), p. 5.
14. *Ibid.*, p. 21.
15. Samuel Bard, *A Discourse upon the Duties of a Physician, with Some Sentiments on the Usefulness and Necessity of a Public Hospital* (New York: Printed by A. & J. Robertson, 1769).
16. "The New York Hospital" (editorial), *The Medical Record*, XII (1877), p. 184.
17. John Jones, *Plain Concise Practical Remarks, on the Treatment of Wounds and Fractures* . . . (Philadelphia: Robert Bell, 1776), p. 103.
18. Quoted in *supra*, note 16, pp. 185–86.

6. *DISSECTION AND ANATOMY*

1. *The Statutes at Large from the Thirty-Second Year of King Henry VIII to the Seventh Year of King Edward VI Inclusive.* Ed. by D. Pickering (Cambridge, England: Joseph Bentham (for Charles Bathurst), 1763), Vol. V, p. 60.
2. Quoted in Packard, *History of Medicine in the United States,* Vol. I, p. 54.
3. *Ibid.*, pp. 54–55.
4. Frederick C. Waite, "The Development of Anatomical Laws in the States of New England," *The New England Journal of Medicine,* CCXXXIII: 24 (Dec. 13, 1945), p. 718.
5. Quoted in Edward M. Hartwell, "The Hindrances to Anatomical Study in the United States, Including a Special Record of the Struggles of Our Early Anatomical Teachers," *Annals of Anatomy and Surgery,* Vol. III (1881), p. 211.
6. Packard, *op. cit.*, pp. 56–58.
7. Edward B. Krumbhaar, "The Early History of Anatomy in the United States," *Annals of Medical History,* IV (1922), p. 272.
8. Waite, *op. cit.*

9. Krumbhaar, *op. cit.,* pp. 272–73; Thacher, *American Medical Biography,* Vol. I, p. 212.

10. Hartwell, *op. cit.,* p. 212.

11. Krumbhaar, *op. cit.,* p. 275.

12. Quoted in Cecilia C. Mettler, *History of Medicine,* ed. by Fred A. Mettler (Philadelphia and Toronto: The Blakiston Company, 1947), p. 88.

13. Francisco Guerra, *American Medical Bibliography, 1639–1783* (New York: Lathrop C. Harper, 1962), pp. 640–42.

14. Mettler, *op. cit.*

15. C. F. Adams, *Works of John Adams* (Boston: Little, Brown and Company, 1853), Vol. II, p. 397.

16. John Jeffries, *A Narrative of the Two Aerial Voyages of Doctor Jeffries with Mons. Blanchard; with Meteorological Observations and Remarks* (London: J. Robson, 1786).

17. William Blackstone, *Commentaries on the Laws of England.* Ed. by E. Christian (Philadelphia: Robert H. Small, 1825), Vol. II, pp. 437, 437 *n.*

18. Frederick C. Waite, "Grave Robbing in New England," *Bulletin of the Medical Library Association,* XXXIII (1945), p. 274; Toner, *Contributions to the Annals of Medical Progress . . . ,* p. 57.

19. Rhoda Truax, *The Doctors Warren of Boston* (Boston: Houghton, Mifflin Company, 1968), p. 47; Mettler, *op. cit.,* p. 89; Edward M. Hartwell, "Anatomical Society in Massachusetts," *Annals of Anatomy and Surgery,* Vol. III (1881), p. 266.

20. Truax, *op. cit.,* pp. 47–49.

21. Whitfield J. Bell, Jr., "Body Snatching in Philadelphia," *Journal of the History of Medicine,* XXIII (Jan. 1968), pp. 108–10.

22. Claude E. Heaton, "Body Snatching in New York City," *New York State Journal of Medicine,* XLIII, Pt. 2 (Oct. 1, 1943), p. 1862.

23. Quoted *ibid.*

24. Whitfield J. Bell, Jr., "Doctors' Riot, New York, 1788," *Bulletin of the New York Academy of Medicine,* XLVII: 12 (Dec. 1971), pp. 1501–1502.

25. Quoted *ibid.,* pp. 1502–1503.

26. Linden F. Edwards, "An Unusual 'Physician's Notice,' " *Ohio State Medical Journal,* XLVII (1951), pp. 739–40.

27. *Address to the Community on the Necessity of Legalizing The Study of Anatomy* (Boston: Perkins & Marvin, 1829), p. 2.

28. *Ibid.,* pp. 4–7.
29. *Ibid.,* pp. 8–9, 26.
30. *Report of the Select Committee of the House of Representatives on So Much of the Governor's Speech, at the June Session, 1830, as Relates to Legalizing the Study of Anatomy* (Boston: Dutton & Wentworth, 1831), pp. 3, 4, 25, 62.
31. *Ibid.,* pp. 73–74, 77, 83–86.
32. Horace Montgomery, "A Body Snatcher Sponsors Pennsylvania's Anatomy Act," *Journal of the History of Medicine,* XXI (Oct. 1966), p. 392.

7. *THE EARLY MEDICAL SCHOOLS*

1. Toner, *Contributions to the Annals of Medical Progress . . . ,* p. 95.
2. Henry E. Sigerist, *American Medicine,* tr. by Hildegard Nagel (New York: W. W. Norton, 1934), p. 41.
3. George W. Corner, *Two Centuries of Medicine* (Philadelphia & Montreal: J. B. Lippincott Company, 1965), p. 13.
4. *Ibid.,* p. 14.
5. *Ibid.,* pp. 18–19.
6. Genevieve Miller, "Medical Schools in the Colonies," *Ciba Symposia,* VIII: 10 (Jan. 1947), p. 526.
7. *Ibid.,* pp. 526–27.
8. Corner, *op. cit.,* p. 20.
9. *Ibid.,* p. 23.
10. *Ibid.*
11. *Ibid.,* p. 25.
12. William Frederick Norwood, *Medical Education in the United States before the Civil War* (Philadelphia: University of Pennsylvania Press, 1944), pp. 65–66.
13. *Ibid.,* pp. 84–85.
14. Quoted in Miller, *op. cit.,* p. 532.
15. Norwood, *op. cit.,* p. 111.
16. *Ibid.,* p. 112.
17. [Samuel Latham Mitchill], *The Present State of Medical Learning in the City of New York* (New York: T. & J. Swords, 1797), p. 3.
18. "Petition of Henry Dunster," *Records of the Colony of New Plymouth in New England,* IX: 95, quoted in Norwood, *op. cit.,* p. 167.

19. Gordon, *Aesculapius Comes to the Colonies,* p. 91.
20. Quoted in Packard, *History of Medicine in the United States,* Vol. I, p. 434.
21. *Ibid.,* p. 435.
22. Norwood, *op. cit.,* p. 174.
23. *Ibid.,* p. 175.
24. Quoted in Packard, *op. cit.,* p. 461.

8. MEDICINE AND WAR

1. Walter R. Steiner, "The Reverend Gershom Bulkeley, of Connecticut, an Eminent Clerical Physician," *Bulletin of the Johns Hopkins Hospital,* XVII: 179 (Feb. 1906), pp. 48–49.
2. *Ibid.,* p. 49.
3. *Ibid.,* p. 50.
4. Stanley B. Weld, "Early Medical Practice in Hartford County," *Connecticut State Medical Journal,* V (1941), pp. 489–90; Gordon, *Aesculapius Comes to the Colonies,* pp. 118, 211–14.
5. From Dr. Nicholas Romayne's annual address to The Medical Society of The State of New York, quoted in Krumbhaar, "The Early History of Anatomy in the United States," p. 274.
6. Ransom, "Beginnings of Hospitals in the United States," p. 70.
7. H. Winnett Orr, "Biographical Notes Regarding Some American Military Surgeons," *Quarterly Bulletin Northwestern University Medical School,* XX (1946), pp. 113–14.
8. William Frederick Norwood, "Medicine in the Era of the American Revolution," *International Record of Medicine,* CLXXI: 7 (July 1958), pp. 396–97.
9. Lawrence Farmer, "The Early Directors of the Medical Services of the American Revolutionary Army," *Bulletin New York Academy of Medicine,* XXXVI: 11 (Nov. 1960), p. 766.
10. *Ibid.,* p. 767.
11. *Ibid.,* pp. 766–67.
12. *Ibid.,* p. 772.
13. Quoted *ibid.*
14. Quoted in Isobel Stevenson, "Beginnings of American Military Medicine, *Ciba Symposia,* I: 11 (Feb. 1940), p. 348.
15. Farmer, *op. cit.,* p. 775.

16. *Ibid.*, pp. 775–76.

17. Quoted in Gordon, *op. cit.*, p. 370.

18. Stevenson, *op. cit.*, p. 354.

19. Farmer, *op. cit.*, p. 776.

20. C. Malcolm B. Gilman, "Military Surgery in the American Revolution," *Journal of the Medical Society of New Jersey*, LVII (1960), pp. 492–93.

21. Quoted *ibid.*, p. 492.

22. P. M. Ashburn, *A History of the Medical Department of the United States Army* (Boston & New York: Houghton, Mifflin Company, 1929), p. 23.

23. Henry R. Viets, "James Thacher and his Influence on American Medicine," *Virigina Medical Monthly*, LXXVI (1949), p. 384.

24. James Thacher, *The American Revolution . . .* (New York: American Subscription Publishing House, 1860), pp. 43–45. The following quotations are from pp. 78, 82–84, 86, 90–91, 97, 103, 145, 147–48, 152, 233, 255–56, 257–58, 307, 309, 325–26.

25. Thacher, *American Medical Biography*, Vol. II, p. 131.

26. James Evelyn Pilcher, "James Tilton, Physician and Surgeon General of the United States Army, 1813–1815," *Journal of the Association of Military Surgeons of the United States*, XIV (1904), pp. 271–72; Thacher, *op. cit.*, p. 132.

27. Pilcher, *op. cit.*, p. 273.

28. Quoted in Stevenson, *op. cit.*, p. 351.

29. Thacher, *op. cit.*, pp. 132–33.

30. Quoted in Stevenson, *op. cit.*, p. 352.

31. Blair O. Rogers, "Surgery in the Revolutionary War, Contributions of John Jones, M.D. (1729–1791)," *Plastic & Reconstructive Surgery*, XLIX: 1 (Jan. 1972), pp. 9–10.

32. Quoted *ibid.*, pp. 1–2.

33. Norwood, *op. cit.*, p. 400; Stevenson, *op. cit.*, p. 354.

9. *MEDICINE BEYOND THE ALLEGHENIES*

1. T. V. Woodring, "Pioneer Physicians and Medicine in Middle Tennessee," *Journal of the Tennessee State Medical Association*, XXXIV (1941), p. 469.

2. Richard Dunlop, *Doctors of the American Frontier* (New York: Doubleday & Company, 1965), p. 1.

3. *Ibid.*, p. 9.

4. *Ibid.*, p. 10.

5. *Ibid.*, pp. 2–3.

6. Sigerist, *American Medicine*, p. 88.

7. Dunlop, *op. cit.*, p. 21.

8. August Schachner, *Ephraim McDowell, "Father of Ovariotomy" and Founder of Abdominal Surgery* (Philadelphia: J. B. Lippincott Company, 1921), p. 67.

9. Samuel D. Gross quoted in Ralph H. Major, *A History of Medicine* (Springfield, Ill.: Charles C Thomas, 1954), Vol. II, p. 741.

10. Fielding H. Garrison, *An Introduction to the History of Medicine* (Philadelphia & London: W. B. Saunders, 1929), p. 441.

11. Quoted in Otto Juettner, *Daniel Drake and His Followers, Historical and Biographical Sketches* (Cincinnati: Harvey Publishing Company, 1909), p. 20.

12. Garrison, *op. cit.*

13. Quoted in Major, *op. cit.*, p. 746.

14. Quoted in Mettler, *History of Medicine*, p. 160.

15. Packard, *History of Medicine in the United States*, Vol. II, p. 1063.

16. *Ibid.*, p. 1064.

10. THE PHENOMENON OF SPECIALIZATION

1. Shryock, *Medicine and Society in America*, p. 7.

2. John Morgan, *A Discourse Upon the Institution of Medical Schools in America* (Philadelphia: William Bradford, 1765), p. xvii.

3. Miller, *Medical Schools in the Colonies*, p. 528.

4. George Rosen, "Changing Attitudes of the Medical Profession to Specialization," *Bulletin of the History of Medicine*, XII (1942), pp. 348–49.

5. Benjamin Tenney, "Obstetrics and Gynecology," in *The Choice of a Medical Career*, ed. by Joseph Garland and Joseph Stokes III (Philadelphia–Montreal: J. B. Lippincott Company, 2nd ed., 1962), pp. 101–102.

6. Shryock, *op. cit.*, p. 132.

7. J. Marion Sims, *The Story of My Life* (New York: D. Appleton, 1889), p. 116.

8. *Ibid.*, pp. 234–35.

9. Richard Harrison Shryock, *Medicine in America, Historical Essays* (Baltimore: Johns Hopkins University Press, 1966), p. 167.

10. Mettler, *History of Medicine*, p. 96.

11. Packard, *History of Medicine in the United States*, Vol. II, p. 1145.

12. William F. Mengert, "The Origin of the Male Midwife," *Annals of Medical History*, n.s. IV (1932), p. 462.

13. H. Thoms, *Chapters in American Obstetrics* (Springfield, Ill.: Charles C Thomas, 1933), p. 60.

14. *Medical Classics*, Vol. I (1936), p. 243.

15. Quoted in Major, *A History of Medicine*, Vol. II, pp. 751–52.

16. J. Snow, *On Chloroform and Other Anaesthetics: Their Action and Administration* (London: J. Churchill, 1858), p. 14.

17. Shryock, *Medicine and Society in America*, p. 133.

18. J. Englebert Dunphy, "Surgery," in *The Choice of a Medical Career*, p. 88.

19. Harvey Cushing, quoted in J. W. Duckett, "The Halsted Heritage," *Surgery*, LV: 6 (June 1964), p. 859.

20. *Ibid.*, p. 864.

21. Quoted *ibid.*

22. Quoted *ibid.*, pp. 864–65.

23. John F. Fulton, "Medicine, Warfare, and History," *Journal of the American Medical Association*, CLIII: 5 (Oct. 3, 1953), p. 483.

24. Circular No. 6 Surgeon-General's Office (March 10) 1864, quoted *ibid.*

25. Edward Warren, *The Life of John Collins Warren; compiled chiefly from his Autobiography and Journals* (Boston: Ticknor & Fields, 1860), Vol. II, p. 13.

26. George Rosen, "Special Medical Societies in the United States after 1860," *Ciba Symposia*, IX: 9 (Dec. 1947), p. 785.

27. *Ibid.*, pp. 785–86.

11. *THE SECTARIANS*

1. Shryock, *Medicine and Society in America*, p. 144.

2. Shryock, *Medicine in America, Historical Essays*, p. 171.

3. Samuel Thomson, *Life and Medical Discoveries of Samuel Thomson . . .* (Columbus, Ohio: Pike, Platt, & Company, 6th ed., 1832), pp. 18–19, 22.

4. John Uri Lloyd, ed., "Life and Medical Discoveries of Samuel Thomson and a History of the Thomsonian Materia Medica," *Bulletin of the Lloyd Library of Botany, Pharmacy and Materia Medica,* No. 11, Reproduction Series No. 7 (1909), p. 6.

5. Thomson, *op. cit.,* pp. 23–25.

6. *Ibid.,* p. 47.

7. Alexander Wilder, *History of Medicine* (New Sharon, Me.: New England Eclectic Publishing Company, 1901), p. 453.

8. Thomson, *op. cit.,* pp. 51–53.

9. Garrison, *An Introduction to the History of Medicine,* p. 237.

10. William Henderson, *Homœopathy Fairly Represented. A Reply to Professor Simpson's "Homœopathy" Misrepresented* (Philadelphia: Lindsay & Blakiston, 1854), p. 166.

11. Sigerist, *American Medicine,* p. 195.

12. Andrew T. Still, "Osteopathy and Truth," in George V. Webster, *Concerning Osteopathy* (Norwood, Mass.: The Plimpton Press, 1919), p. 13.

13. Andrew T. Still, *Autobiography of Andrew T. Still* (Kirksville, Mo.: Published by the Author, 1897), pp. 31–32. The following quotations are from pp. 86, 114, 115, 122.

14. George W. Northup, *Osteopathic Medicine: An American Reformation* (Chicago: American Osteopathic Association, 1966), pp. 16, 71.

15. Sigerist, *op. cit.,* p. 197.

12. REFORMS IN MEDICAL PRACTICE AND EDUCATION

1. William Frederick Norwood, "The Early History of American Medical Societies," *Ciba Symposia,* IX: 9 (Dec. 1947), p. 762.

2. W. B. McDaniel, II, "A Brief Sketch of the Rise of American Medical Societies," *International Record of Medicine,* CLXXI: 8 (Aug. 1958), p. 485.

3. Norwood, *loc. cit.*

4. McDaniel, *loc. cit.*

5. *Ibid.,* p. 487.

6. Norwood, *op. cit.,* p. 766.

7. *Ibid.,* p. 767.

8. William Dosite Postell, "The American Medical Association," *Ciba Symposia*, IX: 9 (Dec. 1947), p. 776.

9. Quoted *ibid.*, p. 780.

10. *Ibid.*, p. 784.

11. William Frederick Norwood, "Medical Education in the United States before 1900," in C. D. O'Malley, *History of Medical Education* (Los Angeles: UCLA Press, 1970), p. 477.

12. William K. Beatty, "Daniel Hale Williams: Innovative Surgeon, Educator, and Hospital Administrator," *Chest*, LX: 8 (Aug. 1971), pp. 175–82.

13. Geoffrey Marks and William K. Beatty, *Women in White* (New York: Charles Scribner's Sons, 1972), pp. 82–83.

14. Abraham Flexner, "Medical Education in the United States and Canada," *Bulletin of the Carnegie Foundation for the Advancement of Teaching*, No. 4 (1910), p. viii.

15. Sigerist, *American Medicine*, p. 139.

16. William H. Welch, "Medical Education in the United States," *Harvey Lectures*, Ser. XI (1915–1916), p. 375.

17. R. K. Merton, "Some preliminaries to a Sociology of Medical Education," *The Student Physician,* ed. by R. K. Merton, G. Reader, and P. L. Kendal (Cambridge, Mass.: Harvard University Press, 1957), p. 18.

18. Nathan Smith Davis, *Contributions to the History of Medical Education and Medical Institutions in the United States of America, 1776–1876* (Washington, D.C.: Government Printing Office, 1877), p. 48.

19. Frederick C. Waite, "Advent of the Graded Curriculum in American Medical Colleges," *Journal of the Association of American Medical Colleges*, XXV (1950), pp. 316, 318.

20. Dean F. Smiley, "History of the Association of American Medical Colleges—1876–1956," *Journal of Medical Education*, XXXIII: 7 (July 1957), p. 515.

21. Flexner, *op. cit.*, pp. 143–45.

22. *Ibid.*, p. 145.

23. Abraham Flexner, *I Remember: An Autobiography* (New York: Simon & Schuster, 1940), p. 115.

24. Abraham Flexner, *Daniel Coit Gilman: Creator of the American Type of University* (New York: Harcourt, Brace & Company, 1946), p. 154; *supra,* note 14, p. 12.

25. Sigerist, *op. cit.*, p. 129.

26. Richard H. Shryock, *Medical Licensing in America* (Baltimore: Johns Hopkins University Press, 1967), pp. 63–64.

27. William H. Welch, "The Medical Curriculum," *Bulletin of the American Academy of Medicine,* XI (1910), p. 720.

13. THE SMALLPOX EPIDEMICS

1. John Duffy, *Epidemics in Colonial America* (Baton Rouge: Louisiana State University Press, 1953), p. 22.

2. *Ibid.*, p. 43; Thomas Hutchinson, *The History of the Colony and Province of Massachusetts Bay,* ed. by Lawrence Shaw Mayo (Cambridge, Mass.: Harvard University Press, 1936), Vol. I, p. 32 *n.*

3. Packard, *History of Medicine in the United States,* Vol. I, pp. 74–75.

4. Philip Alexander Bruce, *Institutional History of Virginia in the Seventeenth Century,* (New York: G. P. Putnam's Sons, 1910) Vol. II, p. 18.

5. Samuel A. Green (ed.), *Diary by Increase Mather, March 1675–December 1676. Together with extracts from another diary by him, 1674–1687* (Cambridge: J. Wilson & Son, 1900), p. 2.

6. Gordon, *Aesculapius Comes to the Colonies,* pp. 83–84.

7. Facsimile published with Nolie Mumey, *Reverend Thomas Thacher; a Biographical Sketch* (Denver: The Author, 1937).

8. Gordon, *op. cit.*, p. 160.

9. Quoted in Duffy, *op. cit.*, p. 49.

10. *The History of Inoculation and Vaccination for the Prevention and Treatment of Disease* (London: Burroughs Wellcome & Company, 1913), p. 14.

11. Mettler, *History of Medicine,* pp. 419–20.

12. *Philosophic Transactions of the Royal Society,* XXIX (1714–16), pp. 72–82, 393–99.

13. Quoted in Frederick C. Kilgour, "The Rise of Scientific Activity in Colonial New England," *Yale Journal of Biology and Medicine,* XXII (Dec. 1949), p. 130.

14. *Ibid.*, p. 131.

15. Packard, *op. cit.*, p. 94.

16. Reginald Fitz, "The Massachusetts Medical Society—From Cow-Path to State Road," *New England Journal of Medicine*, CCXIV: 24 (June 11, 1936), p. 1180.

17. Reginald Heber Fitz, "Zabdiel Boylston, Inoculator, and the Epidemic of Smallpox in Boston in 1721," *Bulletin of the Johns Hopkins Hospital*, XXII: 247 (Sept. 1911), p. 318.

18. Quoted *ibid.*, pp. 318–19.

19. Quoted *ibid.*, p. 319.

20. John B. Blake, *Public Health in the Town of Boston, 1630–1822* (Cambridge, Mass.: Harvard University Press, 1959), p. 57.

21. Whitfield J. Bell, Jr., "Medical Practice in Colonial America," *Bulletin of the History of Medicine*, XXXI (1957), p. 443.

22. Quoted in *supra*, note 17, p. 319.

23. Zabdiel Boylston, *An historical account of the smallpox inoculated in New England*, 2nd ed. cor. (Boston: Reprinted for S. Gerrish and T. Hancock, 1730), p. 34.

24. Quoted in Blake, *op. cit.*, p. 71.

25. Quoted in Henry Lee Smith, "Dr. Adam Thomson, The Originator of the American Method of Inoculation for Small-Pox," *Bulletin of the Johns Hopkins Hospital*, XX: 215 (Feb. 1909), p. 50 *n*.

26. *Ibid.*, p. 50.

27. Quoted *ibid.*

28. *Ibid.*

29. *Ibid.*, p. 51.

30. *Ibid.*

31. Daniel Sutton, *The Inoculator; or Suttonian System of Inoculation* (London: Printed for the Author by T. Gillet, 1796), p. iii.

32. *Ibid.*, pp. 77–78, 82.

33. Thomas Rushton, *An Essay on Inoculation for the Small Pox* (London: Printed for J. Payne, 1767), pp. 1–2.

34. Smith, *op. cit.*

35. Rushton, *op. cit.*, pp. 51, 68, 70.

36. Sutton, *op. cit.*, facing p. 160.

37. Shryock, *Medicine in America, Historical Essays*, p. 258.

38. *Supra*, note 10, p. 59.

39. *Ibid.*, pp. 53–54.

40. Edgar M. Crookshank, *History and Pathology of Vaccination* (Philadelphia: P. Blakiston, Son, 1889), Vol. I, p. 116.

41. Garrison, *An Introduction to the History of Medicine*, pp. 373–74.

42. *North Carolina Medical Journal*, XXXII: 12 (Dec. 1971), pp. 507–508.
43. *Time*, Jan. 24, 1972, p. 46.

14. THE SCOURGE OF YELLOW FEVER

1. Duffy, *Epidemics in Colonial America*, pp. 140–41.
2. John B. Blake, "Yellow Fever in Eighteenth Century America," *Bulletin of the New York Academy of Medicine*, XLIV: 6 (June 1968), p. 677.
3. Thacher, *American Medical Biography*, I, 393.
4. *Ibid.*, pp. 357–58.
5. Garrison, *An Introduction to the History of Medicine*, pp. 404, 833.
6. Mathew Carey, *A Short Account of the Malignant Fever, lately prevalent in Philadelphia:* . . . (Philadelphia: Printed by the Author, 1793), pp. 28–29.
7. Benjamin Rush, *An Account of the Bilious remitting Yellow Fever as it Appeared in the City of Philadelphia, in the Year 1793* (Philadelphia: Thomas Dobson, 2nd ed., 1794), pp. 124–25.
8. George W. Corner, ed., *The Autobiography of Benjamin Rush* (Princeton, N.J.: Princeton University Press, 1948), p. 95 *n*.
9. Carey, *op. cit.*, pp. 16, 18.
10. [Benjamin Rush], *Old Family Letters relating to the Yellow Fever* (Philadelphia: J. B. Lippincott Company, 1892), p. 3.
11. William S. Middleton, "Yellow Fever Epidemic of 1793 in Philadelphia," *Annals of Medical History*, X (1928), p. 437.
12. [Rush], *supra*, note 10, pp. 15, 25.
13. Middleton, *op. cit.*, p. 442.
14. Nathan G. Goodman, *Benjamin Rush Physician and Citizen* (Philadelphia: University of Pennsylvania Press, 1934), pp. 194–95.
15. Chris Holmes, "Benjamin Rush and the Yellow Fever," *Bulletin of the History of Medicine*, XL (1966), pp. 259–60.
16. Sigismund Peller, "Walter Reed, C. Finlay, and their Predecessors Around 1800," *Bulletin of the History of Medicine*, XXXIII: 3 (May–June 1959), p. 198.
17. *Ibid.*, p. 199.
18. *Ibid.*, p. 200.

19. Walter Reed, *et al.*, "The etiology of yellow fever. A preliminary note," *Philadelphia Medical Journal,* VI (1901), p. 796.
20. Wilbur G. Downs, "The Story of Yellow Fever Since Walter Reed," *Bulletin of the New York Academy of Medicine,* XLIV (1968), pp. 725–26.
21. Jo Ann Carrigan, "Yellow Fever in New Orleans, 1905: The Last Epidemic," *Bulletin of Tulane University Medical Faculty,* XXVI: 1 (Feb. 1967), pp. 19–20.

15. THE BATTLE AGAINST WIDESPREAD DISEASES

1. Duffy, *Epidemics of Colonial America,* pp. 222–23.
2. William W. Gerhard, "On the typhus fever which occurred at Philadelphia in the spring and summer of 1836 . . . ," *American Journal of Medicine and Science,* XIX (Nov. 1837), pp. 292, 302, 322.
3. Elisha Bartlett, *The history, diagnosis and treatment of typhoid and of typhus fever* . . . (Philadelphia: Lea & Blanchard, 1842), p. 180.
4. Duffy, *op. cit.,* pp. 214–15.
5. Arthur L. Bloomfield, *A Bibliography of Internal Medicine; Communicable Diseases* (Chicago: University of Chicago Press, 1958), pp. 35–36.
6. *Ibid.,* p. 40.
7. Duffy, *op. cit.,* p. 137.
8. Mettler, *History of Medicine,* pp. 763–64.
9. Duffy, *op. cit.,* pp. 184–85.
10. William Cullen, *First Lines of the Practice of Physic,* 2 vols. (Dublin: W. Jones, 1791), Vol. I, p. 187.
11. Packard, *History of Medicine in the United States,* Vol. II, p. 1109.

16. TOWARD A PUBLIC HEALTH SERVICE

1. Blake, *Public Health in the Town of Boston, 1630–1822,* pp. 18–19.
2. J. Calvin Weaver, "Early Medical History of Georgia," *The Journal of the Medical Association of Georgia,* XXIX, 3 (Mar. 1940), pp. 103–04.

3. William B. DeWitt, "Contributions of the U.S. Public Health Service in Tropical Medicine: Part I," *Bulletin of the New York Academy of Medicine,* XLIV (1968), p. 728.

4. Harold M. Cavins, "The National Quarantine and Sanitary Conventions of 1857 to 1860 and the Beginnings of the American Public Health Association," *Bulletin of the History of Medicine,* XIII (1943), pp. 413–14.

5. John B. Blake, "The Origins of Public Health in the United States," *American Journal of Public Health,* XXXVIII (1948), p. 1540.

6. Shryock, *Medicine and Society in America,* p. 103.

7. Quoted in Cavins, *op. cit.,* p. 415.

8. *Ibid.,* pp. 415–16.

9. Quoted *ibid.,* p. 426.

10. Milton I. Roemer, "Government's Role in American Medicine," *Bulletin of the History of Medicine,* XVIII (1945), p. 156.

17. RESEARCH ON A SOUND FOUNDATION

1. Morris C. Leikind, "The Evolution of Medical Research in the United States," *International Record of Medicine,* CLXXI: 7 (July 1958), pp. 456–57.

2. Richard H. Shryock, *American Medical Research Past and Present* (New York: The Commonwealth Fund, 1947), p. 1.

3. Edward H. Clarke, *A Century of American Medicine, 1776–1876* (Philadelphia: Henry C. Lea, 1876), p. 13.

4. Samuel Jackson, *Address to the Medical Graduates of the University of Pennsylvania* (Philadelphia: T. K. & P. G. Collins, 1840), p. 15.

5. Sigerist, *American Medicine,* p. 268.

6. Leikind, *op. cit.,* p. 458.

7. Quoted in Iago Galdston, "Research in the United States," *Ciba Symposia,* VIII: 3–4 (June–July 1946), p. 364.

8. George Washington, "Farewell Address, Sept. 17, 1796," in James D. Richardson, comp., *A Compilation of the Messages and Papers of the Presidents, 1789–1902* (Washington: Bureau of National Literature and Art, 1904), Vol. I, p. 220.

9. Quoted in Galdston, *op. cit.,* pp. 366–67.

10. Wilder Penfield, *The Difficult Art of Giving* (Boston & Toronto: Little, Brown & Company, 1967), p. 129.

11. Shryock, *op. cit.,* p. 99.
12. *Medical Research: A Midcentury Survey,* (Boston & Toronto: Little, Brown & Company, 1955), Vol. I, pp. 539–40.
13. *Ibid.,* p. 540.
14. John R. Paul, *A History of Poliomyelitis* (New Haven & London: Yale University Press, 1971), p. 312.

18. THE FIGHT AGAINST POLIO

1. Michael Underwood, *A Treatise on the Dieases* [*sic*] *of Children with General Directions for the Management of Infants from the Birth,* 2 vols. in 1 (Philadelphia: T. Dobson, 1793), p. 255.
2. Quoted in Paul, *A History of Poliomyelitis,* p. 68.
3. *Ibid.,* p. 253.
4. James P. Leake, "Poliomyelitis following Vaccination against the Disease," *Journal of the American Medical Association,* CV (1935), p. 2152.
5. Paul, *op. cit.,* p. 233.
6. *Ibid.,* p. 420.
7. Quoted *ibid.,* p. 434.
8. *Ibid.,* p. 450.
9. *Journal of the American Medical Association,* CLXXVIII (Nov. 18, 1961), p. 755.
10. Paul, *op. cit.,* p. 468.

19. INVESTIGATION OF THE BRAIN

1. Walter E. Dandy quoted in Charles Wilson, "American Contributions to Neurosurgery," *New Orleans Medical and Surgical Journal,* XCVI (1943), p. 140.
2. Jefferson Browder, "Advances in Neurological Surgery during the Past Fifty Years," *American Journal of Surgery,* LI (1941), p. 164.
3. John F. Fulton, *Harvey Cushing* (Springfield, Ill.: Charles C Thomas, 1946), p. 257.
4. *Ibid.,* pp. 47–50.
5. *Ibid.,* pp. 257–58.
6. *Ibid.,* pp. 259, 261.

7. *Ibid.,* pp. 104–105.

8. Harvey Cushing, "A method of total extirpation of the Gasserian ganglion for trigeminal neuralgia. . . ." *Journal of the American Medical Association,* XXXIV (April 28, 1900), pp. 1035–41.

9. Fulton, *op. cit.,* p. 163.

10. *Ibid.,* p. 186.

11. *Ibid.,* p. 198.

12. *Ibid.,* pp. 198–99.

13. *Ibid.,* p. 204.

14. *Ibid.,* p. 202.

15. *Ibid.,* p. 266.

16. Edwin Clarke and C. D. O'Malley, *The Human Brain and the Spinal Cord* (Berkeley: University of California Press, 1968), p. 803.

17. "Psychosurgery," *The Lancet,* II: 7767 (July 8, 1972), p. 69.

18. Garfield Tourney, "A History of Therapeutic Fashions in Psychiatry, 1800–1966," *American Journal of Psychiatry,* CXXIV: 6 (Dec. 1967), p. 787.

19. Howard P. Rome, "Psychiatry: Circa 1919–1969–2019," *Annals of Internal Medicine,* LXXI: 4 (Oct. 1969), p. 846.

20. "The Most Common Mental Disorder," *Time,* Aug. 7, 1972, pp. 16–17.

21. Perry London, *Behavior Control* (New York: Harper & Row, 1969), p. 115.

22. Thomas P. Detre and Henry C. Jarecki, *Modern Psychiatric Treatment* (Philadelphia & Toronto: J. B. Lippincott Company, 1971), p. 664.

23. London, *op. cit.,* p. 116.

24. *Supra,* note 20, p. 17.

25. Ashton L. Welsh, *Psychotherapeutic Drugs* (Springfield, Ill.: Charles C Thomas, 1958), p. ix.

26. London, *op. cit.,* p. 119; Wilbur M. Benson and Burtrum C. Schiele, *Tranquilizing and Antidepressive Drugs* (Springfield, Ill.: Charles C Thomas, 1962), pp. 27, 29.

20. IN DEFIANCE OF OBSOLESCENCE

1. Donald Longmore, *Spare-Part Surgery* (New York: Doubleday & Company, 1968), pp. 9–10.

2. David Fishlock, *Man Modified* (New York: Funk & Wagnalls, 1969), p. 87.

3. Longmore, *op. cit.,* p. 75.

4. *Ibid.,* p. 31.

5. Alexis Carrel and C. C. Guthrie, "Anastomosis of Blood Vessels by the Patching Method and Transplantation of the Kidney," *Journal of the American Medical Association,* XLVII: 20 (Nov. 17, 1906), pp. 1648–51.

6. C. C. Guthrie, "Structural Changes and Survival of Cells in Transplanted Blood Vessels," *Journal of the American Medical Association,* L (1908), pp. 1035–36, and "Some Physiologic Aspects of Blood-Vessel Surgery," *Journal of the American Medical Association,* LI (1908), pp. 1658–62; Blair O. Rogers, "Charles Claude Guthrie, M.D., Ph.D.: A Remarkable Pioneer in Tissue and Organ Transplantation," *Plastic & Reconstructive Surgery,* XXIV: 4 (Oct. 1959), p. 380.

7. Alexis Carrel and Charles A. Lindbergh, *The Culture of Organs* (New York: Paul B. Hoeber, 1938), pp. 8–9.

8. *Ibid.,* pp. 216, 220.

9. Longmore, *op. cit.,* pp. 58–59.

10. Samuel Rapport and Helen Wright, eds., *Great Adventures in Medicine* (New York: Dial Press, 2nd revised ed., 1961), pp. 810–11.

11. Alexis Carrel, *Man the Unknown* (New York: Harper & Brothers, 1935), p. 239.

12. Longmore, *op. cit.,* pp. 11–13.

13. *Ibid.,* p. 27.

14. "Transplant Survival," *Time* (April 27, 1970), p. 71.

15. John P. Kemph, "Psychiatry and New Surgical Procedures—A Challenge to the Profession," *American Journal of Psychiatry,* CXXVI: 3 (Sept. 1969), pp. 144–45.

16. Longmore, *op. cit.,* pp. 96, 98.

21. AEROSPACE MEDICINE

1. Harry G. Armstrong, *Aerospace Medicine* (Baltimore: Williams & Wilkins, 1961), p. 1.

2. George Zinnemann, "Aerospace Medicine—Present, Past and Fu-

ture," in Hugh W. Randall, *Aerospace Medicine* (Baltimore: Williams & Wilkins, 2nd ed., 1971), p. 1.

3. *Ibid.,* pp. 2–3.
4. There is an English translation by M. A. and H. A. Hitchcock, *Barometric Pressure* (Columbus, Ohio: College Book Company, 1943).
5. Armstrong, *op. cit.,* p. 5.
6. Zinnemann, *op. cit.,* p. 4.
7. *Ibid.*
8. *Ibid.,* p. 9.

22. NUCLEAR MEDICINE

1. Henry N. Wagner, Jr., "The Rationale of Nuclear Medicine," *Hospital Practice,* VI (Oct. 1971), p. 15.
2. Ruth and Edward Brecher, *The Rays—a History of Radiology in the United States and Canada* (Baltimore: Williams & Wilkins, 1969), p. 332.
3. *Ibid.,* pp. 379–80.
4. H. S. Winchell, "Radioactive Tracers in Medicine," *Hospital Practice,* VI (Oct. 1971), p. 60.

23. THE FUTURE OF MEDICAL PRACTICE

1. Howard W. Haggard, *Devils, Drugs and Doctors* (New York: Blue Ribbon Books, 1929), p. 293.
2. *American Journal of Nursing,* LXXII: 9 (Sept. 1972), p. 1754.
3. Helen Clapesattle, *The Doctors Mayo* (Minneapolis: University of Minnesota Press, 1941), p. 114.
4. *Ibid.,* pp. 114–15.
5. *Ibid.,* pp. 116–18.
6. *Ibid.,* p. 209.
7. *Ibid.,* p. 501.
8. Garrison, *An Introduction to the History of Medicine,* p. 762.
9. Clapesattle, *op. cit.,* p. 534.
10. Michael M. Davis, Jr., "Group Medicine," *American Journal of Public Health,* IX (1919), p. 358.

REFERENCE NOTES

11. Greer Williams, *Kaiser-Permanente Health Plan—Why It Works* (Oakland, Calif.: Henry J. Kaiser Foundation, 1971), p. 3.
12. Paul de Kruif, *Kaiser Wakes the Doctors* (New York: Harcourt, Brace & Company, 1943), pp. 26–27.
13. Williams, *op. cit.*, pp. 3–4.
14. *Ibid.*, p. 4.
15. *Ibid.*, pp. 4–5.
16. *Ibid.*, pp. 66–67.
17. Robert M. Hendrickson, personal communication to authors, Oct. 21, 1972.
18. *Health Maintenance Organization the concept and structure* (Rockville, Md.: Health Services and Mental Health Administration, undated).
19. Robert M. Hendrickson, "There's an HMO in your future," *Physician's Management,* IX (May 1971), p. 64.
20. "Can the HMO puzzle ever be put together?" *American Medical News* (Aug. 7, 1972), p. 10.
21. *Ibid.*, p. 11.
22. *Ibid.*, p. 13.
23. George A. Silver, "A Challenge to the Academic Leopards: or HO, HO, HMO!" *Connecticut Medicine,* XXXVI: 7 (July 1972), p. 417.

SELECTED BIBLIOGRAPHY

❦

Address to the Community on the Necessity of Legislating the Study of Anatomy. Boston: Perkins & Marvin, 1829.

ARMSTRONG, HARRY G. *Aerospace Medicine*. Baltimore: Williams & Wilkins, 1961.

ASHBURN, P. M. *A History of the Medical Department of the United States Army*. Boston & New York: Houghton, Mifflin Company, 1929.

BALL, JAMES M. *The Sack-Em-Up Men*. London & Edinburgh: Oliver & Boyd, 1928.

BARD, SAMUEL. *A Discourse upon the Duties of a Physician, With Some Sentiments on the Usefulness and Necessity of a Public Hospital*. New York: Printed by A. & J. Robertson, 1769.

BEALL, OTHO T., JR., and SHRYOCK, RICHARD H. *Cotton Mather, First Significant Figure in American Medicine*. Baltimore: Johns Hopkins University Press, 1954.

BEATTY, WILLIAM K. "Daniel Hale Williams: Innovative Surgeon, Educator, and Hospital Administrator," *Chest* LX: 8 (Aug. 1971), pp. 175–82.

BEEBE, TANNA. "The Oldest and Biggest HMO," *Human Needs*, I: 1 (July 1972), pp. 12–14.

BELL, WHITFIELD J., JR. "Doctors' Riot, New York, 1788," *Bulletin of the New York Academy of Medicine*, XLVII: 12 (Dec. 1971), pp. 1501–03.

————. "Medical Practice in Colonial America," *Bulletin of the History of Medicine*, XXXI (1957), pp. 442–53.

BENSON, WILBUR M., and SCHIELE, BURTRUM C. *Tranquilizing and Antidepressive Drugs*. Springfield, Ill.: Charles C Thomas, 1962.

BERMAN, ALEX. "The Thomsonian movement and its relation to American pharmacy and medicine," *Bulletin of the History of Medicine*, XXV (1951), pp. 405–28, 519–38.

388

BLAKE, JOHN B. *Public Health in the Town of Boston, 1630–1822.*
Cambridge, Mass.: Harvard University Press, 1959.
————. "The Origins of Public Health in the United States," *American
Journal of Public Health,* XXXVIII (Nov. 1948), pp. 1539–50.
————. "Yellow Fever in Eighteenth Century America," *Bulletin of the
New York Academy of Medicine,* XLIV: 6 (June 1968), pp.
673–86.
BLANTON, WYNDHAM B. *Medicine in Virginia in the Seventeenth Cen-
tury.* Richmond: William Byrd Press, 1930.
BLOOMFIELD, ARTHUR L. *A Bibliography of Internal Medicine: Com-
municable Diseases.* Chicago: University of Chicago Press, 1958.
BRECHER, RUTH and EDWARD. *The Rays—A History of Radiology in
the United States and Canada.* Baltimore: Williams & Wilkins,
1969.
BROWDER, JEFFERSON. "Advances in Neurological Surgery During the Past
Fifty Years," *American Journal of Surgery,* LI (1941), pp. 164–87.
BROWN, ALEXANDER. *The Genesis of the United States.* 2 vols. New
York: Houghton, Mifflin Company, 1897.
BRUCER, MARSHALL. *Vignettes in Nuclear Medicine.* St. Louis: Mal-
linckrodt Chemical Works, 1966–68.
"Can the HMO puzzle ever be put together?" *American Medical News*
(Aug. 7, 1972), pp. 10–14.
CAREY, MATHEW. *A Short Account of the Malignant Fever, Lately Preva-
lent in Philadelphia. . . .* Philadelphia: Printed by the Author, 1793.
CARREL, ALEXIS. *Man the Unknown.* New York: Harper & Brothers,
1935.
————, and GUTHRIE, C. C. "Anastomosis of Blood Vessels by the Patch-
ing Method and Transplantation of the Kidney," *Journal of the
American Medical Association,* XLVII: 20 (Nov. 17, 1906), pp.
1848–51.
————, and LINDBERGH, CHARLES A. *The Culture of Organs.* New
York: Paul B. Hoeber, 1938.
CARRIGAN, JO ANN. "Yellow Fever in New Orleans, 1905: The Last Epidemic," *Bulletin of the Tulane University Medical Faculty,* XXVI: 1
(Feb. 1967), pp. 19–28.
CAVINS, HAROLD M. "The National Quarantine and Sanitary Conventions
of 1857 to 1860 and the Beginnings of the Public Health Association," *Bulletin of the History of Medicine,* XIII (1943), pp.
404–26.

CLAPESATTLE, HELEN. *The Doctors Mayo.* Minneapolis: University of Minnesota Press, 1941.

CLARKE, EDWARD H., *et al. A Century of American Medicine, 1776–1876.* Philadelphia: Henry C. Lea, 1876; reprinted: New York: Burt Franklin, 1968.

CLARKE, EDWIN, and O'MALLEY, C. D. *The Human Brain and Spinal Cord.* Berkeley: University of California Press, 1968.

CORNER, GEORGE W., ed. *The Autobiography of Benjamin Rush.* Princeton, N.J.: Princeton University Press, 1948.

————. *Two Centuries of Medicine.* Philadelphia & Montreal: J. B. Lippincott Company, 1965.

CURRAN, JEAN A. "Medical Correspondence and Other Writings in Seventeenth Century New York," *New York State Journal of Medicine,* LIV (July–Dec. 1954), pp. 3264–72.

DAIN, NORMAN. *Concepts of Insanity in the United States, 1789–1865.* New Brunswick, N.J.: Rutgers University Press, 1964.

DAUZICKAS, PAUL P. JR. "Health Maintenance Organizations," *Medical Bulletin Standard Oil Co. (N.J.) & Affiliated Companies,* XXXII: 2 (July, 1972), pp. 174–80.

DAVENPORT, F. H. "Specialism in Medical Practice; Its Present Status and Tendencies," *Boston Medical and Surgical Journal,* CXLV: 4 (July 25, 1901), pp. 81–86.

DAVIS, N. S. *Contributions to the History of Medical Education and Medical Institutions in the United States of America. 1776–1876.* Washington: Government Printing Office, 1877.

DE KRUIF, PAUL. *Kaiser Wakes the Doctors.* New York: Harcourt, Brace & Company, 1943.

DELGADO, JOSÉ M. R. *Physical Control of the Mind.* New York: Harper & Row, 1969.

DETRE, THOMAS P., and JARECKI, HENRY G. *Modern Psychiatric Treatment.* Philadelphia & Toronto: J. B. Lippincott Company, 1971.

DEWITT, WILLIAM B. "Contributions of the U.S. Public Health Service in Tropical Medicine: Part I," *Bulletin of the New York Academy of Medicine,* XLIV (1968), pp. 728–36.

Dictionary of American Biography, s.v. "Mather, Cotton." New York: Charles Scribner's Sons, 1928–1937.

DOWNS, WILBUR G. "The Story of Yellow Fever since Walter Reed," *Bulletin of the New York Academy of Medicine,* XLIV (1968), pp. 721–27.

SELECTED BIBLIOGRAPHY

DUCKETT, J. W. "The Halsted Heritage," *Surgery,* LV: 6 (June 1964), pp. 859–69.

DUFFY, JOHN. *Epidemics in Colonial America.* Baton Rouge: Louisiana State University Press, 1953.

———— (ed.). *The Rudolph Matas History of Medicine in Louisiana.* 2 vols. Baton Rouge: Louisiana State University Press, 1958.

DUNLOP, RICHARD. *Doctors of the American Frontier.* New York: Doubleday & Co., 1965.

DURANT, THOMAS M. "The Medical Society in America: Past and Present," *Transactions & Studies of the College of Physicians of Philadelphia,* Fourth Series, XXXI: 4 (April 1964), pp. 275–82.

EDWARDS, LINDEN F. "An Unusual 'Physician's Notice,'" *Ohio State Medical Journal,* XLVII (1951), pp. 738–40.

————. "Resurrection Riots during the Heroic Age of Anatomy in America," *Bulletin of the History of Medicine,* XXV (1951), pp. 178–84.

————. "The Ohio Anatomy Law of 1881," *Ohio State Medical Journal,* XLVI (1950), pp. 1190–92; XLVII (1951), pp. 49–52, 143–46.

ESSELSTYN, CALWELL B. "The Next Ten Years in Medicine," *The New England Journal of Medicine,* CCLXVI: 3 (Jan. 18, 1962), pp. 124–29.

FARMER, LAURENCE. "Medical Correspondence in Eighteenth Century New York State," *New York State Journal of Medicine,* LIV (July–Dec. 1954), pp. 2296–99.

————. "The Early Directors of the Medical Services of the American Revolutionary Army," *Bulletin of the New York Academy of Medicine,* XXXVI: 11 (Nov. 1960), pp. 765–76.

FINDLEY, THOMAS. "Sappington's Anti-Fever Pills and the Westward Migration," *Transactions, American Clinical and Climatological Association,* LXXIX (1967), 43–44.

FISHLOCK, DAVID. *Man Modified.* New York: Funk & Wagnalls, 1969.

FITZ, REGINALD. "The Massachusetts Medical Society, From Cow-Path to State Road," *New England Journal of Medicine,* CCXIV: 24 (June 11, 1936), pp. 1178–88.

FITZ, REGINALD HEBER. "Zabdiel Boylston, Inoculator, and the Epidemic of Smallpox in Boston in 1721," *Bulletin of the Johns Hopkins Hospital,* XXII: 247 (Sept. 1911), pp. 315–27.

FLEXNER, ABRAHAM. *Medical Education in the United States and Can-*

ada. New York: The Carnegie Foundation for the Advancement of Teaching, 1910. (Bulletin of the Carnegie Foundation, No. 4.)

[FRANKLIN, BENJAMIN]. *Some Account of the Pennsylvania Hospital from its First Rise to the Beginning of the Fifth Month, Called May, 1754.* Philadelphia: Printed at the Office of the *United States Gazette,* 1817.

FULTON, JOHN F. *Harvey Cushing.* Springfield, Ill.: Charles C Thomas, 1946.

————. "Medicine, Warfare, and History," *Journal of the American Medical Association,* CLIII: 5 (Oct. 3, 1953), pp. 482–86.

GALDSTON, IAGO. "Research in the United States," *Ciba Symposia,* VIII: 3–4 (June–July, 1946), pp. 362–72.

————. "Wanted—A History of Research," *Ciba Symposia,* VIII: 3–4 (June–July 1946), pp. 338–39, 361.

GARLAND, JOSEPH, and STOKES, JOSEPH, III, eds. *The Choice of a Medical Career, Essays on the Fields of Medicine.* Philadelphia & Montreal: J. B. Lippincott Company, 2nd ed., 1962.

GARRISON, FIELDING H. *An Introduction to the History of Medicine.* (Philadelphia) London: W. B. Saunders Company, 4th ed. 1929.

GIBSON, JAMES E. "The Role of Disease in the 70,000 Casualties in the American Revolutionary Army," *Transactions & Studies, College of Physicians of Philadelphia,* 4th ser. XVII: 3 (Dec. 1949), pp. 121–27.

GILMAN, C. MALCOLM B. "Military Surgery in the American Revolution," *Journal of the Medical Society of New Jersey,* LVII: 8 (Aug. 1960), pp. 491–96.

GOLDBERGER, MARY FARRAR, "Dr. Joseph Goldberger, His Wife's Recollections," *Journal of the American Dietetic Association,* XXXII (1956), pp. 724–27.

GOLDSMITH, HARRY S. "Some Historical Aspects of Human Dissection," *The Boston Medical Quarterly,* XI: 3 (Sept. 1960), pp. 89–93.

GOODMAN, NATHAN G. *Benjamin Rush Physician and Citizen.* Philadelphia: University of Pennsylvania Press, 1934.

GORDON, MAURICE B. *Aesculapius Comes to the Colonies.* Ventnor, N.J.: Ventnor Publishers, 1949.

GUERRA, FRANCISCO. *American Medical Bibliography 1639–1783.* New York: Lathrop C. Harper, 1962.

GUTHRIE, CHARLES CLAUDE. *Blood-Vessel Surgery and Its Applications.* New York: Longmans, Green & Company, 1912.

HARRINGTON, THOMAS F. *The Harvard Medical School.* Ed. by James Gregory Mumford. 3 vols. New York and Chicago: Lewis Publishing Company, 1905.

HARTWELL, EDWARD M. "The Hindrances to Anatomical Study in the United States, including a Special Record of the Struggles of Our Early Anatomical Teachers," *Annals of Anatomy and Surgery,* III (1881), pp. 209–25.

HEATON, CLAUDE E. "Body Snatching in New York City," *New York State Journal of Medicine,* XLIII, part 2 (Oct. 1, 1943), pp. 1861–65.

———. "Medicine in New Amsterdam," *Bulletin of the History of Medicine,* IX: 2 (Feb. 1941), pp. 125–43.

———. "Medicine in New York during the English Colonial Period," *Bulletin of the History of Medicine,* XVII (Jan. 1945), pp. 9–37.

HENDERSON, WILLIAM. *Homœopathy Fairly Represented. A Reply to Professor Simpson's "Homœopathy" Misrepresented.* Philadelphia: Lindsay & Blakiston, 1854.

HENDRICKSON, ROBERT M. "There's an HMO in your future," *Physician's Management,* IX (May 1971), pp. 63–67.

HENRY, JAMES P. *Biomedical Aspects of Space Flight.* New York: Holt, Rinehart & Winston, 1966.

History of Inoculation and Vaccination for the Prevention and Treatment of Disease, The, London: Burroughs Wellcome & Company, 1913.

HOFFMAN, BERNARD G. "John Clayton's Account of the Medicinal Practices of the Virginia Indians," *Ethnohistory,* XI: 1 (Winter 1964), pp. 1–40.

HOLMES, CHRIS. "Benjamin Rush and the Yellow Fever," *Bulletin of the History of Medicine,* XL (1966), pp. 246–63.

HOLMES, OLIVER WENDELL. *Medical Essays, 1842–1882.* Boston: Houghton, Mifflin Company, 1883.

HORINE, ERNEST F. *Daniel Drake, M.D.; Pioneer Physician of the Midwest.* Philadelphia: University of Pennsylvania Press, 1961.

ISAAC LORD BISHOP OF WORCESTER. *A Sermon Preached before His Grace Charles Duke of Marlborough, President, The Vice-Presidents and Governors of the Hospital for the Small-Pox, and for Inoculation.* London: Printed by H. Woodfall, 7th ed., 1753.

JARCHO, SAUL. "Medical Education in the United States—1910–1956," *Journal of the Mount Sinai Hospital,* XXVI: 4 (1959), pp. 339–85.

JELLIFFE, SMITH E. "The Dutch Physician in New Amsterdam and His Colleagues at Home," *Medical Library and Historical Journal*, IV: 2 (Jan. 1906), pp. 145–61.

JOHNSON, STEPHEN L. *The History of Cardiac Surgery, 1896–1955.* Baltimore: Johns Hopkins Press, 1970.

JONES, JOHN. *Plain Concise Practical Remarks on the Treatment of Wounds and Fractures.* . . . Philadelphia: Robert Bell, 1776.

JORDAN, PHILIP D. "Treatment of Gun-Shot Wounds in Frontier Ohio," *Ohio State Medical Journal*, XXXIX (1943), pp. 844–46.

JOSSELYN, JOHN. *An Account of Two Voyages to New-England.* London: G. Widdowes, 1675. Reprinted in *Collections of the Massachusetts Historical Society*, Ser. 3, Vol. 3. Cambridge, Mass.: E. W. Metcalf, 1833.

JUETTNER, OTTO. *Daniel Drake and His Followers: Historical and Biographical Sketches.* Cincinnati: Harvey Publishing Company, 1909.

———. "The Medical Records of the Indian Campaigns of Generals St. Clair, Hamar, and Wayne," *New York Medical Journal*, CI (1915), pp. 732–35.

KAUFMAN, MARTIN. *Homeopathy in America: The Rise and Fall of a Medical Heresy.* Baltimore: Johns Hopkins University Press, 1971.

KETT, JOSEPH F. *The Formation of the American Medical Profession.* New Haven: Yale University Press, 1968.

KILGOUR, FREDERICK G. "The Rise of Scientific Activity in Colonial New England," *Yale Journal of Biology and Medicine*, XXII (Oct. 1949–July 1950), pp. 123–38.

KING, LESTER S. "Do-It-Yourself Medicine," *Journal of the American Medical Association*, CC: 1 (April 3, 1967), pp. 23–29.

———. *The Medical World of the Eighteenth Century.* Chicago: University of Chicago Press, 1958.

KIRKPATRICK, J. *The Analysis of Inoculation.* London: J. Buckland & R. Griffiths, 2nd ed., 1761.

KLEBS, ARNOLD C. "The Historical Evolution of Variolation," *Bulletin of the Johns Hopkins Hospital*, XXIV: 265 (March 1913), pp. 69–83.

KNOPF, RICHARD C. "Report on Surgeons of the Indian Wars," *Ohio State Medical Journal*, XLVIII (1952), pp. 1035–38.

KRUMBHAAR, EDWARD B. "The Early History of Anatomy in the United States," *Annals of Medical History*, IV (1922), pp. 271–86.

LEIKIND, MORRIS C. "The Evolution of Medical Research in the United

States," *International Record of Medicine,* CLXXI: 7 (July 1958), pp. 455–68.

LLOYD, JOHN URI, ed. "Life and Medical Discoveries of Samuel Thomson and a history of the Thomsonian Materia Medica. . . ." *Bulletin of the Lloyd Library of Botany, Pharmacy, and Materia Medica,* Bull. No. 11, Reproduction Series, No. 7 (1909).

LONDON, PERRY. *Behavior Control.* New York: Harper & Row, 1969.

LONG, DOROTHY. "Native and Imported Medicines in Eighteenth Century North Carolina," *North Carolina Medical Journal,* XV: 1 (Jan. 1954), pp. 37–38.

LONGMORE, DONALD. *Spare-Part Surgery.* New York: Doubleday & Company, 1968.

LUDOVICI, L. J. *Cone of Oblivion.* London: Max Parrish, 1961.

MARKS, GEOFFREY, and BEATTY, WILLIAM K. *The Medical Garden.* New York: Charles Scribner's Sons, 1971.

———. *Women in White.* New York: Charles Scribner's Sons, 1972.

MATHER, COTTON. *Magnalia Christi Americana.* Hartford, Conn.: S. Andrus Son, 1855.

MCDANIEL, W. B., II. "A Brief Sketch of the Rise of American Medical Societies," *International Record of Medicine,* CLXXI: 8 (Aug. 1958), pp. 483–91.

Medical Research: A Midcentury Survey. 2 vols. Boston: Little, Brown & Company, 1955.

MIDDLETON, WILLIAM S. "The Yellow Fever Epidemic of 1793 in Philadelphia," *Annals of Medical History,* X (1928), pp. 434–50.

MILLER, GENEVIEVE, ed. *Bibliography of the History of Medicine of the United States and Canada, 1939–1960.* Baltimore: Johns Hopkins University Press, 1964.

———. "Medical Education in Colonial America," *Ciba Symposia,* VIII: 10 (Jan. 1947), pp. 502–32.

MONTGOMERY, HORACE. "A Body Snatcher Sponsors Pennsylvania's Anatomy Act," *Journal of the History of Medicine,* XXI (Oct. 1966), pp. 374–93.

MOORE, FRANCIS D. *Transplant; The Give and Take of Tissue Transplantation.* New York: Simon and Schuster, rev. ed., 1972.

MORGAN, JOHN. *A Discourse Upon the Institution of Medical Schools in America.* Philadelphia: William Bradford, 1765.

MORTON, THOMAS G., assisted by WOODBURY, FRANK. *The History of the Pennsylvania Hospital, 1751–1895.* Philadelphia: Times Printing House, 1895.

NEILL, EDWARD D. *History of the Virginia Company of London.* Albany, N.Y.: J. Munsell, 1869.

―――. *Virginia Carolorum.* Albany, N.Y.: J. Munsell's Sons, 1886.

"New York Hospital, The," (editorial), *The Medical Record,* XII (1877), pp. 184–86.

NORTHUP, GEORGE W. *Osteopathic Medicine: An American Reformation.* Chicago: American Osteopathic Association, 1966.

NORWOOD, WILLIAM FREDERICK. *Medical Education in the United States before the Civil War.* Philadelphia: University of Pennsylvania Press, 1944.

―――. "Medicine in the Era of the American Revolution," *International Record of Medicine,* CLXXI: 7 (July 1958), pp. 391–407.

―――. "The Early History of American Medical Societies," *Ciba Symposia,* IX: 9 (Dec. 1947), pp. 762–72.

O'MALLEY, C. D. *History of Medical Education.* Los Angeles: UCLA Press, 1970.

ORR, H. WINNETT, "Biographical Notes Regarding Some American Military Surgeons," *Quarterly Bulletin, Northwestern University Medical School,* XX (1946), pp. 111–27.

PACKARD, FRANCIS R. *History of Medicine in the United States.* 2 vols. New York: Paul B. Hoeber, 1931.

PAUL, JOHN R. *A History of Poliomyelitis.* New Haven: Yale University Press, 1971.

PELLER, SIGISMUND. "Walter Reed, C. Finlay, and their Predecessors Around 1800," *Bulletin of the History of Medicine,* XXXIII: 3 (May–June 1959), pp. 195–211.

PENFIELD, WILDER. *The Difficult Art of Giving—The Epic of Alan Gregg.* Boston & Toronto: Little, Brown & Company, 1967.

PEPPER, WILLIAM. *Higher Medical Education, The True Interest of the Public and of the Profession.* Philadelphia: J. B. Lippincott Company, 1894.

PICKARD, MADGE E., and BULEY, R. CARLYLE. *The Midwest Pioneer, His Ills, Cures, & Doctors.* New York: Henry Schuman, 1946.

PILCHER, JAMES EVELYN. "The Surgeon Generals of the United States Army. VII. James Tilton, Physician and Surgeon General of the United States Army, 1813–1815," *Journal of the Association of Military Surgeons of the United States,* XIV (1904), pp. 271–75.

POSTELL, WILLIAM DOSITE. "The American Medical Association," *Ciba Symposia*, IX: 9 (Dec. 1947), pp. 773–84.

POWSNER, EDWARD R., and RAESIDE, DAVID E. *Diagnostic Nuclear Medicine*. New York & London: Grune & Stratton, 1971.

RANDALL, HUGH W. *Aerospace Medicine*. Baltimore: Williams & Wilkins, 2nd ed., 1971.

RANSOM, JOHN E. "Beginnings of Hospitals in the United States," *Hospitals*, XV (Dec. 1941), pp. 68–71; XVI (Jan. 1942), pp. 74–79.

RAVENEL, MAZŸCK P., ed. *A Half Century of Public Health*. New York: American Public Health Association, 1921.

Report of the Select Committee of the House of Representatives on So Much of the Governor's Speech, at the June Session, 1830, as Relates to Legalizing the Study of Anatomy. Boston: Dutton & Wentworth, Printers to the State, 1831.

RICHARDSON, ROBERT G. *The Scalpel and the Heart*. New York: Charles Scribner's Sons, 1970.

ROEMER, MILTON I. "Government's Role in American Medicine," *Bulletin of the History of Medicine*, XVIII (1945), pp. 146–68.

ROGERS, BLAIR O. "Charles Claude Guthrie, M.D., Ph.D.: A Remarkable Pioneer in Tissue and Organ Transplantation," *Plastic & Reconstructive Surgery*, XXIV: 4 (Oct. 1959), pp. 380–83.

———. "Surgery in the Revolutionary War—Contributions of John Jones, M.D. (1729–1791), *Plastic & Reconstructive Surgery*, XLIX: 1 (Jan. 1972), pp. 1–14.

ROME, HOWARD P. "Psychiatry: Circa 1919–1969–2019," *Annals of Internal Medicine*, LXXI: 4 (Oct. 1969), pp. 845–53.

RORVIK, DAVID M. *As Man Becomes Machine: The Evolution of the Cyborg*. New York: Doubleday Company, 1971.

ROSEN, GEORGE. "Changing Attitudes of the Medical Profession to Specialization," *Bulletin of the History of Medicine*, XII (1942), pp. 343–54.

———. "Special Medical Societies in the United States after 1860," *Ciba Symposia*, IX: 9 (Dec. 1947), pp. 785–92.

ROSENBERG, CHARLES. *The Cholera Years*. Chicago: University of Chicago Press, 1962.

ROTHSTEIN, WILLIAM G. *American Physicians in the Nineteenth Century*. Baltimore: Johns Hopkins University Press, 1972.

RUSH, BENJAMIN. *An Account of the Bilious remitting Yellow Fever, as it Appeared in the City of Philadelphia in the Year 1793*. Philadelphia: Thomas Dobson, 2nd ed., 1794.

[RUSH, BENJAMIN]. *Old Family Letters relating to Yellow Fever*. Philadelphia: J. B. Lippincott Company, 1892.

RUSHTON, THOMAS. *An Essay on Inoculation for the Small Pox*. London: J. Payne, 1767.

SHAFER, HENRY BURNELL. *The American Medical Profession 1783 to 1850*. New York: Columbia University Press, 1936.

SHAPIRO, HENRY D., and MILLER, ZANE L., eds. *Physician to the West: Selected Writings of Daniel Drake on Science and Society*. Lexington, Ky.: University Press of Kentucky, 1970.

SHRYOCK, RICHARD H. *American Medical Research Past and Present*. New York: The Commonwealth Fund, 1947.

————. *Development of Modern Medicine*. New York: Alfred A. Knopf, 2nd ed., 1947. (Reprinted, New York: Hafner, 1969.)

————. "Factors Affecting Medical Research in the United States, 1800–1900," *Bulletin of the Society of Medical History of Chicago*, V: 4 (July 1943), pp. 1–18.

————. *Medical Licensing in America, 1650–1965*. Baltimore: Johns Hopkins University Press, 1967.

————. *Medicine and Society in America, 1660–1860*. New York: New York University Press, 1960.

————. *Medicine in America: Historical Essays*. Baltimore: Johns Hopkins University Press, 1966.

SHUMAN, JOHN W. "Spanish California Medicine," *Medical Record*, CXL (Jan.–June 1939), pp. 230–35.

SIGERIST, HENRY E. *American Medicine*. Tr. by Hildegard Nagel. New York: W. W. Norton, 1934.

SILVER, GEORGE A. "A Challenge to the Academic Leopards: or, HO, HO, HMO!" *Connecticut Medicine*, XXXVI: 7 (July 1972), pp. 417–20.

SIMS, J. MARION. *The Story of My Life*. New York: D. Appleton, 1889.

SMITH, CAPTAIN JOHN. *Travels and Works of Captain John Smith*. Ed. by Edward Arber. Edinburgh: J. Grant, 1910.

SMITH, HENRY LEE. "Dr. Adam Thomson, the Originator of the American Method of Inoculation for Small-pox," *Bulletin of the Johns Hopkins Hospital*, XX: 215 (Feb. 1909), pp. 49–52.

SMITH, ROBERT B. "Alexis Carrel (1873–1944)," *Investigative Urology*, V: 1 (July 1967), pp. 102–105.

SMILEY, DEAN F. "History of the Association of American Medical Colleges—1876–1956," *Journal of Medical Education*, XXXII: 7 (July 1957), pp. 512–25.

STEINER, WALTER R. "The Reverend Gershom Bulkeley, of Connecticut, an Eminent Clerical Physician," *Bulletin of the Johns Hopkins Hospital*, XVII: 179 (Feb. 1906), pp. 48–53.

STEVENS, ROSEMARY. *American Medicine & the Public Interest.* New Haven: Yale University Press, 1971.

STEVENSON, ISOBEL. "Beginnings of American Military Medicine," *Ciba Symposia*, I: 11 (Feb. 1940), pp. 344–59.

STILL, ANDREW T. *Autobiography of Andrew T. Still, with a History of the Development of the Science of Osteopathy.* Kirksville, Mo.: Published by the Author, 1897.

STOOKEY, BYRON. "Found! The Record of the 1767 Medical Society in Litchfield," *Connecticut State Medical Journal*, XXI: 3–4 (March–April 1957), pp. 191–200, 346–54.

STRICKLAND, STEPHEN P. *Politics, Science, and Dread Disease; A Short History of the United States Medical Research Policy.* Cambridge, Mass.: Harvard University Press, 1972.

SUTTON, DANIEL M. *The Inoculator; or, Suttonian System of Inoculation.* London: Printed for the author by T. Gillet, 1796.

THACHER, JAMES. *American Medical Biography.* 2 vols. in 1. Boston: Richardson & Lord and Cottons & Barnard, 1828.

————. *The American Revolution, from the Commencement to the Disbanding of the American Army; Given in the Form of a Daily Journal, with the Exact Dates of all the Important Events; also a Biographical Sketch of all the Most Important Generals.* New York: American Subscription Publishing House, 1860.

THACHER, THOMAS. *A Brief Rule to Guide the Common People of New-England How to Order Themselves and Theirs in the Small Pocks, or Measles,* with an Introductory Note by Henry R. Viets, M.D. Baltimore: Johns Hopkins University Press, 1937.

THOMAS, D. G. "History of the Founding and Development of the First Hospitals in the United States," *American Journal of Insanity*, XXIV (1867–68), pp. 130–54.

THOMSON, SAMUEL. *A Narrative of the Life and Medical Discoveries of Samuel Thomson. . . .* Columbus, Ohio: Pike, Platt, & Company, 6th ed., 1832.

THORWALD, JÜRGEN. *The Patients.* Tr. by Richard and Clara Winston. New York: Harcourt, Brace, Jovanovich, 1972.

TONER, JOSEPH M. *Contributions to the Annals of Medical Progress and Medical Education in the United States before and during the War of Independence.* Washington: Government Printing Office, 1874.

————. *The Medical Men of the Revolution, with a brief history of the*

Medical Department of the Continental Army; containing the names of nearly twelve hundred physicians. Philadelphia: Collins, 1876.

TOURNEY, GARFIELD. "A History of Therapeutic Fashions in Psychiatry, 1800–1966," *American Journal of Psychiatry,* CXXIV: 6 (Dec. 1967), pp. 784–96.

TRUAX, RHODA. *The Doctors Warren of Boston.* Boston: Houghton Mifflin Company, 1968.

TRUSSELL, RAY E. *Hunterdon Medical Center.* Cambridge: Harvard University Press, 1955.

VICTOR, RALPH G. "An Indictment for Grave Robbing at the Time of the 'Doctors' Riot,' 1788," *Annals of Medical History,* 3rd ser., II (1940), pp. 366–70.

VIETS, HENRY R. "James Thacher and His Influence on American Medicine," *Virginia Medical Monthly,* LXXVI (1949), pp. 384–99.

WAITE, FREDERICK C. "Advent of the Graded Curriculum in American Medical Colleges," *Journal of the Association of American Medical Colleges,* XXV (1950), pp. 315–22.

————. "Censors and Medical Colleges," *Ohio State Medical Journal,* L (1954), pp. 1160–62.

————. "Grave Robbing in New England," *Bulletin of the Medical Library Association,* XXXIII (1945), pp. 272–94.

————. "The Development of Anatomical Laws in the States of New England," *The New England Journal of Medicine,* CCXXXIII: 24 (Dec. 13, 1945), pp. 716–26.

WEAVER, J. CALVIN. "Early Medical History of Georgia," *The Journal of the Medical Association of Georgia,* XXIX: 3 (March 1940), pp. 89–112.

WEBSTER, GEORGE V. *Concerning Osteopathy.* . . . Norwood, Mass.: Plimpton Press, 1919.

WELD, STANLEY B. "Early Medical Practice in Hartford County," *Connecticut State Medical Journal,* V (1941), pp. 484–95.

WILLIAMS, GREER. *Kaiser-Permanente Health Plan—Why It Works.* Oakland, Calif.: Henry J. Kaiser Foundation, 1971.

WILSON, CHARLES. "American Contributions to Neurosurgery," *New Orleans Medical and Surgical Journal,* XCVI (1943), pp. 140–47.

Winslow's Relation in *Chronicles of the Pilgrim Fathers.* London: Dent, 1910.

WOMACK, NATHAN A. "The Evolution of the National Board of Medical Examiners," *Journal of the American Medical Association,* CXCII: 10 (June 7, 1965), pp. 817–23.

SELECTED BIBLIOGRAPHY

WOODRING, T. V. "Pioneer Physicians and Medicine in Middle Tennessee," *Journal of the Tennessee State Medical Association,* XXXIV (Dec. 1941), pp. 469–78.

WYLIE, W. GILL. "Hospitals: History of their Origin and Development —Their Progress during the Century of the American Republic," *Transactions of the New York Academy of Medicine,* 2nd ser., II (1874–76), pp. 251–85.

ZAUGG, DAVID. "History of the United States Public Health Service Hospital Situated at Baltimore, Maryland," *Maryland State Medical Journal,* VII: 3 (March 1958), pp. 140–43.

ZEUCH, LUCIUS H. *History of Medical Practice in Illinois, Vol. I: Preceding 1850.* Chicago: Illinois State Medical Society, 1927.

ILLUSTRATION CREDITS

⟋ᘐᘐᘐ⟍

American Osteopathic Association. Page 189

Jacob Bigelow, *American Medical Botany* (Boston: Cummings and Hilliard, 1818). Following page 138: tobacco plant

N. I. Bowditch, *A History of the Massachusetts General Hospital* (2nd ed. Boston: Printed by the Trustees, 1872). Following page 138: Massachusetts General Hospital

Bulletin of the History of Medicine 8 (1940):23. Page 133

Bulletin of the Lloyd Library . . . 2 (1901):7. Following page 138: *Indian Doctor's Dispensatory*

Ciba Symposia 3 (1941–42):1099. Page 41

College of Physicians of Philadelphia Historical Collections. Following page 138: manuscript home remedy book

Abraham Flexner, *I Remember* . . . (New York: Simon & Schuster, 1940). Page 203

John F. Fulton, *Harvey Cushing* (Springfield, Ill.: Charles C Thomas, 1946). Following page 138: Cushing and Dandy

Isis 23 (1935): facing p. 396. Page 25

John James, *The American Household Book of Medicine* . . . (Cincinnati: Carroll, 1869). Page 149

Journal of the Association of Military Surgeons 16 (1905):441. Following page 138: Rush statue

Journal of the Indiana State Medical Association 35 (1942):166. Page 237

Mayo Clinic. *Sketch of the History of the Mayo Clinic and the Mayo Foundation* (Philadelphia: Saunders, 1926). Following page 138: the Mayos

Medical Annals of the District of Columbia 23 (1954):707. Page 329

S. Weir Mitchell, *New Samaria* . . . (Philadelphia: Lippincott, 1904). Page 176

Thomas G. Morton, *The History of the Pennsylvania Hospital 1751–1895* (Philadelphia: Times Printing House, 1895). Following page 138: apothecary's indenture, Pennsylvania Hospital, admission card, bill for chains

ILLUSTRATION CREDITS

Northwestern University Medical Library Portrait Collection. Pages 60, 67, 76, 100, 108, 118, 122, 154, 162, 173, 242; following page 138: McDowell medal, Jefferson Medical College, demonstration of anesthesia, Welch and colleagues

Provident Hospital, Chicago. Following page 138: D. H. Williams

Mazÿck P. Ravenel, ed., *A Half Century of Public Health* (New York: American Public Health Association, 1921). Page 266

Surgery, Gynecology, and Obstetrics 51 (1930): facing p. 740. Page 136

James Thacher, *American Medical Biography* (Boston: Richardson, 1828). Page 128

Samuel Thomson, *The Thomsonian Materia Medica* . . . (12th ed. Albany, N.Y.: Munsell, 1841), Page 183; following page 138: "Thomson's patent"

INDEX

⟨W⟩

Abel, John Jacob, 317
Aberdeen, University of, 82
acceleration / deceleration, 332, 335–336
Adams, John, 81, 127, 263
Adams, John Quincy, 276
Albany, N. Y., 130
Alcott, William A., 179
American Cancer Society, 280
American Heart Association, 280–281
American Hospital Association, 208
American Medical Association, 160, 199–201, 361
American Ophthalmological Society, 180
American Osteopathic Association, 192
American Otological Society, 180
American Philosophical Society, 195–196
American Physiological Society, 179
American Psychiatric Association, 179–180
American Public Health Association, 264–267
American School of Osteopathy, 192
Amoss, Harold L., 286
anatomy, 23, 48, 73–75, 77–86, 89–97, 99, 101–102, 105, 107–109, 111–112, 146, 151, 167, 179, 190–191, 201
anesthesia, 147, 166–171, 173, 192, 292, 305, 352
Angel of Bethesda, 45, 49–54
apothecaries, 3, 4, 20, 99, 120, 151, 160, 263
apprenticeship, 4, 12, 14, 21, 83, 98, 101–102, 151–152, 154, 157, 197, 201
army doctors, 114–135, 137, 153–156, 171–172, 176–177, 191, 242–243, 257
Arnold, Benedict, 130
Arrow Rock, Mo., 157
artificial heart, 329–331
artificial limbs, 310–312
asepsis, 174–175, 292, 294
Association of American Medical Colleges, 205
astronauts, 335–341
Atlee, John Light, 148
Atlee, Washington Lemuel, 148
atom-smasher, 344, 346
Auenbrugger, Leopold, 252
Avery, Oswald T., 253, 280
Avram, Morrell M., 318

bacteriology, 51–52, 174, 248, 250, 255, 257, 279, 286, 335, 338

Baglivi, Giorgio, 50
Bagnall, Anthony, 8
Bailey, Charles B., 313
Bailey, Percival, 293, 301
ballooning, 82, 333–335
Baltimore, 80, 86, 122, 173, 207, 236, 241, 263–264
barber-surgeons, 4–5, 16, 73–74, 81
Bard, John, 78, 195
Bard, Samuel, 67–68, 78, 105–106
Barnard, Christiaan N., 322–323
Barnard Cancer Hospital (St. Louis), 342
Bartholow, Robert, 293–294
Bartlett, Elisha, 247
Barza, J. A., 305
Bassini, Edoardo, 173
Bauer, Johannes H., 244
Bayley, Richard, 86
Beach, Wooster, 186
Beaumont, William, 153–156, 275, 293
Becquerel, Henri, 342
Bell, James, 146–148
Bellevue Hospital (New York), 56, 258; Medical College, 205, 258
Bernard, Claude, 177, 333
Berne, University of, 297–298
Bert, Paul, 333–334
Bigelow, Henry J., 169–170
Bigelow, Wilfred G., 314
Biggs, Herman M., 279
Billings, John Shaw, 171–172
Blaiberg, Philip, 323–324
Black, Joseph, 146
Blackfan, Kenneth Daniel, 301
Blackwell, Elizabeth, 203
Blackwell, Emily, 203

Blancard (Blankaart), Stephen, 50–51
bloodletting, 35, 66, 131, 145, 157, 182, 216, 239
Blumgart, Hermann L., 345
bodies willed for science, 97
Boerhaave, Hermann, 151, 226
Bohun, Lawrence, 8–10, 14, 29
Bond, Thomas, 59–61, 102–104, 195
Boston, 21, 24–27, 41, 44–46, 57, 60, 82, 108, 110, 118, 120, 122, 128–129, 169, 179, 194, 214–215, 217, 219–221, 225, 235–236, 253, 262–264, 312–313, 319–320, 330
Boston Medical Society, 82, 108
Boston Phrenological Society, 179
botanicals, 9, 29–36, 38–39, 48, 101, 132, 142–143, 160, 182–187
Botanico-Medical College (Ohio), 185; (Southern), 185
Boylston, Thomas, 221
Boylston, Zabdiel, 221–226
Bradford, William, 17–18
brain helmet, 341
brain surgery, 292–303, 326
Brewster, William, 15
Brief Rule, 24, 26, 215–216
bubonic plague, 17, 190, 232, 237–238, 268
Bulkeley, Gershom, 114–115
Bunker Hill, 118

Cadwalader, Thomas, 77–78, 99
Calhoun, John Caldwell, 276
California, 193, 266, 268, 303, 356–357

California Institute of Technology, 344

California, University of (Berkeley), 344, 346; (Los Angeles), 341, 348

calomel (mercurious chloride), 132, 228, 230, 239–240

Cambridge, Mass., 23–24, 26, 109–110, 127, 164

Cambridge University, 20, 23, 25, 44

Carey, Mathew, 201, 237–239

Carnegie Foundation, 203

Carnegie Institution, 278

Carrel, Alexis, 280, 314–316, 319, 321, 326

Cassen, Benjamin, 348

central localization, 292–293, 295

central nervous system, 285, 294–296

Chadwick, Edwin, 264–265

Champlain, N.Y., 153

Chapman, Nathaniel, 200

Chaptal, Jean Antoine, 151

Chardack, William, 327

Charleston, S.C., 17, 195, 227, 235

Charlestown, Mass., 17–18, 27, 215

Chauncy, Charles, 23–24, 26

Cheselden, William, 77, 151

Chicago, 202, 278, 314

Chicago Medical College, 202, 204, 353

Chicago Medical School, 175

Chicago, University of, 277–278, 314–315

Chittenden, Russell H., 295

cholera, 121, 190, 268

Chovet, Abraham, 81, 99

Church, Benjamin, 84–85, 117, 119–121, 124

Cincinnati, 92, 143, 151–153, 264, 293

Cincinnati College medical department, 150

Civil War, American, 170, 176, 180, 191, 246–248, 264

Clark, John, 84–85

Clark, William E., 168

Clarke, Edward H., 274

Clayton, John, 29–30, 33–36, 39

clergyman-physician, 16, 27–28, 44

Cleveland Clinic, 318

Clossy, Samuel, 80, 99, 105

cocaine, 166, 173

Cochran, John, 116, 124–125

Cohn, Alfred, 280

Cole, Rufus, 253, 280

College of Physicians (New York), 205; (Philadelphia), 239–240, 296

College of Physicians and Surgeons (Kansas City), 191; (New York), 69, 106–107

Colorado, University of, 325

Columbia University (King's College, New York), 80, 106, 345; medical department, 67–69, 80, 105–107, 135, 204

Columbus, Ohio, 90–91, 185

computer enhancement, 340–341

Congress, 117, 119–125, 127, 172, 266–268, 276, 361

Connecticut, 27, 83, 93, 115–116, 195, 229

Cooley, Denton A., 330–331

Coolidge, William David, 344

Cotton, W. E., 257

cowpox, 230–232

Cox, Herald, 289

Coxwell, Henry Tracy, 334

INDEX

Craik, James, 116
Crawford, Jane Todd, 146–147
Crawford, John, 241
Crocé-Spinelli, Joseph E., 333–334
Cruz, Oswaldo G., 243
Cullen, William, 151, 252
Culpeper, Nicholas, 43
Curie, Irène, 345
Curie, Marie, 342
Curie, Pierre, 342
Curtis, Alva, 186
Cushing, Harvey, 292–301
Cutler, John, 221, 225

Dandy, Walter Edward, 293, 301
Danville, Ky., 145–147
Dartmouth College medical department, 104, 110–112, 148
Davis, Nathan Smith, 199, 204
Davy, Humphry, 167
DeBakey, Michael E., 327, 329–331
Declaration of Independence, 115, 123
Delafield, Francis, 205
De La Warr, Lord, 8
Dexter, Aaron, 109
dialysis, 318
diarrhea, 9, 171, 247–248
diphtheria, 144–145, 249–250, 259, 350
discrimination in schools, 202–203
dissection, 73–79, 83–86, 88–93, 95–97, 108, 191
legislation to aid, 73–74, 93–97
Dix, Dorothea, 302
Dolaeus, Johann, 53
Douglass, William, 194, 220, 222, 224–225
Dover, Del., 133, 135

Drake, Daniel, 149–153, 157, 172, 275
Drake, Isaac, 149–151
Dunglison, Robley, 156
Dunster, Henry, 24, 107
dysentery, 9, 121, 130, 171, 246–249

Edinburgh, University of, 80, 103–104, 106, 145
electrocardiography, 340
electroencephalography, 341
Eliot, Charles, 204–205
Eliot, John, 23, 27, 74–75
Elliot, John Wheelock, 295
Elvehjem, Conrad, 261
Endecott, John, 16–18
Enders, John F., 251
Esmond, William G., 318
ether, 168–170, 295
Evans, Alice, 257
Every Man His Own Doctor, 141

Fajans, Kasimir, 343
Feldman, W. H., 256
Fermi, Enrico, 346
Ferrier, David, 293
Finlay, Carlos Juan, 241–243
Firmin, Giles, Jr., 20–23, 74–75
fistulas, 155, 163, 175–176
Flexner, Abraham, 203–208
Flexner, Simon, 248–249, 276–280, 286
Flexner report, 203–207
Flint, Austin, Jr., 258
Fort Mackinac, Michigan, 154–155
Fothergill, John, 79, 81, 99
Francis, Thomas, Jr., 254, 289–290
Franklin, Benjamin, 58–63, 78, 195, 227, 236

INDEX

Freedmen's Hospital (Washington, D.C.), 202
Freeman, Walter Jackson, 303
French and Indian wars, 115–118, 135
frontier doctors, 141–158, 352
Fritsch, Gustav, 293
Fuller, Matthew, 27
Fuller, Samuel, 16–19, 27, 214
Fulton, John Farquhar, 302

Gage, Andrew, 328
Gager, William, 26–27
Galdston, Iago, 273
Gall, Franz Joseph, 179, 293
Galloway, E. H., 260
Garfield, Sidney R., 355–357
Gasser, Herbert S., 280
Gates, Frederick T., 277–278
Geneva (N.Y.) College of Medicine, 203
Georgetown University Medical Center, 328
Georgia, 168, 259, 263, 274
Gerhard, William Wood, 247
Gibbon, John H., Jr., 316
Gilman, Charles, 126–127
Gilman, Daniel Coit, 207
Ginnat, Post, 6
Glaiseer, James, 334
Goforth, William, 150–152
Goldberger, Joseph, 258–261
Goodhue, Joseph, 110–111
Gordon, Alexander, 165
Gorgas, William Crawford, 243, 245
graded curriculum, 204–205, 208
Graham, Sylvester, 179
Gram, Hans Burch, 188

Granger, George, 351–352
grave robbing, 82–83, 85–88, 90–92, 96–97; legislation against, 91, 93, 95–96
Greenland, Henry, 27
Gregory, James, 146
Gross, Samuel D., 153
Group Health Cooperative of Puget Sound, 358–359
group practice, 351, 353–362
Guthrie, Charles Claude, 315
gynecology, 99, 146–148, 161–164, 166, 208

Hahnemann, Christian Frederick, 186–189, 193
Hahnemann Medical College (Chicago), 188
Halsted, William Stewart, 172–175, 208, 296
Hammond, William Alexander, 170–171, 177
Hardy, James D., 322–323
Harken, Dwight E., 313
Hartford, Conn., 116, 168
Harvard College, 24, 27, 40–43, 82–83, 108–110, 114, 164, 204, 274
Harvard Medical Institution, 82, 104, 107–111, 164, 204–205, 295, 301, 345
Harvey, John, 11–12
Harvey, William, 43–44
Hauptman, August, 50–51
Heale, Giles, 16
health maintenance organization, 359–362
heart bypass pump, 329–330

heart disease, 280, 324, 327, 331
heart surgery, 202, 312–314, 316, 322–325, 329–330
heart-lung machine, 314, 316–317, 325, 329
Hektoen, Ludwig, 250
Henricropolis, Va., 55
Henry, Joseph, 276
Hershey, Ezekiel, 107
Hershey, Thomas, 185
Herter, Christian A., 279
Hevesy, Georg von, 344–345
Hinshaw, H. C., 256
Hippocrates, 149, 164, 284
Hitzig, Eduard, 293
Hoar, Leonard, 24, 43
Hodge, Hugh L., 165
Holmes, Oliver Wendell, 21–23, 75, 109, 164–166
Holt, L. Emmett, 278–279
Home, Francis, 250
Homeopathic Hospital (Philadelphia), 188
Homeopathic Medical College (New York), 188; (Philadelphia), 188
homeopathy, 182, 186–189, 193
Horsley, Victor, 294–295, 297–298, 301
hospitals, 55–70, 171–172, 188, 205, 208, 302, 354, 357–359, 361
Hudson, N. Paul, 244
Hudson River, 15, 130
Hufnagel, Charles A., 325
Hunter, William, 79, 99
Hunterdon (N.J.) Medical Center, 354
Hutchinson, James, 239–240
hypothermia, 314

Illinois, 141, 258
Indian Doctor's Dispensatory, The, 143
Indians (American), 5–6, 8, 11, 13, 17–20, 29–31, 33–39, 47–48, 55, 74, 110, 115–129, 142–143, 146, 190–191, 214–215, 234, 274
infantile paralysis, 280–282, 284–291. See also National Foundation for Infantile Paralysis
influenza, 251–255, 280, 288, 335
Innes, John, 151
inoculation, 54, 125, 128–129, 132, 159, 217–231, 286–290
internal medicine, 16–17, 101, 160–161
Ipswich, Mass., 21, 25, 75
isometric exercises, 337–338
isotopes, 343–344, 347

Jackson, Charles Thomas, 168–169
Jackson, Samuel, 274
Jacobi, Abraham, 160, 249–250
Jacobi, Mary Putnam, 285
Jacobsen, Carlyle F., 302
jalop, 132, 239
James, Thomas C., 148
Jamestown, Va., 3, 5, 8, 15, 30, 55, 215, 248
Jefferson Medical College (Philadelphia), 97, 162, 165, 176, 316
Jeffries, John, 82, 84–85
Jenner, Edward, 230–232
Jesty, Benjamin, 231
Jewell, Wilson, 264
Jobling, James W., 279–280

Johns Hopkins:
  Hospital, 173, 175, 207–208,
    296, 299, 301
  Medical School, 166, 207–209,
    278, 301
  Medical Society, 296
  University, 207–208, 317
Joliot, Frédéric, 345
Jones, John, 69, 105, 135–137
Josselyn, John, 30–33, 39, 75–76

Kaiser, Edgar, 356–357
Kaiser, Henry J., 356–357
Kaiser Foundation, 357
Kaiser-Permanente, 356–358
Kantrowitz, Adrian, 323, 329
Keen, William W., 177, 294, 296,
    300
Kelly, Howard Atwood, 166, 208
Kelly, William D., 320
Kentucky, 141, 143, 146, 149, 151;
    School of Medicine, 113
kidney, 312–313, 317–321, 330,
    347; artificial, 317–318, 325
King's College School of Medicine.
    See Columbia University.
Kinross-Wright, V., 305
Kinyoun, Joseph, 267–268
Kircher, Athanasius, 50–51
Kirksville, Mo., 192
Kitasato, Shibasaburo, 249
Klemperer, Felix, 252–253
Klemperer, Georg, 252–253
Kline, Nathan S., 305
Koch, Robert, 255–256
Kocher, Theodore, 297–298
Kohnke, Quitman, 245
Kolff, William J., 317–318
Koller, Carl, 173

Kolmer, John A., 287
Koplik, Henry, 250–251
Koprowski, Hilary, 289
Kronecker, Hugo, 298
Kuhn, Adam, 103, 240

Laborit, Henri, 305
Ladd, George C., 294–295
Landsteiner, Karl, 286
Lane, William Arbuthnot, 313
Larrey, Dominique Jean, 312
Lauritsen, Charles C., 344
Lawler, Richard H., 319
Lawrence, Ernest Orlando, 344, 346
Lawrence, John H., 346
Lawson, John, 30, 36–39
Leake, James P., 287
Lewis, F. John, 314
Lewis, Paul A., 286
Lexington, Ky., 112, 149
Leyden, University of, 17, 43, 79,
    224, 226
library of medicine, national, 171
Lillehei, C. Walton, 316, 327
Lillehei, Richard C., 320–321
limbs, restoration of severed, 312
Lindbergh, Charles A., 314–316
Lining, John, 236
Lister, Joseph, 174, 294
liver, 312–313, 325, 347
Lizars, John, 148
Lloyd, James, 82, 84–85
lobelia, 183
Loeb, Jacques, 280
London Company, 3, 5–6, 8, 10,
    13–15, 56
Long, Crawford Williamson, 168
Long Island Hospital (New York),
    318

Los Angeles, 338, 356
Louisburg (Canada), 115
Lovell, Joseph, 154
Lower, Richard, 324
lung, 312, 316, 322, 324–325, 347
Lyon, University of, 314

Macewen, William, 294
Magendie, François, 156
Magill, T. P., 254
Maine, 16, 274
malaria, 142, 157–158, 241–242, 350
Malouin, Paul Jacques, 164–165
man-made replacement parts, 310–312, 326–331
Marten, Benjamin, 50, 52
Maryland, 157, 226, 229
Maryland College of Medicine, 198
Maryland, University of, 247, 318
Massachusetts, 16, 20, 27, 30, 41, 46, 74, 82, 93–96, 108, 115, 118, 130, 132, 214, 217, 259, 262, 264, 266, 274
Massachusetts General Hospital, 169, 295–296, 312
Massachusetts Medical Society, 93–94
Massasoit, 19–20
Mather, Cotton, 40–54, 217, 219–225, 235
Mather, Increase, 26, 40–41, 215, 224
Mayo, Charles Horace, 353–354
Mayo, William James, 353–354
Mayo, William Worrell, 351–353
Mayo Clinic, 256, 353–355
Mayo Foundation, 354
McClurg, James, 107, 159

McCormick Institute, 250–251, 278
McDowell, Ephraim, 145–148, 161
McDowell, Joseph Nash, 147
McDowell, William, 148
McGill University (Montreal), 343
McKnight, William James, 96–97
McQuiston, William O., 314
measles, 24, 215, 247, 250–251, 259
Medical Department (U.S. Army), 116–125, 127
Medical Director of the Army (Surgeon-General), 116, 120–125, 134, 154, 171–172, 177
medical journals, 77, 150, 157–158, 163, 170, 185, 201, 232, 290
medical schools, 77, 85, 92, 97–113, 150, 152, 185, 188, 192–193, 198–209, 278, 361
medical societies, 179–180, 185–186, 188, 192, 194–201
Meigs, Charles D., 165
meningitis, 190, 279, 294
mental illness, 45, 50, 57, 59, 61–62, 64–67, 263, 302–306, 349–350, 359
mercury-antimony, 226–228, 230
Merrill, John P., 319
Michigan, University of, 205, 289; medical school, 353
Middleton, Peter, 68, 78, 105
midwives, 4, 14, 17, 99, 165, 263
military hospitals, 116, 119–125, 129–131, 133–135, 172, 177
Miller, David, 319
Minnesota, University of, 314, 316, 321
Mississippi, University of, Medical Center, 322
Mississippi Valley, 157–158

Missouri, 141, 190–191
Mitchell, John, 236
Mitchell, S. Weir, 176–178
Moniz, Egas, 302
Monro, Alexander (Primus), 79
Monro, Alexander (Secundus), 79–80, 146
Monteggia, Giovanni Battista, 285
Morehouse, George Reed, 177
Morgan, John, 79, 99–103, 105, 110, 121–123, 124, 160, 195
Morrison, Norman, 116
Morton, William T. G., 168–170
mosquitoes, 142, 158, 240–245
Mosso, Angelo, 298
Murray, Joseph E., 319

National Foundation for Infantile Paralysis, 280–282, 287–290
National Institutes of Health, 268, 282, 329
National Tuberculosis Association, 280–281
neurology, 176–179, 296
neuropsychiatry, 301–304
neurosurgery, 292–303
New Amsterdam. See New York
New England, 16–17, 20, 26, 28–31, 49, 77, 83, 110, 214–215, 234, 263
New Hampshire, 16, 83, 115, 182, 217
New Jersey, 122, 134, 142, 149, 151, 197–198; Medical Society of, 196–197
New Orleans, 152, 235–236, 244–245, 263–264
Newport, R.I., 79, 86
New York (New Amsterdam), 29, 56, 77–78, 82, 93, 116, 175, 179–180, 188, 195–197, 199, 217, 227, 235–236, 250, 253, 256, 258, 264, 268, 279, 282, 288, 331
New York, City College of, 258
New York Doctors' Riot, 86–90
New York Hospital, 55, 67–70, 86, 88–89
New York Medical Society, 106–107, 198
New York State, 115–116, 254, 263, 265, 277, 281, 328; Medical Society, 160, 198, 204
nitrous oxide, 167–169
Noguchi, Hideyo, 280
noise, 332, 339
North Carolina, 30, 232
Northwestern University medical department, 202, 204, 353
Nott, Josiah Clark, 241
nurses, 14, 55–56, 59, 175, 238, 263

Oak Ridge, Tenn., 342, 346
obstetricians (obstetrics), 14, 99, 126, 144, 146, 148, 160–161, 164–166, 201, 350, 359
O'Connor, Basil, 282
Ohio, Medical College of, 150, 172
organ transplantation, 280, 310, 314–316, 318–326, 331
Osler, William, 164, 208, 264, 300
osteopathy, 182, 189–193
ovariotomy, 147–148
Oxford University, 24, 44

pacemaker, 327–329
Paracelsus, 187

Park, William Hallock, 250, 286–287
Pasteur, Louis, 174
pathology, 101, 151, 208, 248, 250, 277–279, 348, 353
Pawlett, Robert, 13–14
pediatrics, 99, 160–161, 251, 278, 285
pellagra, 257–261
Penn, William, 100
Pennsylvania, 96–97, 100, 115, 134, 258, 263, 288
Pennsylvania Hospital, 55, 57–64, 79, 81, 102, 247, 263
Pennsylvania, University of, School of Medicine, 104–105, 148, 152, 157, 165–166, 200, 204, 251, 274, 277
Perkins, Cyrus, 111–112
Perrine, Henry, 157
pesthouses, 57
pharmacology (materia medica), 101, 103, 109, 151–152, 159–160, 189, 200–201, 279, 305–306, 315
Philadelphia, 57–58, 60, 64, 77, 80–82, 96, 99, 101, 110, 117, 119, 121–122, 152, 157, 159–160, 179, 199, 226, 235–240, 264, 273–274, 276, 287, 294, 313
Philadelphia, College of, 99–106, 133
Philadelphia Hospital, 57–58
Philadelphia Medical Society, 195–196
Phips, William, 41–42
phrenology, 179, 293
physicians, 3–4, 14, 52–53, 159–160

Physick, Philip Syng, 147–148
physiology, 48, 101, 105, 151, 156–157, 176–177, 179, 279, 295, 297–298, 302, 315, 333, 349
Pinel, Philippe, 65–66
pleurisy, 31, 251–252
Plummer, Henry, 353
Plymouth, Mass., 15–20, 24, 27, 214
pneumonia, 121, 144, 251–253, 280, 319, 330, 356
Pott, John, 10–14
prefrontal lobotomy, 302–303, 305
prepaid medical care, 263, 355–362
Princeton University, 142, 279, 344
Provident Hospital (Chicago), 202
Prudden, T. Mitchell, 278
puerperal fever, 164–166
purging, 35, 66, 145, 157, 182, 216, 228, 230, 239
Puritans, 15–16, 18, 20, 41, 48
Putnam, Israel, 130–131
Pylarini, Giacomo, 218–219

quacks, 41, 136, 179, 181, 186, 227
quarantine, 16, 57, 235–236, 241, 244–245, 259, 262–264, 267, 335
quinine, 136–137, 157–158, 226

radiation, 332, 336, 339, 342–346
radioisotopes, 328, 342, 345–348
radiology, 292, 295–296, 320, 341, 346–348, 359
resurrection wars, 90–92
Revolution, American, 14, 27, 69, 82, 88, 98, 102, 105, 108, 115, 117–137, 141, 154, 196, 214
Reed, Walter, 241–243
regulatory measures, 62, 103–104,

regulatory measures (*continued*) 106, 196–201, 204–206, 208–209

Rehn, Ludwig, 313

Rhode Island, 134, 247

Ricketts, Howard Taylor, 259

Ridgely, Frederick, 112

Rivers, Thomas M., 282

Rochester, Minn., 351–354

Rockefeller, John D., 276–278

Rockefeller Foundation, 243–244, 278, 280

Rockefeller Institute, 253, 276–280, 282, 286, 315

Romayne, Nicholas, 106–107

Roosevelt, Franklin D., 281–282

Rosenau, Milton J., 268

Rous, Peyton, 280

Rowntree, Leonard George, 317

Rush, Benjamin, 64–67, 103, 123–124, 135, 152, 157, 181, 236–241

Rush Medical College (Chicago), 175–176

Rushton, Thomas, 229–230

Russell, Louis B., Jr., 324

Russell, Walter, 5, 7, 14

Rutherford, Ernest, 343–344

Sabin, Albert B., 281, 288, 290; polio vaccine, 281, 290–291

Sakel, Manfred, 304

Salem, Mass., 16–18, 25, 42, 57

Salk, Jonas E., 281, 288–289, 291; polio vaccine, 281, 288–291

Salt Lake City, 331

San Francisco, 253, 268, 357

sanitation, 245, 264–267

Sappington, John, 157–158

scanners, 345, 347–348

scarlet fever, 187, 249–250

Schroeder, Ernest Charles, 257

Schwann, Theodor, 156

Scudder, Nathaniel, 126

scurvy, 6–7, 9, 16–17, 32

Senn, Nicholas, 175–176

Senning, Ake, 327

Shattuck, Lemuel, 264–265

Sherrington, Charles Scott, 297–299

Shippen, William, Jr., 77, 79–81, 85, 99–103, 110, 121–124

Shippen, William, Sr., 77, 79, 122

shock therapy, 66, 303–305

Shumway, Norman E., 323

Silliman, Benjamin, 156

Simons, David G., 334

Sims, James Marion, 161–164

Sivel, H. Theodore, 333–334

smallpox, 17, 24, 121, 125, 128–129, 132, 144, 190, 213–233, 246–247, 249–250

Smith, James, 105

Smith, John, 5, 7–8, 13, 15

Smith, Joseph M., 69–70

Smith, Nathan, 110–112, 148

Smith, Peter, 142–143

Smith, Stephen, 265, 267

Smith, Theobald, 279

Smith, William, 103

Smithson, James, 275–276

Smithsonian Institution, 275–276

Soddy, Frederick, 343

Soper, Fred L., 244

South Carolina, 162, 242

Souttar, Henry Sessions, 313

space program, 334–341

Spaulding, Lyman, 111

Spiller, William G., 296

INDEX

spinal cord, 285–286, 294, 297, 300–301
Spunkers, 83–85
Spurzheim, Johann Caspar, 179, 293
Stanford University, 323
Starzl, Thomas E., 325
Steck, H., 304
Sternberg, George M., 243
stethoscope, electronic, 339
Stiles, Charles Wardell, 268
Still, Andrew Taylor, 189–193
St. Martin, Alexis, 154–156
St. Mary's Hospital (Rochester, Minn.), 352–354
Stokes, Adrian, 244
Stokes, Joseph, Jr., 251
surgeons (surgery), 3–4, 8, 14, 56, 69, 89, 92–93, 95, 99, 102, 105, 108–112, 118, 120, 122–123, 125–127, 129–132, 134–137, 143–144, 146–147, 153, 159–164, 166–176, 193, 201–202, 208, 279, 292–301, 309–314, 318–326, 328–330, 338–339, 350, 352–355, 359
Sutton, Daniel, 228–230
Sutton, Robert, 228
Swan, Henry, 314
sweatings, 30, 34, 39, 142
Swift, Homer, 280
Sydenham, Thomas, 149, 215

Tennant, John V. B., 105
Tennent, John, 141
Tennessee, 141, 143, 190
Thacher, James, 18, 127–133
Thacher, Thomas, 24–26, 215–216
Theiler, Max, 244
Thompson, Alexander, 199

Thomson, Adam, 159, 226–230
Thomson, Samuel, 182–186, 193
Thomsonianism, 182–186, 193
Thornton, Matthew, 115–116
Tilton, James, 133–135
Timoni, Emanuel, 218–219, 223
Tissandier, Gaston, 334
tissue rejection, 319–322
tobacco, 10, 32–33
Townsend, David, 129
Townshend, Richard, 12–13
Transylvania University (Kentucky), medical department, 112–113, 152
Trudeau, Edward Livingston, 256
tuberculosis, 30, 52–53, 255–256, 350
Tufts, Cotton, 195
Tuke, William, 65
Tunnicliff, Ruth, 250–251
Turner, B. B., 317
typhoid, 179, 246–248
typhus, 17, 121, 134, 246–248, 259

Underwood, Michael, 285
Urey, Harold C., 345
U.S. Public Health Service (Marine Hospital Service), 172, 232–233, 258–259, 263, 267, 269, 287, 290, 319

vaccination, 109, 228, 230–233, 244, 250–251
vaccine:
    influenza, 254–255
    measles, 251
    yellow fever, 244
Van de Graaff, Robert J., 344
van Leeuwenhoek, Anton, 50–51

415

van Swieten, Gerald B., 151
Varrevanger, Jacob Hendricksen, 56
Vermont, 192, 284
vibration, 332, 339, 341
Virginia, 88, 141, 145, 159, 190, 214, 229, 236, 263, 266; colony, 3, 6–7, 10, 14, 28, 248, 251
vomiting (induced), 35, 66, 145, 157, 183, 216
von Behring, Emil, 249
von Bergmann, Ernst, 174
von Haller, Albrecht, 151, 226
von Heine, Jacob, 285
von Meduna, Ladislaus, 303

Warm Springs, Ga., 281
Warren, John, 82, 83, 84, 108–109, 127, 169
Warren, John C., 93, 169–170, 179
Warren, Joseph, 83, 108, 117–118
Washington, D.C., 172, 266, 268, 275, 278, 303
Washington, George, 116, 119–121, 122, 124–127, 131, 275
waste body products, 336, 339–340
Waterhouse, Benjamin, 109
Watts, James Winston, 303
weightlessness, 332, 336, 338, 341
Weiss, Soma, 345
Welch, William H., 205, 208–209, 273, 278
Wells, Horace, 168–169

West, James W., 319
West Indies, 9–10, 121, 234–235, 262
Weymouth, Mass., 18, 26, 195
Wheelock, Eleazar, 111
Wheelock, John, 111–112
White, Charles, 165
Wiener, Norbert, 311
Wiesenthal, Charles F., 80
Williams, Daniel Hale, 202, 312–313
Willkinson, Will, 4
Wilmington, Del., 134
Winslow, Edward, 19–20
Winthrop, John, 27, 74, 214
Winthrop, John, Jr., 27, 49
witches, 40–42
Wolcott, Alexander, 115–116
Woodward, Theodore E., 247–248
Wooton, Thomas, 4–5
wounds and fractures, 118–119, 126, 130–131, 135–137, 144–145, 154–155, 171, 175, 177, 296

Yale University, 156, 294, 302
Yeardley, George, 9–10
yellow fever, 234–246, 259, 262, 280
Yellow Fever Commission (Rockefeller Foundation), 243–244; (U.S. Army), 243–244
Yens, Otto C., 345

ABOUT THE AUTHORS

Geoffrey Marks was born in Australia and received his B.A. (1928) and his M.A. (1940) from Trinity College, Oxford. Now a United States citizen, he was formerly associate editor of *Physicians Management* and is a frequent contributor to medical periodicals, as well as the author of *The Medieval Plague* and *The Amazing Stethoscope*.

William K. Beatty was born in Canada and received his B.A. (1951) and his M.A. (1952) from Columbia University. Since 1962 he has been librarian and professor of medical bibliography at Northwestern University Medical School. He has written articles for library and medical journals and contributed to books published in this country and in England.

Mr. Marks and Mr. Beatty are also co-authors of *The Medical Garden* and *Women in White*.